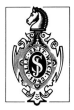

Advances in
Forensic Haemogenetics
4

14th Congress of the
International Society for Forensic Haemogenetics
(Internationale Gesellschaft for forensische Hämogenetik e.V.)
Mainz, September 18–21, 1991

Edited by C. Rittner and P. M. Schneider

Springer-Verlag
Berlin Heidelberg New York
London Paris Tokyo
Hong Kong Barcelona
Budapest

Prof. Dr. Christian Rittner
Dr. rer. nat. Peter M. Schneider

Institut für Rechtsmedizin
Johannes Gutenberg-Universität Mainz
Am Pulverturm 3
W-6500 Mainz, FRG

With 227 Figures

ISBN 3-540-55194-8 Springer-Verlag Berlin Heidelberg New York
ISBN 0-387-55194-8 Springer-Verlag New York Berlin Heidelberg

© Springer-Verlag Berlin Heidelberg 1992
Printed in Germany

The use of general descriptive names, registered names, trademark, etc. in this publication does not imply, even in the absence of a specific statement, that such names are exempt from the relevant protective laws and regulations and therefore free for general use.

Product liability: The publishers cannot guarantee the accuracy of any information about dosage and application contained in this book. In every individual case the user must check such information by consulting the relevant literature.

Typesetting: Camera ready by author
19/3130-543210 – Printed on acid-free paper

Preface

Due to the ever-increasing progress in molecular genetics on the one hand and the necessity to obtain evidential proof on the other, the velocity of change in forensic haemogenetics has been on the increase for decades. Ten years ago discoveries took years before they were introduced into forensic work; nowadays this often happens after just a few months.

The presentations at this Congress dealt mainly with the forensic application and applicability of recent DNA technology. The invited papers dealt with topics such as amplified fragment length polymorphisms, short tandem repeats, and elucidation of micro-heterogeneity within "classical" VNTRs. Original contributions concentrated on standardization, artifacts, and identification of human remains. Legal and ethical implications were also included.

PCR-related systems have become one of the areas of greatest progress, and nearly overtaking classical RFLP analysis. New information was presented regarding technology, new systems, and important features of practical application. "Classical" VNTR technology seems to have moved into a new dimension, mainly due to Jeffreys' new approach (meanwhile published in *Nature* 354:204–209 (1991)). New results deal with classical marker systems, biostatistics, and basic methodology. Thanks to the contributors and the sterling work of Christian Rittner and Peter Schneider, this Congress turned out to be one of the most successful events in the history of forensic haemogenetics.

Bernd Brinkmann

Contents

Speech of the Minister of Justice of Rheinland-Pfalz (Germany)
Peter Caeser at the occasion of the opening of the 14th Congress
of the International Society of Forensic Haemogenetics 1

1 PCR Systems

1.1 General

Some Considerations for use of AMP-FLPS for Identity Testing
(B. Budowle, F. S. Baechtel, and C. T. Comey) 11

Forensic Use of Short Tandem Repeats via PCR
(C. T. Caskey and H. A. Hammond) 18

Automation of the Amplification and Sequencing
of Mitochondrial DNA (K. M. Sullivan, R. Hopgood, and P. Gill) ... 26

1.2 Methodology

The Development and Evaluation of New Genetic Markers
for the Application of PCR to Forensic Casework
(R. Reynolds, R. Saiki, M. Grow, N. Fildes, G. McClure, S. Scharf,
S. Cosso, S. Walsh, and H. Erlich) 29

Investigations to Improve Allele Definition
in the "Collagen 2A1" System (AMP-FLP)
(C. Puers, P. Wiegand, and B. Brinkmann) 32

Automated Analysis
of Fluorescent Amplified Fragment Length Polymorphisms
for DNA Typing (J. Robertson, T. Schaefer,
M. Kronick, and B. Budowle) 35

Sex Identification of Forensic Samples Using PCR Analysis
for the Presence of Y-Chromosome Specific DNA Sequences
(S. Nørby and B. Eriksen) 38

Automation of DNA Profiling by Fluorescent Labelling
of PCR Products *(K. M. Sullivan, S. Pope, C. Kimpton, P. Gill,
and J. Sutton)* 41

PCR Typing Including High Resolution Gel Electrophoresis
Reveals new Alleles in the COL2A1 VNTR *(E. S. Berg and B. Olaisen)* 44

The Usefulness of Chelating Resins for DNA Extraction
from Forensic Material Prior to PCR Amplification
(M. V. Lareu, M. S. Rodriguez-Calvo, F. Barros, and A. Carracedo) ... 47

The Isolation of DNA for Forensic PCR Analysis.
An Evaluation of Available Methodologies *(R. Coquoz)* 50

Detection of Three Different VNTR's by DNA-Amplification
*(A. Kloosterman, R. Vossen, D. Wust, W. de Leeuw,
and A. Uitterlinden)* 53

1.3 Practical Application

Validation of the Use DNA Amplification for the Analysis
of Forensic Samples by Comparison with Tests Using
Non-Amplified DNA Polymorphisms *(L. Perlee and I. Balazs)* 57

Investigations on the Forensic Application
of 4 AMPFLP Systems *(P. Wiegand, S. Rand, and B. Brinkmann)* .. 60

SDS-Page Typing of HLA-DQA1 and PMCT118
after PCR Amplification *(F. Barros, M. C. Vide,
M. V. Lareu, and A. Carracedo* 64

Gene Frequencies of ApoB Alleles in a Sample of Random
Italian Individuals (Central and Southern Italy)
(E. d'Aloja, M. Dobosz, M. Pescarmona, A. Moscetti, and V. L. Pascali) 67

Study of the HLA DQα Polymorphism in the Population
of Catalonia (Spain) *(M. Gené, E. Huguet, A. Carracedo,
and J. Mezquita)* 70

Use of PCR for Forensic Analysis of DNA from Formaldehyde
Fixed and Paraffin Embedded Human Tissues
(B. Ludes, M. C. Tortel, and P. Mangin) 72

Comparison of Population Data Using 3 AMPFLP Systems
(K. Skowasch, M. Schürenkamp, and S. Rand) 75

The Amplified Fragment Length Polymorphism Study
of Locus PMCT118 and its Application in Forensic Biology
(Li Boling, Ding Yan, Ni Jintang, Chen Song, Hu Lan, and Ye Jian) 78

DNA Typing from Formalin-Fixed, Paraffin-Embedded Tissues
(*H. Fukushima, M. Ota, K. Tanaka, A. Ichinose, K. Sato,
and K. Honda*) 81

HLA-DQA1 and HLA-DPB1 Gene Polymorphisms
in the Japanese Populations (*A. Ichinose, M. Ota, H. Inoko,
K. Sato, K. Tanaka, K. Kiyono, K. Honda, and H. Fukushima*) 84

The Study of ApoB Locus AMP-FLP and its Application
in Forensic Sciences (*Li Boling, Ding Yan, Ni Jintang, Chen Song,
Hu Lan, and Ye Jian*) 87

Application of HLA-Class II Genotyping by the Modified
PCR-RFLP Method to the Forensic Science (*M. Ota, H. Inoko,
T. Seki, A. Ichinose, K. Honda, K. Tsuji, and H. Fukushima*) 90

Simultaneous DNA Analysis of HLA-DPB and DQB Loci
from Single Hairs: A Criminal Case Report
(*S. Pelotti, V. Mantovani, G. Angelini, F. Barboni, and G. Pappalardo*) 93

Sex Determination by Genomic Dot Blot Hybridization
and HLA-DQα Typing by PCR from Fixed Tissues
(*L. Pötsch, L. Penzes, M. Prager-Eberle, P. M. Schneider, and C. Rittner*) 96

HLA-DQα Typing of Human Fingernails
(*L. Pötsch, L. Penzes, M. Prager-Eberle, and C. Rittner*) 99

Identification of Fire Victims by Using DNA Amplification (PCR)
(*A. Sajantila, M. Ström, B. Budowle, P. J. Karhunen,
and L. Peltonen*) 102

Polymerase Chain Reaction: Typing of DNA Isolated
from Various Forms of Biological Evidence (*J. Schnee and S. Aab*) 106

Analysis of D1S80 (PMCT 118) Locus Polymorphism
in an Italian Population Sample by the Polymerase Chain Reaction
(*A. Tagliabracci, R. Giorgetti, A. Agostini, M. Cingolani,
and S. D. Ferrara*) 109

Sex Determination in Bloodstains and Single Hairs
(*K. Tanaka, H. Fukushima, M. Ota, A. Ichinose, K. Sato, K. Honda,
and S. Kiyono*) 112

Analysis of Forensic Stains via PCR Amplification
of Polymorphic Simple (gata)$_n$ Repeats
(*L. Roewer, J. Arnemann, and J. T. Epplen*) 115

Species Identification by Polymerase Chain Reaction
and Direct Sequencing (*S. Tsuchida, F. Umenishi, and S. Ikemoto*) .. 118

2 DNA (RFLP, VNTR) Systems

2.1 General

Paternity Investigations Based on DNA-Analysis only
(*W. Bär and A. Kratzer*) 123

Achievement of Interlaboratory Uniformity – A Summary of Work
Carried out by the EDNAP Group (*P. Gill, S. Woodroffe, W. Bär,
B. Brinkmann, A. Carracedo, B. Eriksen, S. Jones, A. D. Kloosterman,
B. Ludes, B. Mevag, V. L. Pascali, M. Rudler, H. Schmitter,
P. M. Schneider, and J. A. Thomson*) 126

Cloning and Characterisation of Novel Single Locus Probes
for Forensic Purposes (*C. P. Kimpton, R. Hopgood, S. K. Watson,
P. Gill, and K. Sullivan*) 129

2.2 Methodology

The Use of a Chemiluminescent Detection System for Paternity
and Forensic Testing. Verification of the Reliability
of the Oligonucleotide-Probes Used for Genetic Analysis
(*J. Neuweiler, J. Venturini, I. Balazs, S. Kornher, D. Hintz, and J. Victor*) 132

A Multi-Locus Probe for Human DNA Fingerprinting Based
on *CHI*-like Sequences (*N. Z. Ehtesham and S. E. Hasnain*) 137

The Effects of Using Different Molecular Weight Markers
in DNA Profiling (*M. J. Greenhalgh*) 140

Influence of Agarose Concentration and Electric Field Strength
on the Separation of DNA-Fragments During Electrophoresis
(*B. L. Guo, M. Prinz, and M. Staak*) 143

Size Calculations of Restriction Fragments:
Comparison Between Two Laboratories
(*L. Henke, P. H. van Eede, J. Henke, and G. G. de Lange*) 146

Matching Criteria for Paternity Testing with VNTR Systems
(*N. Morling and H. E. Hansen*) 149

Computer-Aided Fragment Size Determination
of Single Locus DNA Probes (*M. Muche*) 153

Chemiluminescent Detection of Single Locus and
Multilocus Hybridization Patterns (*M. Prinz, C. Loch, and M. Staak*) 156

Precision and Accuracy in the Analysis
of VNTR Polymorphisms for Paternity Testing
(*S. C. Reavis, T. Schlaphoff, R. Martell, and E. D. du Toit*) 159

A Simple Method to Prevent Inhibition of TAQ Polymerase
and HINFI Restriction Enzyme in DNA Analysis of Stain Material
(W. Pflug, G. Mai, G. Wahl, S. Aab, B. Eberspächer, and U. Keller) ... 163

Optimal Size Calling Methods for Electrophoretic Analysis
Utilizing Internal Size Standards (K. Corcoran, E. Mayrand,
J. Robertson, T. Shaefer, and M. Kronick) 166

Extraction of DNA from Coagulated Blood Samples
(R. Scheithauer and H. J. Weisser) 169

Investigation of Variation in Fragment Size Determinations
Found when Using Single Locus DNA Probes
(J. A. Thomson, T. Fedor, M. Gouldstone, P. J. Lincoln, C. P. Phillips,
D. Syndercombe Court, V. Tate, and P. H. Watts) 172

Optimization of the Digoxigenin/Chemiluminescence Method
for the VNTR Detection (N. Dimo-Simonin, C. Brandt-Casadevall,
and H. R. Gujer) 175

2.3 Practical Application

Paternity Analysis Using the Multilocus DNA Probe MZ 1.3
(P. M. Schneider, R. Fimmers, U. Schacker, and C. Rittner) 179

Analysis of Australian, Black, Caucasian, Chinese
and Amerindian Populations with Hypervariable DNA Loci
(I. Balazs, J. Neuweiler, R. C. Williams, and C. Lantz) 182

The Application of DNA-Polymorphisms in Paternity Testing
(M. Basler, W. Sprecher, M. Rink, and K.-S. Saternus) 184

Allele Frequency in the Population of Spain
Using Several Single Locus Probes
(E. Valverde, C. Cabrero, A. Diez, A. Carracedo, and T. Borrás) 187

DNA Fingerprints of Families from Bejsce/South-East Poland
(T. Dobosz, P. Koziol, K. Sawicki, M. Szczepaniak, J. Jagielski,
C. Vogt, and S. Szymaniec) 190

Paternity Testing with Five VNTR System in Danes
(H. E. Hansen, and N. Morling) 192

Comparison of Population Genetics of the Single Locus Probes
PS 194 and PL427-4 (W. Martin, H. H. Hoppe, and M. Muche) 195

Comparison of Minisatellite DNA Probes and Blood Group,
Protein, and Enzyme Markers in Paternity Cases
(G. Mauff, G. Pulverer, E. Mühlenbrock, L. Kochhan, A. Klein,
K. Volz, A. Bräutigam, K. Hummel, R. Fimmers, and M. P. Baur) 198

Allele Frequency Distribution of Two VNTR Polymorphisms
(YNH24/D2S44; Alpha Globin 3'HVR/D16) in Italy
(V. L. Pascali, M. Dobosz, M. Pescarmona, E. d'Aloja, and A. Fiori) .. 201

DNA-Profiling with PHINS310, PMUC7, PMR24/1, PYNH24
and PMS43A for Paternity Testing *(T. Rothämel, H. J. Krüger,
W. Keil, and H. D. Tröger)* 204

Frequency Databases for the DNA Probes MS1, MS31, MS43A,
and YNH24, Derived from Caucasians, and Afrocaribbeans
in the London Area *(C. Buffery, F. Burridge, M. Greenhalgh,
S. Jones, and G. Willott)* 207

An Evaluation of Single Locus Probes in Casework
(F. J. Burridge, M. J. Greenhalgh, and G. M. Willott) 210

On DNA Typing of Hard Tissues
(U. Hammer, U. Bulnheim, and R. Wegener) 213

Use of the Minisatellite Probe MZ 1.3 for Identification
and Relation of Dismembered Corpses
(W. Huckenbeck and H. Müller) 216

RFLP in Conjunction with Anatomical Traits in Individualisation
of Bone *(G. V. Rao and V. K. Kashyap)* 219

Application of DNA Fingerprinting to Problematical Paternity
Cases *(T. Kishida, M. Fukuda, and Y. Tamaki)* 222

Application of Conventional Polymorphisms and
Single Locus DNA Probes in Cases of Disputed Paternity
*(P. J. Lincoln, C. P. Phillips, D. Syndercombe Court,
J. A. Thomson, and P. H. Watts)* 225

MS1, MS31 and MS43A Single Locus Probes: A Preliminary
Study in the Basque Population and its Application
in Paternity Testing *(S. Alonso, A. Castro, A. García-Orad, P. Arizti,
G. Tamayo, and M. Martínez de Pancorbo)* 228

DNA Fingerprinting with Probes 33.15 and 33.6 in Population
from the Basque Country *(S. Alonso, A. Castro, A. García-Orad,
P. Arizti, G. Tamayo, and M. Martínez de Pancorbo)* 231

Casuistic: The Use of DNA-Fingerprinting
in Cases of Affiliation Without Mother
(W. Huckenbeck, H. Müller, and M. Prinz) 234

Results of DNA Analysis from Six Forensic Science Laboratories
in Germany *(W. Pflug, J. Teifel-Greding, S. Herrmann, M. Gerhard,
R. Wenzl, and H. Schmitter* 237

Allele Frequencies for Five Different Single Locus Probes
in a Population of South-West Germany *(W. Pflug, G. Bäßler,
G. Mai, U. Keller, S. Aab, B. Eberspächer, and G. Wahl)* 240

Distribution of Variable Number of Tandem Repeat (VNTR)
DNA Polymorphism at D2S44 Locus in Tuscany (Italy)
*R. Domenici, I. Spinetti, M. Nardone, M. Pistello,
and L. Ceccherini-Nelli)* 243

Experiences with Six Single Locus Probes in Paternity Testing
(B. Brüggemann, D. Teixidor, M. Kilp, and S. Seidl) 246

Detection of DNA Polymorphisms by Using α Satellite Probes:
Application to the Forensic Identification
(M. Yamada, Y. Yamamoto, T. Fukunaga, Y. Tatsuno, and K. Nishi) .. 249

Population Genetic Studies of Six Hypervariable DNA-Loci
(A. Wilting, U. Hintzen, M. O. Völker, and J. Bertrams) 252

Minisatellite DNA Probe MZ1.3: Band Sharing Rates Among
Siblings and the Part of Informative Bands Among Children
(D. Padeberg, U. Hintzen, and J. Bertrams) 255

DNA Fingerprinting in Paternity Testing in Lithuania
(V. Naktinis, V. Popendikyte, G. Khvatovitch, and G. Garmus 258

DNA Typing in Forensic Casework in Norway:
Strategies and Experiences
(B. Mevåg, S. Jacobsen, B. Eriksen, and B. Olaisen) 260

Determination of Incest in Forensic Casework
Using Multi-Locus DNA Profiling *(P. L. Ivanov, L. V. Verbovaya,
and M. B. Maljutov)* 263

3   Biostatistics and Databases

The Robustness of Models for Evaluating Patterns
of DNA Multi-Locus Probes *(Ch. Brenner)* 269

Comparison of Different Methods for the Calculation
of Indices for Paternity *(R. Fimmers, P. M. Schneider, and M. P. Baur)* 277

How to Deal with Mutations in DNA-Testing
(R. Fimmers, L. Henke, J. Henke, and M. P. Baur) 285

The Relationship of the HLA Phenotype Frequency
of the Alleged Father to the Resulting Paternity Index
in Caucasian Non-Exclusion Paternity Cases
(R. H. Walker and A. B. Eisenbrey) 288

DNASYS: A User-Friendly Computer Program for Evaluating
Single Locus Probe Data in Forensic Casework
(I. W. Evett, R. Pinchin, and J. Scranage) 291

Series Sexual Crimes Identified
by a DNA Computerised Database *(J. E. Allard)* 295

Experiences with a Computerised Database of DNA Profiles
in Forensic Casework *(M. J. Greenhalgh and J. E. Allard)* 298

4   Conventional Systems

4.1   General

Genetic and Molecular Aspects of the Human Red Cell Acid
Phosphatase Polymorphism *(J. Dissing)* 303

A de novo Mutation in the Alpha-1-Antitrypsin Gene Detected
in a Case of Disputed Paternity by DNA Sequence Analysis
*(S. Weidinger, J.-P. Faber, U. Bäcker, F. Schwarzfischer,
and K. Olek)* 306

Isoelectric Focusing of Inter-Alphatrypsin-Inhibitor (ITI)
(C. Luckenbach, J. Kömpf, A. Amorim, J. Rocha, and A. Trein) 309

Human ZN-Alpha 2-Glycoprotein Phenotyping
in Several Populations *(N. Nakayashiki, I. Yuasa, K. Umetsu,
K. Suenaga, K. Omoto, T. Ishida, S. Misawa, and S. Katsura)* 311

Comparative Typing of Orosomucoid Variants and Proposal
for a New Nomenclature *(I. Yuasa, S. Weidinger, and K. Umetsu)* .. 314

Intragenic Recombination Within the Alpha-1-Antitrypsin Locus
(G. Wetterling) 317

4.2   Methodology

Blotting Techniques for the Detection of Protein Polymorphisms
in Stains *(S. Rand)* 320

Two-Dimensional Isoelectric Focusing Analysis of Rare
and Silent Esterase D Types. Description of a New ESD Variant
Phenotype *(A. Alonso, S. Weidinger, G. Visedo, M. Sancho,
and J. Fernandez-Piqueras)* 329

A Simple Technique for the Determination of GGTP Types
(M. Oya, Y. Kimura, N. Komatsu, and A. Kido) 332

New Variation in Low-Sulphur Keratins Detected
by Hybrid Isoelectric Focusing (HIEF)
(M. S. Rodriguez-Calvo, I. Muñoz, and A. Carracedo) 335

The Influence of Infused Erythrocytes on the Detection
of Individual Membrane-, Enzyme- and DNA-Systems
*(W. Huckenbeck, B. Mainzer, P. Lipfert, H. Müller, A. Wehr,
and V. Stancu)* 338

Serum Protein Typing/ -Subtyping by IEF in PAG
(G. Geserick, H. Schröder, A. Correns, P. Otremba, and H. Waltz) 341

Dot Blot Immunoassay for Detection of HLA Antigens
in Forensic Stains *(D. V. Rao and V. K. Kashyap)* 344

The Use of Microtiter Techniques for the Determination
of Red Blood Cell Phenotypes in Paternity Testing
(D. Mayr and W. R. Mayr) 347

D^u Detection by an Automated Direct Agglutination Method
that Equals Detection by Indirect Antiglobulin Test *(J. Obst)* 350

Absorption-Elution Test for AB0-Determination of Secretor
and Nonsecretor Saliva Stains *(J. Bolt and J. Lötterle)* 353

Determination of ORM Phenotypes Using Gels Precotes 4–6^R
and Phastsystem™ *(M. De la Iglesia, A. Gremo,
M. A. Martínez-Aguilera, and J. M. Ruíz De la Cuesta)* 356

Fast Determination of TF Phenotypes Using Minigels Gradient
4–6,5 Modificated *(M. De la Iglesia, M. A. Maretínez-Aguilera,
A. Gremo, J. M. Ruíz De la Cuesta)* 359

The Use of Microtiter Plates and the Apparatus Dynatech for
Automation of the Routine Determination of AB0-Group
from Body Fluids (or Stains) and Hair
(P. Makovec, M. Laupy, and M. Brezina) 362

P1, C2, GC, ATIII, PLG Typing in Bloodstains
by Hybrid Isoelectric Focusing (HIEF) *(I. Muñoz, A. Carracedo,
L. Concheiro, and V. L. Pascali)* 364

4.3 Practical Application

Parentage Testing Using DBP Subtyping in South African (SA)
Populations *(W. Petersen, T. Schlaphoff, R. Martell, and E. du Toit)*   367

Iso-Electric Focusing Study of Serum Proteins (GC, TF, PI
and ORM) in Four Endogamous Groups of Maharashtra,
Western India: Application in Paternity Testing
(S. S. Mastana, V. Ray, S. S. Bhattacharya, and S. S. Papiha) 370

PGM1 System: A Rare Allele and an Intragenic Recombination
in Two Cases of Disputed Paternity *(M. L. Pontes, M. F. Pinheiro,
and A. C. Gomes)* 373

Genetic Markers (HP, TF, GC and PI) in Two Polish Population
Samples. Preliminary Report *(H. Walter, H. Danker-Hopfe,*
M. Lemmermann, and M. Lorenz) 376

Haptoglobin Subtypes in Lower Saxony (Germany)
(M. Basler, G. Lang, and K.-S. Saternus) 379

C4 Phenotype and Gene Distribution in a Population
of Eastern Lombardy (Italy) *(N. Cerri, F. de Ferrari, G. Carella,*
A. Malagoli, and R. Cattaneo) 382

Distribution of Transferrin (TF), Red Cell Acid Phosphatase (EAP),
Esterase D (ESD) and Group Specific Component (GC)
Phenotypes in China *(Guo Da Wei, Xui Xiao Li, Xing Xiao Ping,*
and Wang Lin) 385

Null and Rare Alleles in Paternity Testing *(A. C. Gomes,*
M. F. Pinheiro, M. L. Pontes, A. Santos, and J. Pinto da Costa) 389

Comparative Subtyping of ACP-1, PGM-1 and ESD in Human
Placenta and Cord Blood by Isoelectric Focusing:
Practical Considerations of Forensic Significance *(M. J. Iturralde,*
M. Montesino, A. Alonso, I. Montesino, and M. Sancho) 391

Distribution of Adenosine Deaminase (EC 3.5.4.4) Phenotypes
in a Series of HIV-Seropositive Patients *(W. Huckenbeck,*
B. Jacob, B. M. E. Kuntz, and H. T. Brüster) 394

Determination of C1R Types in Bloodstains
(A. Kido, N. Komatsu, Y. Kimura, and M. Oya) 397

Coagulation Factor XIIIB Phenotyping in a Japanese Population
and in Bloodstains *(N. Komatsu, A. Kido, Y. Kimura, and M. Oya)* .. 400

Formal Genetic Data on ORM1 Subtypes
(C. Luckenbach, J. Kömpf, H. Ritter, J. Rocha, and A. Amorin) 403

Species Identification from Tissue Particles Using Lectin-
and Immuno-Histochemical Methods *(K. Nishi, T. Fukunaga,*
Y. Yamamoto, M. Yamada, M. Kane, N. Ito, and S. Kawahara) 407

Polymorphism of Plasminogen in Sardinia (Italy)
(R. Domenici and I. Spinetti) 410

Haptoglobin Subtypes in a Population from South West Germany
(U. Härle, W. Reichert, R. Mattern, and G. Pfaff) 413

Plasma Protein Polymorphism in HIV-Seropositive Patients:
GC- and TF*C-Subtypes and PI-System
(W. Huckenbeck, V. Stancu, B. M. E. Kuntz, and H. T. Brüster) 416

Determination of PGM, ESD, GLO (1) and EAP Polymorphs
from Human Dental Pulp *(A. Sharma, V. K. Arora, and V. Bhalla)* ...419

Haptoglobin Subtyping by Polyacrylamide Gel Isoelectric
Focusing of Serum, Hemolyzed Blood and Bloodstains
(A. Correns, D. Patzelt, P. Otremba, H. Schröder, and G. Geserick) 422

Detection of Blood Group H Antigens of Red Cells, Blood
and Saliva Stains, and Hairs by Anti-H Reagents (K. Furukawa,
T. Nakajima, T. Matsuki, and K. Kubo) 425

Evaluation of Sperm Specific Lactate Dehydrogenase Isoenzyme
C4 (LDH C4). Application to Semen Detection in Stains
(R. Pawlowski and B. Brinkmann) 428

PGM1 Subtyping by Isoelectric Focusing (IEF)
in Parentage Testing in South African (SA) Populations
(V. Borrill, W. Petersen, R. Martell, and E. du Toit) 431

Orosomucoid (ORM) Phenotyping by Isoelectric Focusing
in Immobilized PH-Gradient Followed by Immunoblotting
(W. Huckenbeck, S. Weidinger, and V. Stancu) 434

AB0 Blood Grouping and Species Identification of Bloodstains
by Sandwich ELISA Using Monoclonal Antibody Specific
for Human Erythrocyte Band 3 (A. Kimura, T. Uda, S. Nakashima,
M. Osawa, H. Ikeda, S. Yasuda, and T. Tsuji) 437

Monoclonal Antibodies to Blood Group Substances
in Vaginal Secretions (A. Kimura, M. Osawa, H. Ikeda, S. Yasuda,
T. Tsuji, S. Rand, and B. Brinkmann) 440

GC in Human Saliva Stains (J. Lötterle and J. Bolt) 443

Immunoblotting and Immunofixation Techniques
for Subtyping GC in Old Bloodstains and Semen Stains
(I. López-Abadía, A. Gremo, and J. M. Ruiz De la Cuesta) 446

Old Bloodstain and Semen Stain Characterization
in the Transferrin Typing System Using Minigels and Phastsystem
(I. López-Abadía, A. Gremo, and J. M. Ruiz De la Cuesta) 449

List of Senior Authors

Allard, J.E. 295
Alonso, A. 329
Alonso, S. 228, 231

Balazs, I. 182
Bär, W. 123
Barros, F. 64
Basler, M. 184, 379
Berg, E.S. 44
Bolt, J. 353
Borrill, V. 431
Brenner, Ch. 269
Brüggemann, B. 246
Budowle, B. 11
Buffery, C. 207
Burridge, F.J. 210

Caskey, C.T. 18
Cerri, N. 382
Coquoz, R. 50
Corcoran, K. 166
Correns, A. 422

d'Aloja, E. 67
De La Iglesia, M. 356, 359
Dimo-Simonin, N. 175
Dissing, J. 303
Dobosz, T. 190
Domenici, R. 243, 410

Ehtesham, N.Z. 137
Evett, I.W. 291

Fimmers, R. 277, 285
Fukushima, H. 81
Furukawa, K. 425

Gené, M. 70
Geserick, G. 341
Gill, P. 126
Gomes, A.C. 389
Greenhalgh, M.J. 140, 298

Guo Da wei, 385
Guo, B.L. 143

Hammer, U. 213
Hansen, H.E. 192
Härle, U. 413
Henke, L. 146
Huckenbeck, W. 216, 234, 338,
   394, 416, 434

Ichinose, A. 84
Iturralde, M.J. 391
Ivanov, P.L. 263

Kido, A. 397
Kimpton, C.P. 129
Kimura, A. 437, 440
Kishida, T. 222
Kloosterman, A. 53
Komatsu, N. 400

Lareu, M.V. 47
Li Boling 78, 87
Lincoln, P.J. 225
López-Abadia, I. 446, 449
Lötterle, J. 443
Luckenbach, C. 309, 403
Ludes, B. 72

Makovec, P. 362
Martin, W. 195
Mastana, S.S. 370
Mauff, G. 198
Mayr, D. 347
Mevåg, B. 260
Morling, N. 149
Muche, M. 153
Muñoz, I. 364

Nakayashiki, N. 311
Naktinis, V. 258
Neuweiler, J. 132
Nishi, K. 407

Nørby, S. 38

Obst, J. 350
Ota, M. 90
Oya, M. 332

Padeberg, D. 255
Pascali, V.L. 201
Pawlowski, R. 428
Pelotti, S. 93
Perlee, L. 57
Petersen, W. 367
Pflug, W. 163, 237, 240
Pontes, M.L. 373
Pötsch, L. 96, 99
Prinz, M. 156
Puers, C. 32

Rand, S. 320
Rao, D.V. 344
Rao, G.V. 219
Reavis, S.C. 159
Reynolds, R. 29
Robertson, J. 35
Rodriguez-Calvo, M.S. 335
Roewer, L. 115
Rothämel, T. 204

Sajantila, A. 102
Scheithauer, R. 169
Schnee, J. 106
Schneider, P.M. 179
Sharma, A. 419
Skowasch, K. 75
Sullivan, K.M. 26, 41

Tagliabracci, A. 109
Tanaka, K. 112
Thomson, J.A. 172
Tsuchida, S. 118

Valverde, E. 187

Walker, R.H. 288
Walter, H. 376
Weidinger, S. 306
Wetterling, G. 317
Wiegand, P. 60
Wilting, A. 252

Yamada, M. 249
Yuasa, I. 314

Speech of the Minister of Justice of Rheinland-Pfalz (Germany)
Peter Caeser
at the occasion of the opening of the 14th Congress of the International Society of Forensic Haemogenetics

Dear Congress President,
Ladies and Gentlemen,

I am pleased to welcome you here in the Electoral Palace of Mainz to the opening of the 14th congress of the International Society for Forensic Haemogenetics. As a member of the Government of Rheinland-Pfalz I am very glad that you have chosen our beautiful state capital as the meeting place for your convention. It is a city in which the past - the traces of antique and medieval history and the present - art, science, media and economy - form a harmonic entity.

Mainz represents also for you and your society the past and the present. You return this year to the starting point of your scientific society. Back in the year 1968 a group of forensic experts from Rheinland-Pfalz and Saarland have met in the University Clinic of Mainz. In the beginning these scientists have founded the German Society for Forensic Haemogenetics. Today you have returned to your birthplace as an international society renowned throughout the world with members from more than thirty countries.

This year's congress will deal with a number of important questions and current problems in the field of forensic haemogenetics. I am sure that all participants will spend three interesting and profitable days.

Almost thirty years ago the late swiss author Friedrich Dürrenmatt wrote the comedy "The Physicists". In a brilliant way he deals with the responsibility of the scientist for the results of his research. Is a scientist responsible for what other people do with the results of his research? Dürrenmatt convincingly rejects moral and ethical nihilism: It is the very own responsibility of the scientist himself whether other people create a desaster based on the results of his research. Therefore the scientist is urged to take care of practical and human consequences of his research.

I am not sure if Dürrenmatt would put physicists in the centre of such a comedy today. In my opinion the question of responsibility has a particular relevance to the results of genetic research especially today.

Advances in Forensic Haemogenetics 4
Edited by Ch. Rittner and P. M. Schneider
© Springer-Verlag Berlin Heidelberg 1992

Gene technology will be one of the topics of your congress. This subject concerns not only the physicians and biologists. Responsibility is a normative size. Legislation and jurisdiction are urged together with biologists, physicians, philosophers and theologists to reach a consens in dealing responsibly with the results of gene technology.

The work of the International Society for Forensic Haemogenetics as well as this scientific congress and the entire forensic medicine as I presume are strongly influenced by the specific possibilities of the genome analysis and especially the DNA fingerprinting technique. This is an important topic also for the jurisdiction. For me as the Minister of Justice of this state are not only the specific questions of the application of this technique in jurisdiction a major question. The problems which are posed by DNA fingerprinting and genome analysis in general have to be seen in the framework of problems related to gene technology as a whole.

Since the beginning of the eighthies in the Federal Republic of Germany, prospects and risks of gene technology are positive signals

- for challenges and new questions in the whole field of natural sciences,

- for experiments and new developments in applied sciences,

- for innovation processes, calculations and decisions for major investments in economy and industry,

- and for the expectations and hopes of patients and those who take care of them.

Prospects and risks of gene technology are as well negative signals

- for worries, fears and worst expectations of numerous scientists and especially of a significant part of the population.

The expression "prospects and risks of gene technology" represents one of the most important and dynamic topics of our time. No one doubts that gene technology has opened up major opportunities. On the other hand many are well aware of its horrendous risks.

The rapid development and the dynamics of research in gene technology, the speculative description of possible results and developments, have created fear of the future, the so called "Zukunftsangst". Sometimes the risks have been exaggerated. It has been said that abuse by unscrupolous scientists and business people, and even environment catastrophes will become possible.

This wrong picture has emerged, although the relationship between prospects and risks of gene technology have been studied and presented with great responsibility throughout the world. It may be possible, however, that the experts in science and industry have restricted their knowledge on the risk potential of gene technology to their own circles for too long. This had to provoke speculations.

Meanwhile, there has been decisive change concerning this point. The scientific results of gene technology, their possible implications and the judgements by the different disciplines in science are widely presented and discussed in the general public. For example, in Germany a report has been published on "In-Vitro-Fertilisation", genome analysis and gene therapy. This report has been presented in 1985 by a joint working group of the Federal Ministries of Research and Technology and of Justice. It has made a major contribution to form an objective basis for this discussion. This report has pointed out the topics that are relevant for all ethical and legal implications and judgements of these new techniques. In addition, seperate recommendations were also made to the legislature. It is interesting for the application in forensic medicine, that it has been declared legal to study human cells, for example for the identification of a suspect. The suspect has to allow the physical examination as well as the taking of a blood sample according to the rules of the German code of criminal procedures.

The results of the Enquête Commission of the German parliament by the name "Prospects and Risks of Gene Technology" had an even greater impact. Members of all fractions of the German parliament, as well as representatives of science research, theology, legal sciences, molecular genetics and biochemistry, and personalities of the industry of the German trade unions and from the association of German physicians were included in this Enquéte Commission.

The commission was founded on August 14th, 1984. It had the task to present prospects and risks of research in gene technology and biotechnology, in the context of its application in the areas of health, nutrition, production of energy and raw materials as well as environment protection. In addition, criteria had to be worked out for the limitation of the application of cell biological and gene technological methods on human cells and the human individium as a whole.

In the beginning of 1987 the results of the Enquête Commission were presented containing more than 170 proposals. The question of genome analysis in the context of legal procedures is discussed in detail. The commission has expressed the expectation that the recommendations will be accepted and implemented by the responsible experts as soon as possible. A framework shall be created for this new technology before all possible applications are put to work. The chances of gene technology shall be used responsibly and in a socially acceptable manner, and care shall be taken against possible risks, and dangers should be excluded, as far as possible.

The report of the Enquête Commission has initiated a broad discussion about the social and legal implications of the new technologies. The relevant authorities have studied the recommendations and have put forward political consequences. In some areas legislation has already been adopted. An example is the embryo protection law, which prohibits experiments on human embryos.

The State Government of Rheinland-Pfalz has accepted to contribute to the solution of questions and tasks posed by gene technology very early. On the background of the report of the Enquête Commission, the State Government has ordered the State Commission on Bioethics, to work out ethically and legally responsible guidelines for political decisions regarding the application of gene technology in man.

Members of this bioethics commission, of which I am the chairman, are as well scientists of numerous disciplines, representatives of the churches, the industry, the trade unions as well as politicians and members of the respective state ministries. Our starting point is a close linkage between the ethical and political evaluation of modern human genetics with its prospects and risks. The analysis of the human genome is not simply basic research without any moral implication. But even in this context, this research would not be ethically neutral, because of all possible applications that have to be taken into account.

The intervention into the right of the individial has to be considered in the context of the constitution. An example is the right of man not to know anything about his own genes or his genetic predispositions. This is true in the Federal Republic of Germany, in particular regarding the important right of informational self determination. It has to be considered that there is a danger that a man will be classified or even discriminated on basis of certain standards. We have also seen the potential danger that as a result of gene technological methods the acceptance of disease or disabled people in our society will be reduced. We have also discussed the danger that the disclosure of a given genetic predisposition may lead to the loss of job of certain working people. We have studied if genome analysis in the area of insurance may lead to increased risk premiums or even to the exclusion of people expected to be at a certain risk. Concern was expressed that man will only be seen in a biologistic context, so that he is reduced to his genetic composition. The relevance of these concerns is emphasized by recent studies on genetic discrimination of individials by insurances and companies in the United States.

The commission has also covered the problem of genome analysis in the context of legal procedures. Since this topic is of particular interest for you, I will explain it in more detail.

The major results have been published in 1989 in the second report of the Bioethics Commission of Rheinland-Pfalz with the title "Human Genetics, Theses for Genome analysis and Gene Therapy". This report is the basis for decisions of the State Government. The report has also been used by the federal working group on genome analysis. As the result, detailed recommendations regarding the genome analysis in legal procedures have been made last year.

A number of different and often controversial opinions are found in this often spectacular area of application of genome analysis. A number of people are doubting the reliability of these methods and of the results of DNA fingerprinting procedures.

It has been stated that the genome analysis gives a most exact proof of identity compared to conventional procedures. One of the foremost criminalistic experts of the Federal Republic of Germany, Dr. Steinke, head of the departement of forensic technology at the Federal Criminalistic Office (BKA), had recently spoken of a "revolution" in the field of forensic bloodgroup serology and stain analysis, and that a new dimension in forensic medicine has been entered. Spectacular successes have been reported. Recently, a case was published on a fifteen year old girl that had been killed ten years ago. Her body was found only 8 years after the crime. Now the identity of the victim has been revealed using DNA analysis. The work has been carried out by the English scientist Alec Jeffreys, who ist participating in this conference.

I do not intend to discuss the probative valve of DNA analysis at this point. No one will doubt after the recent decisions by state and federal Courts, that DNA analysis has introduced a considerable progress for the identification of a suspect. In addition it is important for the field of forensic medicine that the German federal high court, the so called "Bundesgerichtshof", has accepted the application of DNA analysis and its use as evidence for civil and for crime cases on the basis of the already existing laws.

This opinion is explicitly shared by the Commitee of Interior Affairs of the German parliament by including recommendations of the Enquête Commission. In my opinion the majority of the German state administrations of Justice also share this view. In this context, however, it is important to emphasize that this is only true for the noncoding part of the human genome. The utilization of DNA evidence is based on the assumption that coding sequences and information exceeding the purpose of identification or segregation analysis will not be obtained. In other words - DNA analysis has to be neutral for the personality of the person being investigated.

The Bioethics Commission of Rheinland-Pfalz has studied this problem in great detail. The president of this congress, Professor Rittner, has informed us extensively on the scientific background and the state of knowledge at that time.

The commission did not see a scientific basis for the assumption, that individual traits of character and personality could be obtained from genetic information.

Nevertheless, the commission has made a clear statement on the potential risk that genome analysis could contribute to establishing the ability of being guilty, or the credibility, or for a final evaluation of the offenders personality. The commission has emphasized that this type of genetic investigation would be in violation of privacy rights and man's dignity. Therefore, the commission has put up the guideline that without consent of the affected person, genome analysis may only be used in civil cases and cases only for the purpose of identification or segregation analysis. The use of any information which exceedes this purpose for the case or including the information in the case proceedings, should not be allowed.

In addition the commission has emphasized that for the admissible application of DNA analysis, it is necessary to obtain court orders and to take strict measures for data protection. I fully support these guidelines. Therefore it is my opinion, and this opinion is supported by court practice, that the DNA finterprinting method is already admissible on the basis of the existing law.

Based on the fast development in the field of molecular genetics, concerns have been raised that a limitation of DNA analysis to the areas neutral to the personality can not be guaranteed. I can not disregard these fears. Would it one day be possible, that the worldwide efforts decoding the human genome and the mapping of all human genes will go beyond the obtaining identification from DNA analysis, which should have served only the simple purpose of identification? That even the noncoding part of DNA will become readable and its information being used? That genetic data bases could be established in the near future?

It ist a well known fact that any progress in this area will open up new possibilities of obtaining information and if this information is available, then maybe in practice, it will be used as well. This has to be taken into account! The transparent man or, if you prefer, the genetic inquisition should not become possible in a democratic country. We are operating the switchboard of this development. Once the facts are created and the pratices are established, it will be difficult to reverse this development.

Therefore we need legal regulations for the application of gene technology in man. Misuse has to be stopped and irresponsible developments in research and sciences have to be avoided. The protection of privacy rights and man's dignity have to be guaranteed. To make it clear: It is not my point to stop progress. However, we have to point to an ethically responsible way. Appropriate solutions need an open dialogue between the public, politicians, and scientists.

At the end I want to give an example on the difficulties of the legislation in the area of gene technology. The German code of criminal procedures allows the taking of a bloodsample by a physician even without the consent of the suspect for the purpose of establishing facts which maybe of significance for the trial, already on the basis of existing law.

Last year the Federal Ministry of Justice has presented a first draft for a legal framework of DNA fingerprinting within the criminal procedures. Principally a detailed and specific basis has to be welcomed in the interest of legal safety.

A complete regulation has not yet been achieved by this draft: Results of DNA fingerprinting could be a start of a data base and could be used for a systematic search of suspects. No recommendations are proposed on a regulation in this field. These problems are yet not regulated in German law: It is allowed to use identification procedures on suspects. However, according to the examples given in the law we can see that the legislature means in particular photographs, classical fingerprints and measurements of body weight and size.

In my opinion this does not include the possibility to store results of DNA analysis in a data base. These differ significantly in quality from the storage of a photograph or a fingerprint.

In the light of the basic decision of Dezember 15th 1983 of the Federal Constitutional Court, the general privacy law includes the protection of the individial against an unlimited collection and procession of his personal data. This basic law guarantees the right of the individium to decide himself on the use of his personal data. This is called the right of informational selfdetermination of man.

Based on this decision the processing of DNA fingerprinting data in a data base represents an additional interference with positions protected by the constitution. This could only become possible with a specific authorization not yet existing.

This is particularly true if the results of the analysis should be stored beyond the end of the court case. On the other hand, it is true that the storage of DNA typing results by the police could be quite helpful in solving future crime cases.

A legal authorisation for data storage would be obviously in the interest of the prosecution authorities. I think it is very important that this authorisation would make it clear to the citizen in which way the state is handling personal data. We need this open approach especially, since we want to reduce concerns and fears related to gene technology.

On the other hand, a genetic "pattern" search would be an offence against man's dignity. The individial would be degraded to an object of actions taken by the state. This would be the first step towards the transparent man.

I think that with your congress you will be able to explain these problems to the public. You will make a significant contribution to the acceptance of responsible gene technology. Thus I wish that your convention will take a successful course

1 PCR Systems

1.1 General

SOME CONSIDERATIONS FOR USE OF AMP-FLPS FOR IDENTITY
TESTING

Bruce Budowle, F. Samuel Baechtel, and Catherine T. Comey
FSRTC Laboratory Division, FBI Academy, Quantico, Virginia
22135, USA

INTRODUCTION

AMP-FLP (i.e., amplified fragment length polymorphism)
technology can offer a high degree of discrimination among
individuals when evaluating the potential origin of
biological materials (Boerwinkle et al 1989, Budowle et al
1991, Horn et al 1989, Kasai et al 1990, Ludwig et al
1989). The technique combines the sensitivity of detection
and specificity afforded by the polymerase chain reaction
with the information content of variable number of tandem
repeats (VNTR) loci to provide an efficacious approach to
identity testing. A favorable attribute of the AMP-FLP
approach to identity testing is that loci currently under
study possess alleles that can be resolved readily by gel
electrophoresis into discrete fragment bands (Budowle et al
1991, Allen et al 1989). Such resolution is not possible
with restriction fragment length polymorphism (RFLP)
analysis currently used for the examination of DNA
recovered from biological materials.

Major considerations associated with the use of AMP-FLPs
for identity testing include the approach to profile
comparisons and the manner by which quantitative weight is
placed upon profile occurrences. This short communication
provides a brief discussion of possible approaches for
these areas of AMP-FLP analysis. Validation and population
genetic studies currently underway will determine whether
or not any of these proposed approaches actually will come
to fruition.

ALLELE DESIGNATIONS

With AMP-FLP systems, alleles can be evaluated without
determining their base pair sizes. Unknown samples can be
compared with an "allelic ladder" that is a composite of
common alleles of a particular VNTR locus (Budowle et al
1991). Thus, phenotyping and designation of the various
alleles are similar to the approach used for conventional
protein genetic marker systems. Moreover, when possible,
the allele classifications generally can be based upon the
number of tandem repeats relative to an allelic ladder
(Sajantila et al, in press).

Advances in Forensic Haemogenetics 4
Edited by Ch. Rittner and P. M. Schneider
© Springer-Verlag Berlin Heidelberg 1992

INTRA-LABORATORY COMPARISONS
Matching

While the resolution of AMP-FLP alleles is more
readily possible than with RFLP systems, as with many
genetic marker systems (including protein markers), the
alleles are discrete only to a point. As shown in figures
1 and 2, microvariability in allele sizes can occur in a
population. Such behavior is observed as apparently
different sized allele which cluster around a step in the
allele ladder. This microvariability that occurs among
individuals could be due to sequence variation or slight
differences in the size of alleles.

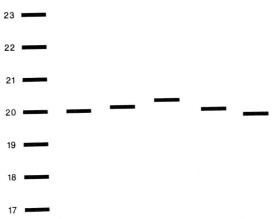

Figure 1. A diagram of alleles from different individuals
displaying microvariability around allele 20.

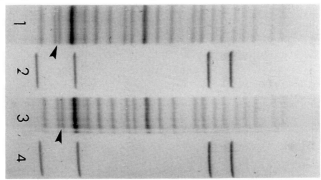

Figure 2. An AMP-FLP gel displaying a D1S80 allelic ladder
in lanes 1, 3, and 5. The ladder is a composite of alleles
from various individuals. Thus, the ladder serves as a
mixing or co-electrophoresis experiment. The arrow points

to a doublet at allele 17. Both alleles of the doublet would be designated generically as a 17, but are clearly resolved in the mixing experiment. In lanes 2 and 4 are bands from the 1 Kb ladder (BRL, Gaithersburg, MD). From top to bottom the sizes of the 1 Kb ladder bands are 517, 506, 396, and 344 base pairs. It is evident that the 1 Kb ladder bands displayed do not migrate according to their true size.

However, this phenomenon should have little impact on determining whether or not two samples' profiles match (i.e., included or excluded as potentially originating from the same source). Although an allelic ladder is placed on the gel, it has little if any impact on the matching process. An inclusion or exclusion is determined by profile comparison and/or co-electrophoresis experiments (figures 3 and 4).

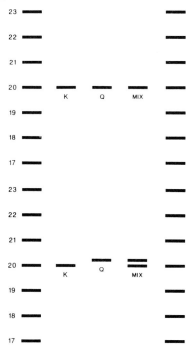

Figure 3. The diagram at the top displays an inclusion (or match), while the bottom diagram displays an exclusion. K is a known sample. Q refers to an unknown or questioned sample. MIX referes to a co-electrophoresis experiment of K and Q for resolving whether or not the two samples are considered similar by the analysis.

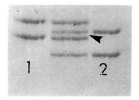

Figure 4. An AMP-FLP gel displaying a Collagen 2A1 VNTR marker. The center lane is a co-electrophoresis experiment of samples 1 and 2. Although samples 1 and 2 can be resolved visually without mixing and co-electrophoresis, the center lane demonstrates the effectiveness of mixing samples for comparison purposes. The arrow points to the two closest bands in the center lane which on the original gel are only 1 mm apart from each other.

WEIGHT CONSIDERATION

The allelic ladder is used after a match has been determined to assist in assigning proper quantitative weight to the occurrence of a profile. The common alleles which should be contained within an allelic ladder will have frequencies assigned to them based on empirical population studies. Gaps or areas in a ladder where there is no direct allele for comparison with the unknown sample, or a rare allele which lies outside the extremes of an allelic ladder, can be assigned an appropriate allele frequency.

Again, microvariability will not be a limitation for assigning the weight of a match. In the case of figure 1, where some of alleles in the sample population align with allele 20 and some are cathodal or anodal to allele 20, the frequencies of all these alleles can be totaled to provide a frequency for a generic allele 20. Thus, all alleles demonstrating microvariability around the step of an allelic ladder, although they could be resolved as different by a matching evaluation, will be given an overestimate of their true frequency in the sample population. Because generic allele frequencies will be used for estimating the frequency of occurrence of observed genotypes for highly polymorphic VNTR loci, classifications for population genetic data will be based on the generic allele classifications.

INTER-LABORATORY COMPARISONS

One of the advantages afforded by using AMP-FLP compared
with RFLP technology is an increased ease of accomplishing
inter-laboratory comparisons of DNA profiles. The nature
of RFLP analysis is such that changes in some aspects of
the technical procedure could result in slightly different
size determinations of bands from the same DNA. This is of
little concern for intra-laboratory comparisons, since the
same protocol generally is used to compare sample profiles;
however, it is not trivial for comparing DNA profiles
developed in different laboratories. Thus, to make
possible inter-laboratory comparisons of RFLP results there
has been a concerted effort by a number of laboratories
towards standardization of methodology. Requirements have
included using the same restriction endonuclease, probes,
and allelic controls. In fact, there are ongoing studies
by the European DNA Profiling (EDNAP) Group and the
Technical Working Group on DNA Analysis Methods (TWGDAM) to
assess the inherent variation among laboratories using
similar methodologies so that compatibility of data can be
made possible (Schneider et al 1991, Hicks 1991).

In contrast, AMP-FLP techniques permit standardization
based on the result instead of the method, as was possible
with protein genetic marker systems. With an allelic
ladder composed of alleles of the locus of interest and the
ability to resolve DNA fragments discretely, the
designation of alleles can be consistent among laboratories
regardless of the analytical method used. For example, it
would be anticipated that allele "18" of the D1S80 locus
should be an "18" in all laboratories involved in the
exchange of data. Of course the caveat that must be
considered is the possibility of different resolving powers
of the various electrophoretic systems employed by
laboratories. A system of lower resolution will not be as
effective for discriminating among individuals, but would
be expected to provide higher frequencies for the alleles.
However, the feasibility of standardizing on the AMP-FLP
result has been demonstrated by Robertson et al (1991).
They obtained similar AMP-FLP results for the D1S80 locus
when using either a discontinuous polyacrylamide gel
electrophoresis technique and silver staining or a
continuous zone agarose gel electrophoresis approach in a
gene scanner and fluorescently tagged primers.

CONCLUSION

This short communication is a brief statement of
considerations for the effective use of AMP-FLP technology.
It should be stressed that intra-laboratory comparisons of

AMP-FLPs will require standards within a laboratory but not standardization with other laboratories. These quality assurance standards are described elsewhere (Kearney et al 1991). While, methodological variation can be tolerated for situations such as identifying a potential serial rapist or the establishment of a DNA database identification system (Hicks 1991), a degree of standardization is essential. To ensure AMP-FLP compatibility between laboratories a nomenclature system for the alleles at each VNTR locus will have to be established. Moreover, the exchange or dissemination of allelic ladders (even if based on different primer sequences between laboratories) and/or known samples for corroborative testing should be encouraged.

REFERENCES

Allen RC, Graves G, Budowle B (1989) Polymerase chain reaction amplification products separated on rehydratable polyacrylamide gels and stained with silver. BioTechniques 7: 736-744

Boerwinkle E, Xiong W, Fourest E, Chan L (1989) Rapid typing of tandemly repeated hypervariable loci by the polymerase chain reaction: application to the apolipoprotein B 3^1 hypervariable region. Proc Natl Acad Sci USA 86: 212-216

Budowle B, Chakraborty R, Giusti AM, Eisenberg AJ, Allen RC (1991) Analysis of VNTR locus D1S80 by the PCR followed by high resolution PAGE. Am J Hum Genet 48: 137-144

Hicks JW (1991) Joint hearing on forensic DNA analysis. Crime Lab Dig 18: 97-100

Horn GT, Richards B, Klinger W (1989) Amplification of a highly polymorphic VNTR segment by the polymerase chain reaction. Nucleic Acids Res 17: 2140

Kasai K, Nakamura Y, White R (1990) Amplification of a variable number of tandem repeats (VNTR) locus (pMCT 118) by the polymerase chain reaction (PCR) and its application to forensic science. J For Sci 35: 1196-1200

Kearney JJ, Mudd JL, Hartmann JR, et al (1991) Guidelines for a quality assurance program for DNA analysis. Crime Lab Dig 18: 44-75

Ludwig EH, Friedl W, McCarthy BJ (1989) High-resolution analysis of a hypervariable region in the human apolipoprotein B gene. Am J Hum Genet 45: 458-464

Robertson J, Schaefer T, Kronick M, Budowle B (1991) Automated analysis of fluorescent amplified fragment length polymorphisms for DNA typing. Advances in Forensic Haemogenetics (in press)

Sajantila A, Budowle B, Strom M, Johnsson V, Lukka M, Peltonen L, Enholm C (1992) Amplification of alleles at the D1S80 locus by the polymerase chain reaction: Comparisons of Finnish and North American Caucasians and forensic casework evaluations. Am J Hum Genet (in press)

Schneider PM, Fimmers R, Woodroffe S, et al (1991) Report of a European collaboration exercise comparing DNA typing results using a single locus VNTR probe. For Sci Int 49: 1-15

Forensic Use of Short Tandem Repeats *via* PCR

C.T. Caskey and H.A. Hammond

Institute for Molecular Genetics and Howard Hughes Medical Institute, Baylor College of Medicine, Houston, TX 77030

INTRODUCTION

The DNA sequence of man's chromosomes has the potential for wide variation from individual to individual since only 1% encodes functional elements, *i.e.* genes. Sequence differences were first detected by restriction fragment length polymorphisms (RFLPs) using the Southern method (Southern, 1975). These two-allele polymorphisms were used for mapping Huntington disease locus and diagnosis of both ß-thalassemia and sickle cell disease. Jeffreys (1985b) and Nakamura (1987) subsequently described a new class of RFLPs which arise from repeated sequences occurring in different copy numbers from individual to individual. They were referred to as satellite sequences or variable number of tandem repeats (VNTR). These highly informative repeat sequence polymorphisms have been used extensively in the mapping of human disease genes such as cystic fibrosis (CF) and neurofibromatosis (NF), and more relevant to this meeting, for personal identification (Jeffreys *et al.* 1985a) (Gill *et al.* 1985). The method of identification was Southern analysis. At many of these loci, the repeat sequences are smaller than the resolving power of agarose gels, so discrete alleles will not be differentiated. Despite this shortcoming, the large number of alleles provides a very powerful DNA-based personal identification method. A summary of how such alleles are measured and grouped for the purpose of determining RFLP matching and significance of match has been discussed in numerous articles (Budowle, 1990; Budowle *et al.* 1991; Devlin *et al.* 1991). Occasionally a forensic DNA specimen may migrate in the gel faster or slower than expected, thus assigning an allele to an incorrect molecular weight and possibly leading to incorrect matching or mismatching. While it has been suggested that internal molecular weight markers could allow for correction of "band shifts", a general method for this correction is not validated. The uncontrollable character of the forensic specimen has also limited the VNTR/Southern technology, since high molecular weight DNA is required in substantial quantity (Budowle *et al.* 1990; McNally *et al.* 1989; Baechtel, 1988). Consequently as high as 25% of forensic specimens are useless for analysis.

We observed in our sequencing of the HPRT gene a single tetramer repeat (AGAT) which was found to vary from person

Advances in Forensic Haemogenetics 4
Edited by Ch. Rittner and P. M. Schneider
© Springer-Verlag Berlin Heidelberg 1992

to person in the number of tetramer repeats (Edwards *et al.* 1990). From this initial observation we have proceeded to develop and characterize a series of highly polymorphic loci whose polymorphisms occur on the basis of single tri-, tetra-, and pentanucleotide repeats. We believe these short tandem repeats (STRs) to be extremely useful genetic markers for personal identification and have shown them to be useful for forensic analysis.

ACQUISITION OF LOCI

The genetic loci listed in Table 1 are now under study since we know them to be highly polymorphic. For some, the repeated sequence was discovered by DNA sequencing of genes being studied in our laboratory. For others, the sequences were identified by scanning Genbank entries. Finally, we have now developed methods for specifically seeking out such polymorphic loci. There appears to be no limitation on the identification of many polymorphic loci.

Table 1. Current STR loci for forensic use

Locus and STR	Chromosome
HUMRENA4[ACAG]	1q32
HUMFABP[AAT]	4q31
HUMTH01[AATG]	11p15.5
HUMPLA2A1[AAT]	12q
HUMCD4[AAAAT]	12p
HUMHPRTB[AGAT]	Xq26
HUMARA[AGC]	Xcen-q13

Two methods are now being used for identification of new STR loci. Since we do not seek a specific chromosome localization of an STR and we are early in development of markers, a shotgun approach continues to be the most rapid. Sheared human DNA is cloned into a DNA sequencing vector, plated at low density and those containing one of five repeats identified by hybridization of a radioactive oligomer of 30 bases in length. Using stringent conditions only those predicted to have more than eight repeats in tandem are detected. Sequencing the ends of the clone provides the flanking sequence to the STR, necessary for fashioning a pair of primers for polymerase chain reaction (PCR) amplification. While the method is useful, it has the disadvantage that the sequence information may be inadequate to develop small PCR elements, *i.e.* the primers may be distant to the repeat. For this reason we developed a general method which provides sequence data immediately flanking the STR (Edwards *et al.* 1991a). We have used the method to obtain 16 new STR loci. Each was identified in λ clones. Our success at amplifying both sides of the AAT repeat is greater than 70%. We have obtained sequence information for 8 pairs of PCR primers and found the repeat sequence to amplify in all cases. Presently 1 of 6 is polymorphic as determined by survey of a panel of 10 unrelated female individuals. Examples of a highly polymorphic and a monomorphic STR are given in Fig. 1.

POPULATION GENETIC FEATURES

The establishment of reliable databases for STRs is operationally easier than for VNTR loci, since the method is PCR-based, alleles are distinguished by sequencing gel analysis, and the allele number is generally smaller. An example of four databases for the AGC repeat within the coding of the androgen receptor is given in Fig. 2. In a separate communication we reported the population genetic features of five loci. There have been no new mutations observed for these loci when over 900 meioses were studied in families provided by Centre d'Etude du Polymorphisme Humain (CEPH). Thus the inheritance of our STRs is stable and they are suitable for parentage studies. We have had the experience of observing new mutation events in CA repeats at the Duchenne muscular dystrophy locus (DMD) and therefore have reservations regarding their stability and utility for parentage studies. Four ethnic population databases have been examined for HUMFABP[AAT], HUMHPRTB[AGAT], HUMARA[AGC], HUMTH01[AATG] and HUMRENA4[ACAG] to determine their population genetic features. The details of these studies are given elsewhere (Edwards *et al.* 1991b). We conclude, however, that the frequencies of alleles measured reflect a genetic marker system which is conforming to Hardy-Weinberg equilibrium and thus allele frequency measurements can be used to calculate the significance of allele matches between two DNA specimens. Furthermore, we find no evidence of linkage disequilibrium between loci and thus the value at each loci identification can be multiplied to estimate the significance of match. These features indicate that these loci can be used in forensic studies based on their genetic properties.

MULTIPLEX AMPLIFICATION OF STRs

We have shown that multiplex amplification of as many as 9 target loci (exons) within the DMD gene can be achieved with fidelity (Chamberlain *et al.* 1988). The multiplex amplification of three STRs is readily achieved using radioisotopic

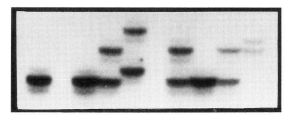

Fig. 1A. PCR results of a polymorphic locus with the STR repeat AAT for ten unrelated female individuals

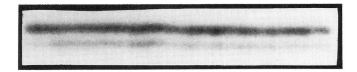

Fig. 1B. PCR results of a monomorphic locus with the STR repeat AAT for ten unrelated female individuals

detection. We sought to co-amplify 9-12 loci and thus turned to a fluorescent detection system. This analysis was facilitated by use of the ABI 373 automated DNA sequencer which uses sequencing gels for resolution and provides 4 different fluorescent tags within the same lane. By judicious choice of fluorescent labelled primers, knowledge of allele sizes, and primer spacing we have achieved a 3 locus co-amplification and related the products to internal allele standards (Edwards *et al.* 1991a). More recently, ABI has developed a GeneScanner which appears to have advantages for this type of analysis. This device uses a molecular weight ladder from prokaryotic sources which allows allele identifications and molecular weight determinations. This appears to be the proper direction to move, toward a user friendly, automated analytic instrument. The A.L.F. unit manufactured by Pharmacia/LKB also has features making it amenable to gel analysis. We are adapting our most informative loci to a multiplex PCR amplification procedure with fluorescent products.

FORENSIC APPLICATIONS

We have applied our STR personal identification system to several medical diagnostic and forensic circumstances. We

Frequency Distribution of HUMARA[AGC] Alleles

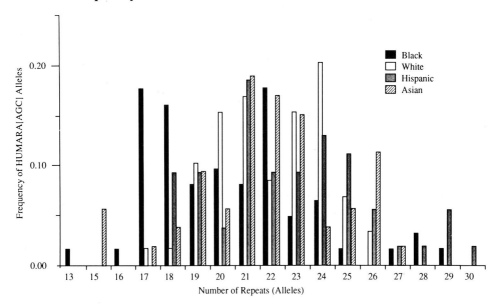

Fig. 2. Allele frequency graph of caucasian, black, hispanic, and asian populations for the HUMARA[AGC] locus

have been able to provide quick resolution of questions in zygosity testing, maternal or fetal origin of chorionic villus biopsies, and pedigree validation for linkage analysis. It has been surprising how quickly we have received a number of request for prenatal paternity testing. Our program has thus far only provided prenatal paternity testing for those case related to documented sexual assaults. We have completed four such cases to date. Counseling in all cases revealed the desire to continue the pregnancies in the event that the fetus was their husband's. One case, shown in Fig. 3, indicated that the fetus of a victim of gang rape was not the progeny of the husband, and termination of the pregnancy was elected. In another case counseling as to the power of the method resulted in the victim dropping the rape charges and identifying a consensual partner.

Forensic identification services have been provide to the Armed Forces Institute of Pathology by a Collaborative effort with Cellmark Diagnostics. The circumstances of aircraft crew submersion (1 month), scud and weapon explosions and the return of air crew remains allowed for the use of PCR based testing to help verify identifications. Fig. 4 shows an

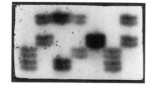

HUMTH01[AATG]

Fig. 3. Results from one of six STR loci analyzed for a paternity trio. The mother was the victim of a gang rape. The husband was excluded as being the father of the fetus using STRs. This exclusion information was the basis for terminating the pregnancy

example of studies performed to verify assignment of body parts by forensic pathologists. Two of the six genetic markers used are illustrated. Note that we observed three genotypes within samples that had been associated with one victim. Calculation of the frequency of six genotypes observed ranged from 1 in 12,000 to 1 in 450,000.
The United States had approximately 450,000 troops involved in the Desert Storm operation, however, all samples were from small combat groups. Had reference samples been available identification would have been greatly simplified. Paternity testing was also employed to verify the remains of a pilot who had been classifies as Missing in Action (MIA). Parental blood specimens were associated with the genotype for the mia remains verifying that the correct body had been returned.

Our laboratory currently provides RFLP-VNTR results to the U.S. Court system, and has reported a significant number (42%) of exclusions in criminal sexual assault cases. We have initiated a policy of screen cases with STRs for rapid identification of exclusions, although are not yet introducing STR data into the courts. All cases and particularly matches with STRs will continue to be studied in parallel with VNTR loci. This experience will strengthen our objective of replacing Southern-based technology, with PCR based analysis of STR loci.

FORENSIC IDENTIFICATION OF HUMAN REMAINS

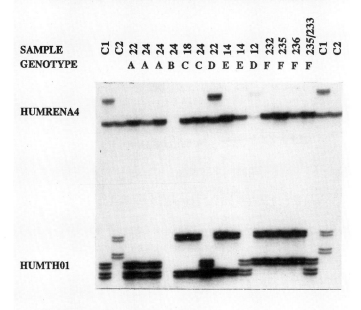

GENOTYPE FREQUENCIES FOR SIX LOCI   (CAUCASIAN)

A - 1 IN 450000	B - 1 IN 126500	C - 1 IN 12000
D - 1 IN 83000	E - 1 IN 357000	F - 1 IN 62500

Fig. 4. Results for 2 STR loci on samples from Operation Desert Storm. Numbers above the samples indicate the assignment of samples by the Army. Letters represent the genotypes represented by STR analysis for six loci for each sample

REFERENCES

Budowle B, Baechtel FS, and Adams DE (1990) Validation with regard to environmental insults of the RFLP procedure for forensic purposes. American Chemical Society Symposium Series (in press)

Budowle B, Giusti AM, Waye JS, Baechtel FS, Fourney RM, Adams DE, Presley LA, Deadman HA, and Monson KL (1991) Fixed BIN analysis for statistical evaluation of continuous distributions of allelic data from VNTR loci for use in forensic comparisons. Am J Hum Genet 48:841-855

Budowle BF (1990) Data for forensic matching criteria for VNTR profiles. In: Data acquisition and statistical analysis for DNA typing laboratories. Promega Corporation, Madison, WI, pp. 103-115

Baechtel FS (1988) Recovery of DNA from human biological specimens. Crime Laboratory Digest 15:95-96

Chamberlain JS, Gibbs RA, Ranier JE, Nguyen P-N, and Caskey CT (1988) Deletion screening of the Duchenne muscular dystrophy locus *via* multiplex DNA amplification. Nucleic Acids Res 16:11141-11156

Devlin B, Risch N, and Roeder K (1991) Estimation of allele frequencies for VNTR loci. Am J Hum Genet 48:662-676

Edwards A, Voss H, Rice P, Civitello A, Stegemann J, Schwager C, Zimmermann J, Erfle H, Caskey CT, and Ansorge W (1990) Automated DNA sequencing of the human HPRT locus. Genomics 6:593-608

Edwards A, Civitello A, Hammond HA, and Caskey CT (1991a) DNA typing and genetic mapping with trimeric and tetrameric tandem repeats. Am J Hum Genet, in press

Edwards A, Hammond HA, Caskey CT, and Chakraborty R (1991b) Population genetics of trimeric and tetrameric tandem repeats in four human ethnic groups. Genomics, submitted

Gill P, Jeffreys AJ, and Werrett DJ (1985) Forensic application of DNA "fingerprints". Nature 318:577-579

Jeffreys AJ, Wilson V, and Thein SL (1985a) Individual-specific "fingerprints" of human DNA. Nature 316:76-79

Jeffreys AJ, Wilson V, and Thein SL (1985b) Hypervariable 'minisatellite' regions in human DNA. Nature 314:67-73

McNally L, Shaler, RC, Baird M, Balazs I, De Forest P, and Kobilinsky L (1989) Evaluation of deoxyribonucleic acid (DNA) isolated from human bloodstains exposed to ultraviolet light, heat, humidity, and soil contamination. J Forensic Sciences 34:1059-1069

Nakamura Y, Leppert M, O'Connel P, Wolff R, Holm T, Culver M, Martin C, Fujimoto E, Hoff M, Kumlin E, and White R (1987) Variable number of tandem repeat (VNTR) markers for human gene mapping. Science 235:1616-1622

Southern EM (1975) Detection of specific sequences among DNA fragments separated by gel electrophoresis. J Mol Biol 98:503-517

Automation of the Amplification and Sequencing of Mitochondrial DNA

K.M. Sullivan, R. Hopgood, and P. Gill

Central Research and Support Establishment, The Forensic Science Service, Aldermaston, Reading, Berkshire, RG7 4PN, UK

INTRODUCTION

Analysis of mitochondrial DNA sequence is an effective method for determining genetic individuality for the purposes of forensic investigation (Reynolds et al. 1991). It is a more sensitive test than the analysis of chromosomal loci since there are between 1000 and 10000 copies of the mitochondrial genome per human cell, and it is also useful in determining familial relationships because mitochondria are of maternal origin (Orrego and King 1990). Much of the observed sequence variation between individuals is concentrated in two hypervariable sections within the mitochondrial control region, which can be readily sequenced and is of high information content (Greenberg et al. 1983; Aquadro and Greenberg 1983).

For DNA sequencing to be used as a routine technique in forensic analysis, it is essential that the process is highly automated to maximise sequence throughput, minimise errors in data handling, and to streamline database management (Sullivan et al. 1991). This paper briefly describes the optimisation of sequence data generation from mtDNA by combining PCR amplification with solid-phase automated sequencing.

DNA AMPLIFICATION

A 2 stage amplification process was utilised. In the first stage, a 1.3Kb fragment spanning the entire non-coding region was amplified using primers L15926 (5'-TCAAAGCTTACACCAGTCTTGTCTTGTAAACC) and H00580 (5'-TTGAGGAGGTAAGCT-ACATA). The PCR reaction comprised the following: primers at 1μM; dATP, dGTP, dCTP and dTTP each at 200μM, 1.25U Taq polymerase; 1x'PARR' buffer (CamBio), in a total volume of 25μl. DNA template amplified included in this mixture varied from 10ng of total DNA extracted from blood, to non-quantifiable amounts isolated from sections of single hair shafts. Cycling conditions were as follows: 94°C for 45 seconds, 50°C for 1 min then 72°C for 5.5 min, for 35 cycles.

0.5μl aliquots of the PCR product were added directly to a second reaction using a pair of primers internal to those used in the first PCR round: M13(-21)H16401 (5'-TGTAAAACGACGACGGCCAGTTGATTTCACGGAGGATGGTG) and L15997 (5'-CACCATTAGCACCCAAAGCT). The former primer is chimaeric comprising the M13(-21) universal sequencing primer sequence at the 5' end plus the H16401 sequence at the 3' end which is complementary to part the mtDNA D-Loop sequence. The latter primer (L15997) was biotinylated at the 5' end. The PCR reaction mix comprised 2.5U Taq polymerase, 0.5μM final concentration of each primer, 1xPARR buffer and 20μM final concentration each dNTP in a final volume of 50μl.

Advances in Forensic Haemogenetics 4
Edited by Ch. Rittner and P. M. Schneider
© Springer-Verlag Berlin Heidelberg 1992

SEQUENCING REACTIONS

The biotinylated PCR product was added to 50µl LiCl and 50µl streptavidin-coated Dynal™ beads, followed by incubation at 48°C for 15 mins to immobilise the DNA. The double-stranded DNA was denatured in 0.15M NaOH for 4 mins and the non-biotinylated strand was eluted from the beads by removing the supernatant, leaving single-stranded sequencing template attached to the beads. The bead pellet was then resuspended in 60µl dH$_2$O.

By tagging the 5' end of one primer of each pair prior to amplification with the universal -21M13 primer sequence it was possible to use the immobilised PCR product in sequencing reactions using dye-labelled universal sequencing primers. Sequencing ladders were generated with an Applied Biosystems Sequenase Sequencing Kit as follows: for the dideoxyadenosine sequencing reaction, 8µl of the beads were immobilised with a magnet, and the supernatant was removed. To the beads 0.4pmol buffered -21M13 primer (labelled with dye 'JOE') was added in a final volume of 4µl. Primers were annealed to the DNA by heating to 65°C then slowly cooling to room temperature. 2U Sequenase T7 DNA polymerase (USB) plus 1µl of appropriate dideoxyadenosine extension mix were added, and the mixture was incubated at 37°C for 20 mins. Set up in parallel were the three other sequencing reactions for dideoxycytosine, dideoxyguanosine and dideoxythymidine, using FAM, TAMRA and ROX-labelled primers respectively, and under effectively identical conditions except that all quantities were doubled for the dideoxyguanosine and dideoxythymidine reactions. The four reactions were terminated by the addition of stop-salt solution; then they were pooled and the supernatant was removed from the beads. The extension products were eluted from the beads by incubation in deionized formamide for 4 mins at 37°C. The supernatant was then loaded on a 6% acrylamide gel and run in an Applied Biosystems 373A sequencer. Sequence manipulations and comparisons were performed with the SEQED software program (Applied Biosystems).

Alternatives to solid-phase sequencing of biotinylated PCR products have been evaluated for the generation of single-stranded sequence template, but have proven inferior in both reproducibility and sequence quality (data not shown). These included asymmetric PCR in the second round of amplification, lambda exonuclease digestion of one product strand which has been generated from a kinased primer, sequencing of double-stranded template, and Taq cycle sequencing.

This amplification and sequencing strategy enables high quality data to be generated from mtDNA (Figure 1). The entire sequence-generation process is highly automated; full-length amplification products (468bp) and sequence ladders can be readily generated from this hypervariable region. 10ng total DNA template is generally used for amplification and sequencing, but successful amplification has been achieved with mtDNA extracted from just 0.5cm of hair shaft.

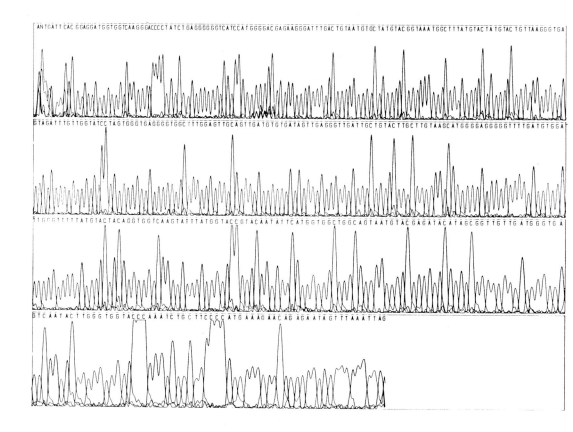

Figure 1. Mitochondrial DNA sequence: PCR product was generated with primers M13(-21)H16401 and L15997 then bound to Dynal beads and sequenced with Sequenase

REFERENCES

Aquadro CF and Greenberg BD (1983) Human mitochondrial DNA variation and evolution: Analysis of nucleotide sequences from seven individuals. Genetics 103: 287-312

Greenberg BD, Newbold JE and Sugino A (1983) Intraspecific nucleotide sequence variability surrounding the origin of replication in human mitochondrial DNA. Gene 21: 33-49

Orrego C and King MC (1990) Determination of familial relationships. In: Innis MA, Gelfand DH, Sninsky JJ, White TJ (eds) PCR Protocols, Academic Press, London, p416

Reynolds R, Sensaburgh G, Blake E (1991) Analysis of genetic markers in forensic DNA samples using the polymerase chain reaction. Analytical Chemistry 63: 2-15

Sullivan KM, Hopgood R, Lang B, Gill P (1991) Automated amplification and sequencing of human mitochondrial DNA. Electrophoresis 12: 17-21

1.2 Methodology

The Development and Evaluation of New Genetic Markers for the Application of PCR to Forensic Casework

R. Reynolds, R. Saiki, M. Grow, N. Fildes, G. McClure, S. Scharf, S. Cosso, S. Walsh, and H. Erlich

Cetus Corporation, 1400 Fifty-Third Street, Emeryville, California, 94608, USA

INTRODUCTION

The forensic group at Cetus Corporation is developing a variety of PCR-based genetic markers for the analysis of forensic evidence samples. We also are working on a system that enables you to assess the quality or "amplifiability" of extracted DNA samples.

SEQUENCE POLYMORPHISM MARKERS

PolyMarker Amplification and Typing System

The Amplitype HLA DQα system was the first PCR-based marker applied to forensic casework samples. This reverse dot blot typing system distinguishes six DQα alleles which result in 21 genotypes. The Pd for this single marker system is 0.94 for Caucasians.

To increase the power of discrimination obtained from a single sample test, we developed a system in which five genetic markers are coamplified with DQα. The six PCR products amplified by this PolyMarker system are listed below along with the sizes of the products, the number of alleles distinguished, and the chromosomal locations of the markers:

Markers	PCR product (bp)	Alleles	Chromosomes
LDL^r	254	2	19
DQα	239/242	6	6
gypA	190	2	4
$^G\gamma$-globin	172	3	11
D7S8	151	2	7
Gc	138	3	4

The combined Pd value for these six markers are greater than 0.999 for Caucasian, Black and Hispanic individuals in the United States.

The five markers containing two or three alleles are typed on a single strip using the reverse dot blot technology; the DQα type is determined on a separate strip. Both sets of strips are hybridized and processed under identical conditions.

We are completing our forensic validation studies which address each of the validation issues in the TWGDAM DNA Quality Assurance Guidelines.

Advances in Forensic Haemogenetics 4
Edited by Ch. Rittner and P. M. Schneider
© Springer-Verlag Berlin Heidelberg 1992

Gender Identification

We have developed a gender identification system in which a single primer pair is used to amplify a polymorphic region of a homologous zinc protein found on the X and Y chromosomes. This region contains a HaeIII site common to both the X and Y chromosome sequences and a polymorphic HaeIII site that is present only on the Y chromosome. Digestion of PCR products with HaeIII reveals the presence of X and Y chromosomes in the extracted DNA sample.

The advantages of this gender identification system over previously described systems are:

1. A product is generated for both the X and Y chromosomes such that the presence female DNA is signalled by a positive response rather than a lack of Y chromosome amplification.

2. Only one primer pair is utilized to generate X and Y specific products of the same size. Potential problems due to preferential priming between X and Y primer pairs and preferential amplification of smaller products are eliminated.

3. The polymorphic, homologous zinc finger protein is present in only one copy on each chromosome, allowing quantitation of X and Y chromosomes.

LENGTH POLYMORPHISM MARKERS

DIS80

We have developed and released a reagent set for the amplification and sizing of DIS80 alleles. We developed a DIS80 ladder containing 15 of the 29 alleles we have identified. Alleles containing 14, 16, and 18 repeat units have been sequenced in both directions, allowing the ladder to be registered and allele designations to be made according to the number of repeat units they contain.

We also are developing reagents sets for the YNZ22, apoB and col2AI loci. We have tested all of these AMP-FLP systems in the TC480 and TC9600 Perkin Elmer-Cetus thermal cyclers, and we have obtained comparable results from both instruments.

AMP-FLP Validation Studies

Frequently forensic DNA samples are degraded to some extent. It has been demonstrated previously that amplification of severely degraded DNA samples yields either the correct HLA DQα type or no type. More recent studies indicate that it is possible to obtain ambiguous and even incorrect DIS80 types from moderately degraded DNA samples.

Ambiguous types are obtained when the smaller of two observed alleles is amplified to a significantly greater extent than the other allele. This type of result can arise from amplification of a partially degraded DNA sample or from amplification of one of a variety of mixed samples.

Incorrect types are obtained when the degraded DNA sample can support amplification of products in the size range of the smaller allele but not in the size range of the larger allele. As a result, a sample from a heterozygous individual can be analyzed incorrectly as a homozygous type. More severely degraded DNA samples simply yield no DIS80 type.

Given some of the inherent properties of amplifying PCR products of significantly different lengths, it is likely that AMP-FLP markers will not be as robust as amplified sequence polymorphism markers. Consequently, great care will have to be taken to interpret AMP-FLP results.

DNA Quality Indicator

It is important to assess the quality of a DNA sample so that the most discriminating information can be obtained from AMP-FLP systems. However, it is not always possible to use agarose gel electrophoresis to analyze the quality of an extracted sample. For example, a portion of DNA extracted from hairs or small stains is too limited to visualize on an ethidium bromide stained gel. Also, single stranded DNA samples resulting from Chelex extraction cannot be visualized on ethidium bromide stained gels.

Clearly, another method for assessing quality is needed. While the term "quality" generally refers to the degradation state of DNA, it also must reflect the "amplifiability" of a DNA sample when PCR based systems are being employed. This aspect of a sample is important to consider because 10 ng of a high molecular weight sample will amplify more efficiently than 10 ng of a significantly degraded sample and 10 ng of a sample containing trace amounts of inhibitors.

We are developing a DNA Quality Indicator system designed to indicate how well a DNA sample will amplify HLA DQα and PCR products in the size range of the DIS80, YN722, apoB and col2AI AMP-FLP alleles. Our first generation indicator contains HLA DQα primers and two additional pairs of primers that yield 1 and 2 kilobase PCR products. The presence and absence of these three products on a gel will indicate which AMP-FLP systems can be amplified reliably from the DNA sample in question. We are modifying the sizes of the PCR products in the Quality Indicator to be more applicable to the AMP-FLP systems listed above.

Since the DNA Quality Indicator system contains HLA DQα primers, samples yielding a HLA-DQα product band on the gel can be typed directly on the HLA-DQα probe strips. This feature of the system allows discriminating information to be obtained from the sample in addition to the information regarding which AMP-FLP systems can be typed, and provides an advantage over agarose gel electrophoresis.

INVESTIGATIONS TO IMPROVE ALLELE DEFINITION IN THE "COLLAGEN 2A1" SYSTEM (AMP-FLP)

C. Puers, P. Wiegand, B. Brinkmann

Institut für Rechtsmedizin, Westfälische-Wilhelms-Universität,
Von-Esmarch-Str. 86, 4400 Münster, Germany

INTRODUCTION

Continuous distributions of fragments are still characteristic of the highly polymorphic single locus VNTR systems (Puers et al. 1991). To solve these problems different bin approaches and match criteria have been elaborated (Baird et al. 1986, Brenner and Morris 1990, Gill et al. 1990). Another inherent problem lies in the use of λ-DNA as marker DNA whose sequences differ considerably from those to be measured. The electrophoretic mobility of DNA is also influenced by sequence and composition. Therefore, λ-DNA is basically not suitable for estimating size of (human) fragments. One concept for a more exact estimation of allele size is to compare the unknown human fragment with a human DNA standard composed of as many alleles from the system under investigation as possible (Puers et al. 1991).
The construction of such a standard is also possible with AMP-FLPs (Amplified Fragment Length Polymorphism) where PCR can be used to construct an allelic ladder.

One such system is "COL 2A1" (12 q 14.3) which is located in the 3'-flanking region of the Collagen gene and was initially sequenced by Stoker et al. (1985). Two types of primers have been applied to amplification (Wu et al. 1990, Priestley et al. 1990), therefore fragments recovered by Priestley et al. are 72 bp longer than those of Wu et al.. Priestley et al. described 5 alleles, in the range between 650 and 890 bp while Wu et al. described 4 alleles in the range 600 - 700 bp. The repeat sequence can be 31 or 34 bp long (Stoker et al. 1985) and is inherited in a mendelian fashion. This situation can therefore lead to fragments which are different in composition but identical in their electrophoretic mobility.
In spite of these considerations the aim of this investigation was to construct a human DNA standard to achieve better comparability.

MATERIALS AND METHODS

Blood samples were extracted as previously described (Brinkmann et al. 1991). The amplification was carried out in a Thermocycler (Biometra) with primers (20mers) described by Wu et al. (1990) under the following conditions: Denaturing: 94°C, 1 min. Annealing: 60°C, 1 min. Extension: 72°C, 1.5 min. Cycles: 25
Each amplification sample contained 100 ng human genomic DNA, 200 μM dNTP, 1x Taq buffer (Promega), 2 U Taq polymerase (Promega) and primers (0.5 μM). The total assay volume was 50 μl and this was covered by 30 μl mineral oil.

The first electrophoretical separation of the amplified fragments (Fig. 1) was carried out in PA-gels (PA = polyacrylamide) (6% T, 3% C; 400 μm; 10 cm; horizontal) with piperazine diacrylamide as cross-linker. The leading buffer was 140 mM borate solution and the tracking buffer was 35 mM sulfate solution. The final separations (Figs. 2 - 5) were performed in PA-gels (5% T, 2,5% C; 400 μm; 20 cm; horizontal) with piperazine diacrylamide as cross-linker, leading buffer 280 mM borate solution and tracking buffer 80 mM formate solution (Budowle, pers. com. 1991). All buffers were adjusted with TRIS to pH 9.0. To eliminate any artefacts due to amplification efficiency, equimolar mixtures of human DNA amplifications were prepared.

RESULTS AND DISCUSSION

The first standard (Fig. 1) consisted of 6 alleles taken from amplified DNA from 6 individuals using 6 % PAG for separation. However, using this gel, the separation was insufficient. The band no. 4 (lane S) was a combination of corresponding alleles from individuals I-IV but 2 individual samples (III, IV) exhibit 2 alleles in this region (Fig. 1). It was therefore necessary to improve the electrophoretic conditions for separation. A modification of the running conditions led to the production of a second standard ladder (Figs. 2; see materials and methods).

Advances in Forensic Haemogenetics 4
Edited by Ch. Rittner and P. M. Schneider
© Springer-Verlag Berlin Heidelberg 1992

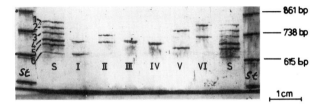

Fig. 1: First standard for the AMP-FLP system "COL 2A1" (S) and PCR amplified human DNA samples (I - IV) from which it was constructed. Separation of DNA fragments was performed in a 6 % PA-Gel using 140 mM borate solution as leading buffer and 35 mM sulfate solution as tracking buffer. TRIS was used in both buffers to adjust the pH to 9.0. The gel was silver stained (Budowle et al. 1991). The original distance between the smallest and largest standard fragment (lane M) was 1.9 cm. St = 123 bp ladder (Gibco)

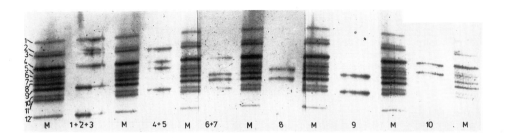

Fig. 2: Magnified section of the PA gel showing the second improved standard for the AMP-FLP system "COL 2A1" (M) and the PCR amplified human DNA samples (1-10) from which it was constructed. Separation of DNA fragments was performed in a 5 % PA gel using 280 mM borate solution as leading buffer and 80 mM formate solution as tracking buffer adjusted with TRIS to pH 9.0 (Budowle, pers. com. 1991). The gel was silver stained (Budowle et al. 1991). 1+2+3: Mixture of the "COL 2A1" DNA fragments of the individuals 1,2 and 3; 4+5: Mixture of the "COL 2A1" DNA fragments of the individuals 4 and 5; 6+7: Mixture of the "COL 2A1" DNA fragments of the individuals 6 and 7; 8,9,10: Separate "COL 2A1" DNA fragments of the individuals 8,9 and 10. The original distance between the smallest and largest standard fragment (lane M) was 1.9 cm

One criterion for the quality of separation is the distance between the smallest and largest standard fragment. This measurement of 1 cm (Fig. 1) could be improved to 1,9 cm using the final method of separation (Fig. 2; see materials and methods).

The second standard finally contained 13 definable alleles (Fig. 3) but sometimes only 12 could be differentiated (Fig. 2).

Figure 3 impressively demonstrates the problems with this type of electrophoresis.

It can be seen that the separate DNA fragments in lane A and B cannot be clearly assigned to the corresponding bands of the allelic ladder, although they are components of this ladder.

PA gels cannot yet be produced with a unified quality so that the results are not reproducible.

It is necessary to obtain an even higher quality of PAG electrophoresis and resolution of fragments in this system from which a larger number of alleles can be assumed.

The smallest distance between the fragment lengths which can be distinguished by the BioImage Video measuring system (Millipore) is only 3 bp but this is difficult to resolve.

One possible improvement would be to label the "COL 2A1" fragments radioactively and to separate them on a sequencing gel (40 cm PAG, denaturing conditions). Sequencing of the individual alleles to verify the gene model would also be desirable.

The "COL 2A1" system seems to be much more complex than was originally assumed in previous publications (Stoker et al. 1985; Priestley et al. 1990; Wu et al. 1990).

Nevertheless this system can be a useful tool for identification and paternity analysis using a binning approach.

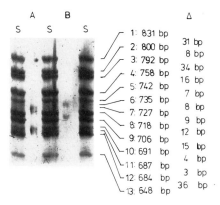

Fig. 3: Magnification of the second improved human DNA standard (S) separated in a second gel using the same method as presented in Figs. 2 - 4. Here it is possible to differentiate 13 alleles instead of 12 in the standard. The DNA fragment lengths were estimated by comparison to the 123 bp ladder using the BioImage system. In lanes **A** and **B** amplified "COL 2A1" fragments from the separate individuals from which the standard is constructed are only recognizable with difficulty. The fragments in lane **B** demonstrate the problems with the gels presently in use. The correct assignment of unknown alleles in such gels is impossible, although they give a high resolution for the human standard

REFERENCES

Baird M, Balazc I, Giusti A, Miyazaki L, Nicholas L, Wexler K, Kanter E, Glassberg J, Allen F, Rubinstein, P. and Sussman, L. (1986) Allele frequency distribution to two highly polymorphic DNA sequences in three ethnic groups and its application to the determination of paternity. Am J Hum Genet, 29, 489-501

Brenner C and Morris JW (1990) Paternity index calculations in single locus hypervariable DNA probes: Validation and other studies. The International Symposium on Human Identification - published by Promega Corporation, 21-55

Brinkmann B, Rand S and Wiegand P (1991) Population and family data of RFLP's using slected single - and multilocus systems, Int J Leg Med 104: 81-86

Budowle B, Chakraborty R, Giusti AM, Eisenberg AJ and Allen RC (1991) Analysis of the variable numer of tandem repeat locus D1S80 by the polymerase chain reaction followed by high resolution polyacrylamide gel elctrophoresis. Am J Hum Genet 48: 137-144

Gill, P., Sullivan, K. and Werrett, D.J. (1990) The analysis of hypervariable DNA profiles: problems associated with the objective determination of the probability of a match. Hum Genet 85: 75-79

Nakamura Y., Leppert M., O'Connell P., Wolff R., Holm T., Culver M., Martin C., Fujimoto E., Hoff M., Kul min E. and White R. (1987a) Variable number of tandem repeat (VNTR) markers for human gene mapping. Science 235: 1616-1622

Nakamura Y, Gillilan S, O'Connell P, Leppert M, Lathrop GM, Lalouel J-M, White R (1987b) Isolation and mapping of a polmorphic DNA sequence pYNH24 on chromosome 2 (D2S44). Nucleic Acids Res 15: 10073

Puers C, Rand S and Brinkmann B (1991) Concept for a more precise definition of the polymorphism YNH24. In: Berghaus G, Brinkmann B, Rittner C and Staak M (eds.), DNA-technology and its forensic application, Springer Verlag / Heidelberg (in press)

Priestley L, Kumar D and Sykes B (1990) Amplification of the COL2A1 3'variable region used for segregation analysis in a family with Stickler syndrome. Hum Genet 85: 525-526

Stoker NG, Cheah KS, Griffin JR, Pope FM and Solomon E (1985) A highly polymorphic region 3' to the human type II collagen gene. Nucleic Acids Res 13: 4613-4622

Wu S, Seino S and Bell GI (1990) Human collagen, type II, alpha 21, (COL2A1) gene: VNTR polymorphism detected by gene amplification. Nucleic Acids Res 18: 3102

Automated Analysis of Fluorescent Amplified Fragment Length Polymorphisms for DNA Typing

J. Robertson*, T. Schaefer**, M. Kronick*, and B. Budowle***

*Applied Biosystems, Inc., Foster City, CA, U.S.A.
**Applied Biosystems GmbH, Weiterstadt, Germany
***FSRTC, FBI Academy, Quantico, VA, U.S.A.

SUMMARY

We have utilized fluorescently labeled PCR primers to amplify 20 ng of genomic DNA at three different VNTR loci.   By using an instrument capable of discriminating the fluorescence emitted from four different dyes, it was possible to analyze the fluorescent PCR products from the three VNTR loci along with an in-lane fluorescently labeled size standard.   The instrument software established a calibration curve for each lane of the gel based on the mobility of the standard in the lane, and then automatically calculated the length of the nucleic acid molecules in base pairs from the calibration curve.   24 individuals could be analyzed per gel for 3 VNTR loci within 6 hours on 2% agarose gels capable of resolving 15 base pair repeats with a high degree of precision and accuracy.   In a validation study, approximately 100 samples were examined at the D1S80 locus, and the data compared perfectly with published results obtained by electrophoresis on polyacrylamide gels and detection by silver staining.

INTRODUCTION

Analysis of electrophoretic gels in the molecular biology laboratory has often been limited to visual inspection of the bands for differences in shape, intensity, and position.   The desire for numerical values has led to the use of scanning densitometers and software to integrate the area associated with a band.   However, these instruments are not always useful for establishing a match in the length of two DNA fragments.   Some of the problems in determining a match in fragment size have been eliminated by switching from RFLP analysis to the PCR, but there still exists the possibility of lane-to-lane differences in DNA mobility.   In order to alleviate this problem, we have used a size standard, which can be co-electrophoresed in the same lane as the sample.   By this technique, the size of a sample is determined by the way it migrates in relation to the known sizes of the fragments of the standard that are subject to the same effects in the electrophoretic lane as the sample.   In this communication, we describe the features of an instrument for automatic DNA fragment analysis that is both convenient to use and capable of high throughput.   The performance of the instrument is discussed in terms of its analytical qualities.

AUTOMATION OF DNA FRAGMENT ANALYSIS

The use of fluorescence for DNA sequence analysis is well established, and the principles of this method can be found in numerous reviews.   In this work, we have utilized the Applied Biosystems 362 GENE SCANNER, which incorporates fluorescent DNA sequencing technology in a horizontal gel configuration for agarose gels.   The fluorescent DNA fragments are excited by a laser beam and the emitted fluorescence is collected as the fragments move past a window that allows the light to pass.   The DNA fragments are thus detected in real time as the bands move through the gel during electrophoresis.   The optics are mounted on a stage

Advances in Forensic Haemogenetics 4
Edited by Ch. Rittner and P. M. Schneider
© Springer-Verlag Berlin Heidelberg 1992

that moves back and forth in a direction perpendicular to the direction of electrophoresis, permitting the analysis of 24 lanes per gel. A filter wheel is placed in the optical pathway and made to rotate in synchrony with the scanning stage to permit the discrimination of the fluorescence emission bands of multiple dyes. The filtered emitted light is collected by a photomultiplyer and converted to digital data. Analysis software can correct for the spectral overlap of the blue, green, yellow, and red fluorescence emitted by the dyes and yields a collection file, from which one obtains a presentation of the data as a familiar gel image. Thus, bands of different color, representing different alleles, appear as individual entities. The sizes of the sample bands are then automatically determined from the calibration curve obtained from the co-electrophoresed standard size ladder. We used a second order least squares curve fit to the size ladder to obtain the calibration curve. The analyzed data are stored in a tabular form suitable for export to database management software.

METHODS OF VNTR ANALYSIS

We have analyzed 94 blind, pristine DNA samples from unrelated Caucasians for the VNTR loci D1S80 (Kasai et al., 1990), D17S5 (Horn et al., 1989), and COL 2A1 (Wu and Bell, 1990) using published sequences for the primers, generally using 20 ng DNA in the PCR. In addition, we examined Chelex (BioRad) extractions of bloodstains on cotton fabric for the same loci using 10 µl of the supernatant in the PCR. We used two methods for obtaining the allele size data. In one, we loaded per lane a pool of 1 µl of the amplification products of three individual PCRs obtained from the same DNA sample using primers fluorescing in blue for D17S5, in green for D1S80, and in yellow for COL 2A1. In the second method, we analyzed three different DNA samples per lane for the same VNTR locus, using a different color for each sample. We added 3 µl of a 2X load buffer containing a red fluorescing size standard, which had a fragment of 946 bp as the longest band. 5 µl of the mixture were loaded in the well of a 2.1% SeaPlaque (FMC) agarose gel at a distance of 4 cm from the detection window. The gel was subjected to electrophoresis at 4 volt/cm for 6 h. In some cases, we re-utilized gels from previous runs and compared the data with that obtained with freshly prepared gels. Used gels generally run faster than fresh ones, so that the electrophoresis and analysis could be reduced by 1 h. Samples found homozygous for the D17S5 locus were re-run on a 1.6% SeaPlaque gel for 5 h with a size standard having bands with lengths of at least 1740 bp.

RESULTS OF THE VALIDATION STUDY

To test the instrument performance, a validation study was carried out using samples that had been analyzed for their D1S80 locus allele frequency on polyacrylamide gels (Budowle et al., 1990) The samples had been binned at the FBI Academy, but the numbers associated with the samples for the Applied Biosystems 362 GENE SCANNER validation study gave no indication of the allele size. The analysis with the GENE SCANNER of these blind samples gave an identical allele frequency as that reported previously, thus demonstrating good precision for the data set. In multiple runs with the same sample, the precision was greater than 99.5%. The repeat length of 16 bp was readily apparent from the difference in size between adjacent bands. Allele 18 was called by the software as 428 bp in length, which must be composed of 16X18 = 288 bp from the repeated segment and 145 bp from the flanking regions established by the primer sites (Kasai et al., 1990). The difference between the size calculated from the electrophorectic analysis, 428 bp, and the expected size of 433 bp is only 5 bp, yielding an accuracy of 98.8%. This degree of accuracy was typical for all allele sizes found in the sample set. A higher degree of accuracy would be expected with a D1S80 allelic size ladder, since DNA fragments composed of specific sequence repeats should migrate differently than restriction fragments composed of a random base composition.

Since the DNA fragments run off the gel during electrophoresis, the gel may be re-used for further separations. However, we noted that the DNA fragments migrate faster on the re-used gels, and it was necessary to determine whether an alteration of the gel matrix affects the size calling precision. Upon analysis of 20 randomly selected samples, we obtained the same allele frequency as we had determined from the electrophoresis through fresh gels. The observation that a difference in the gel matrix does not affect the allele assignment is probably derived from the fact that the size ladder also migrates faster in the used gels.

Sizes determined for the alleles were the same whether three differently colored samples of the same VNTR were loaded in a lane or whether one sample of three differently colored VNTRs of the same sample were loaded in a lane. In other words, it is possible to process 72 samples for the same VNTR when three colors are used for the primers during the PCR. This proves that the software can distinguish three fragments of different color co-migrating on the gel.

COMPARISON OF THE ALLELE FREQUENCIES OF THREE VNTR LOCI

In the 94 samples, we found alleles ranging in size from 428 to 776 bp for D1S80, from 168 to 1040 bp for D17S5, and from 584 to 779 bp for COL 2A1. The repeat lengths between adjacent bands were 16 and 70 bp for the D1S80 and D17S5 loci, respectively. For these two loci, it was easy to assign the DNA fragments to bins upon consideration of two factors: (1) the median value of a set of DNA fragments and (2) the observed repeat lengths. The DNA fragments for the COL 2A1 VNTR could be assigned to bins from the data base, but because there are two repeat lengths for this VNTR (31 bp and 34 bp), it was difficult to establish the bin boundaries. A wide range of lengths are possible for each COL 2A1 fragment, depending on the way the fragment is constructed from the two repeat segments. With a second order least squares curve fitting procedure for the data analysis, we generally found a repeat length of 33 base pairs for COL 2A1. The use of polyacrylamide gels might be preferable for this VNTR.

From the foregoing discussion, it is clear that the use of the PCR and the fluorescence analysis method should make it easy to obtain population data bases accurately and with a high degree of precision. However, the use of the fluorescence technique is not limited to pristine DNA samples. Bloodstains on cotton cloth (3 mm square), extracted with 5% Chelex (Walsh et al., 1991) yielded results of the same quality as those obtained with pristine DNAs. This result suggests that fluorescence methods can be useful in casework analysis. We plan to test cigarette butts, hairs, and mixed body fluids for DNA typing in the future.

REFERENCES

Budowle B, Chakraborty R, Giusti A, Eisenberg AJ, and Allen RC (1990) Analysis of the VNTR Locus D1S80 by the PCR Followed by High-Resolution PAGE. Am J Hum Genet 48: 137-144

Horn GT, Richards B and Klinger KW (1989) Amplification of a Highly Polymorphic VNTR Segment by the Polymerase Chain Reaction. NAR 17: 2140

Kasai K, Nakamura Y, and White R (1990) Amplification of a Variable Number of Tandem Repeats (VNTR) Locus (pMCT118) by the Polymerase Chain Reaction (PCR) and Its Application to Forensic Science. J Foren Sci 35: 1196-1200

Walsh PS, Metzger DA and Higuchi R (1991) Chelex 100 as a Medium for Simple Extraction of DNA for PCR-Based Typing from Forensic Material. BioTechniques 10: 506-513.

Wu S, Seino S and Bell GI (1990) Human Collagen, Type II, alpha 1, (COL2A1) Gene: VNTR Polymorphism Detected by Gene Amplification. NAR 18: 3102

SEX IDENTIFICATION OF FORENSIC SAMPLES USING PCR ANALYSIS FOR THE PRESENCE OF Y-CHROMOSOME SPECIFIC DNA SEQUENCES

S. Nørby and B. Eriksen

Institute of Forensic Genetics, University of Copenhagen
Frederik V's Vej 11, DK-2100 Copenhagen, Denmark

INTRODUCTION

Analysis for Y-chromosome specific DNA sequences can be used to determine the sex of donors of biological samples containing nuclear DNA. In a case in which a child had died in a fire accident, and the abdomen was charred beyond recognition of the sex, we analysed DNA from an intact vertebra for the presence of the following Y-specific sequences, using PCR: alpha satellite repeat (DYZ3), part of the testis determining gene (SRY), and part of the Y-specific zinc-finger protein gene (ZFY).

MATERIALS AND METHODS

A large yield of high molecular weight DNA was obtained from the vertebra by routine methods. Control samples were either isolated DNA or stabilized whole blood from normal adults. For all three systems PCR was carried out on a programmable thermoblock (Hybaid) in 100 µl, containing 200 µM of each dNTP and 2.5 units of Taq DNA polymerase (Promega). The PCR products were analysed by agarose gel electrophoresis (2 % Nusieve + 1 % Bio-Rad) with HinfI digested φX174 as size marker.
DYZ3. Primers: 5'-ATGATAGAACGGAAATATG-3' and 5'-AGTAGAATGCAAA-GGGCTCC-3' (PCR product 170 bp; Witt and Erickson 1989). Isolated DNA from normal adults (two males and a female) served as controls. Primers 0.4 µM each; DNA either 1.0 or 0.1 µg.
35 cycles were performed as follows: 1 min at 90°C (3 min in the first cycle), 1 min at 50°C, and 1.5 min at 70°C (6.5 min in the last cycle).
SRY. Primers: 5'-GAATATTCCCGCTCTCCGGAG-3' and 5'-ACCTGTTGTCCA-GTTGCACT-3' (PCR product 418 bp; Sinclair et al. 1990). Blood samples from normal adults (a male and a female) served as controls. A 321 bp fragment of the Factor IX gene (F9) was amplified as an internal control. Primers: 5'-AACATAGGTGAAAGTCA-ATTAAG-3' and 5'-TTCTCAATCACAGTACCAGTAAT-3' (Yoshitake et al. 1985).
Primers 0.1 µM each; DNA per reaction was 0.1 µg from the forensic sample, and 2 µl whole blood from each of the controls. With the forensic sample 35 cycles were performed as described for DYZ3. With control blood samples the first PCR cycle was skipped, and the reaction mixture for the remaining 34 cycles was prepared as follows (Schwartz 1991): 2 µl blood were incubated with Taq polymerase buffer (Promega) for 1 h at room tp. followed by 10 min denaturation at 99°C, and subsequent addition of primers, dNTPs, and Taq polymerase.

Advances in Forensic Haemogenetics 4
Edited by Ch. Rittner and P. M. Schneider
© Springer-Verlag Berlin Heidelberg 1992

ZFY. Primers: 5'-CATCCTTTGACTGTCTATCCTTG-3' and 5'-CATTATGTGC-
TGGTTCTTTTCTG-3' (PCR product 1131 bp; Schneider-Gädicke et al.
1989, Palsbøll et al. 1991).
PCR was carried out as described for SRY except that annealing
was at 60°C, and elongation was 4 min per cycle (14 min in the
last cycle).
After amplification 5 µl reaction mixture were incubated with
10 units TaqI restriction enzyme in 20 µl at 65°C for 1.5 h.

RESULTS AND DISCUSSION

Photographs of the three PCR gels are shown in Fig.s 1 and 2.

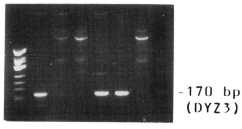

Figure 1. Analysis for Y-specific alpha repeat (DYZ3).
M: size marker (φX174/HinfI). Lane 1: previously ampli-
fied 170 bp alpha repeat fragment (normal male).
Lanes 2 and 3: female control. Lanes 4 and 5: male con-
trol. Lanes 6 and 7: forensic sample.
Even no.s: 1.0 µg DNA. Odd no.s: 0.1 µg DNA

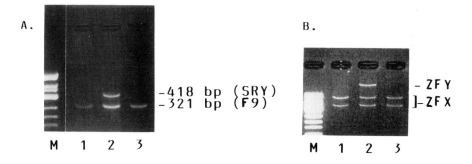

Figure 2. Panel A: Analysis for SRY, with F9 fragment
as internal control. Panel B: Analysis for ZFY.
M: size marker (φX174/HinfI).
Lanes no. 1: forensic sample, 0.1 µg DNA.
Lanes no. 2: male control (2 µl blood).
Lanes no. 3: female control (2 µl blood)

DYZ3 (Fig. 1). DNA from the male controls gave a high yield of the expected 170 bp repeat fragment (lanes 1, 4 and 5), whereas both the female control (lanes 2 and 3) and the forensic sample gave weaker and larger fragments, which served as convenient internal controls.

SRY (Fig. 2A). The F9 fragment was amplified in all three reactions, but only the male control (lane 2) gave the SRY-specific 418 bp fragment.

ZFY (Fig. 2B). The primers used in these reactions amplify fragments of identical size from homologous genes on the X (ZFX) and Y (ZFY) chromosomes. The present analysis exploits the fact, that the ZFX fragment has a TaqI site (bp no. 670-673), which is absent in the ZFY fragment. Another TaqI site (bp no. 49-52) is present in both fragments. TaqI thus cleaves off a 50 bp fragment from both PCR products and cuts the ZFX product once more giving two larger fragments of approx. 620 and 460 bp, while leaving the corresponding 1080 bp ZFY fragment intact.
In the present analysis only the male control (lane 2) gave PCR products both with and without the TaqI site in question.

It is evident from these results, that the DNA from the forensic sample did not contain any of the three Y-chromosome specific DNA sequences, in agreement with the police report of a missing two-year old girl.

REFERENCES

Palsbøll PJ, Vader A, Bakke I, El-Gewely MR (1991). Gender determination in cetaceans by PCR. Can. J. Zool. (submitted)

Schneider-Gädicke A, Beer-Romero P, Brown LG, Nussbaum R, Page DC (1989). ZFX has a gene structure similar to ZFY, the putative human sex determinant, and escapes X inactivation. Cell 57:1247-1258

Schwartz M (1991). Rapid PCR for the screening of ΔF508. Newslett. Europ. Concerted Action on Cystic Fibrosis 4:3

Sinclair AH, Berta P, Palmer MS, Hawkins JR, Griffiths BL, Smith MJ, Foster JW, Frischauf A-M, Lovell-Badge R, Goodfellow PN (1990). A gene from the human sex-determining region encodes a protein with homology to a conserved DNA-binding motif. Nature 346:240-244

Witt M, Erickson RP (1989). A rapid method for detection of Y-chromosomal DNA from dried blood specimens by the polymerase chain reaction. Hum. Genet. 82:271-274

Yoshitake S, Schach BG, Foster DC, Davie EW, Kurachi K (1985). Nucleotide sequence of the gene for human factor IX. Biochemistry 24:3736-3750

ACKNOWLEDGMENTS

We thank Dr. Per Palsbøll for helpful discussions as well as for kindly providing the ZFX/ZFY primers. The skilful technical assistance of Ms. Aase Palvig is also greatly acknowledged.

Automation of DNA Profiling by Fluorescent Labelling of PCR Products

K.M. Sullivan, S. Pope, C. Kimpton, P. Gill and J. Sutton

Central Research and Support Establishment, The Forensic Science Service, Aldermaston, Reading, Berkshire, RG7 4PN, UK

INTRODUCTION

Variable number tandem repeat (VNTR) and short tandem repeat (STR) loci display considerable variation within human populations and are useful markers for both the construction of human linkage maps (Nakamura et al. 1987) and for individual identification in forensic investigations (Hagelberg et al. 1991). PCR amplification of these loci has greatly improved the sensitivity of DNA profiling, and the amplified alleles from small VNTR loci such as D17S5, D1S80 and ApoB can be directly visualised and resolved on ethidium bromide-stained agarose or acrylamide gels (Horn et al. 1989, Kasai et al. 1990, Boerwinkle et al. 1989), whilst STRs are characterised on denaturing sequencing gels using sequence extension products as a size standard (Litt and Luty 1989; Weber and May 1989).

We describe here the use of fluorescent tagging of the PCR products coupled with their detection by laser scanning during electrophoresis to increase the precision and automation of VNTR/STR characterisation. Such technology is routinely used in sequence analysis and has been recently applied to the quantitative determination of Duchenne Muscular Dystrophy status and amplification of VNTR/STR loci (Mayrand et al. in press; A Edwards unpublished results). The utility of this approach is demonstrated in the analysis of incorrectly labelled fixed surgical specimens.

AMPLIFICATION OF VNTR LOCI

Locus D1S80 was amplified in the following reaction mix: 200µM each dNTP, 4U Taq polymerase 1X Amplification buffer, and 0.1µM each primer labelled with fluorescent dye 'JOE' (Applied Biosystems). Samples were denatured at 94°C for 4 mins, followed by 27 cycles of 94°C for 1 min, 56°C for 1 min and 70°C for 1.5 mins, with a final extension at 70°C for 5 mins. For locus D17S5 the reaction mix included 0.4µg each primer labelled with dye 'TAMRA'. Samples were denatured at 94°C for 5 mins, followed by 27 cycles of 94°C for 0.5 mins, 53°C for 0.5mins and 65°C for 4 mins, with a final extension at 65°C for 7 mins. The hypervariable region 3' to the ApoB locus was amplified using 0.1µM each primer labelled with dye 'FAM'. Samples were amplified through 26 cycles at 94°C for 1 min, followed by 58°C for 6 mins. Amplification products were analysed on an Applied Biosystems 362A Genescanner by combining 1µl of each PCR product with 6fmol internal size standard labelled with dye 'ROX', then loaded in a 2% SeaPlaque agarose gel with a well-to-read distance of 4cm. Electrophoresis was for 5.5 hours at 100V. The fragment sizes were automatically determined by the software generating a curve of best fit from the internal standard in each lane.

Advances in Forensic Haemogenetics 4
Edited by Ch. Rittner and P. M. Schneider
© Springer-Verlag Berlin Heidelberg 1992

More than 100 British Caucasians have been analysed at loci D17S5, D1S80 and
ApoB by this method. Alleles differing by a single 15bp repeat (ApoB) were
readily resolved. By using 3 different dyes for the three different loci
it was possible to combine the amplification products and analyse them
simultaneously in the same lane thereby providing a rapid and highly
discriminating test. The automatically called band sizes fall in discrete
groups which define the alleles and the results are summarised as follows:

Table 1. Discrimination power of three VNTR loci

Locus	No. Observed Allele Sizes	Heterozygosity	Prob. of random Match (pM)	Commonest Genotype
D17S5	15	87%	0.035	0.10
D1S80	20	81%	0.065	0.16
ApoB	15	64%	0.081	0.16
		Combined:	2×10^{-4}	2.8×10^{-3}

All 3 VNTR loci show broadly similar levels of amplification efficiency, with
results obtainable from less than 1ng genomic DNA. The absolute limit for
reliable VNTR amplification and analysis is between 100pg and 1ng. At low
initial copy numbers of template DNA, there is a danger of only amplifying
one allele in heterozygotes. To date we have had preliminary success with a
duplex MCT118/ApoB reaction and a triplex MCT118/ApoB/Col 2A1 (Wu et al. 1990)
reaction. The choice of compatible loci will be widened as more systems
become available.

STR AMPLIFICATION

STR HUMTHO1 was amplified using primers cited by Edwards (unpublished results)
one of which was dye-labelled: 29 cycles of 94°C for 45 seconds, 60°C for
30 seconds and 72°C for 30 seconds. Amplification products were
electrophoresed with an internal standard in a 6% denaturing acrylamide gel
using an Applied Biosystems 373A Automated Sequencer, and fragment sizes were
determined automatically with ABI 675 software. In a limited survey of 69
unrelated British Caucasians 5 different alleles were detected with an
overall heterozygosity of 81%. Amplification products were accurately sized
to the nearest 1bp. In addition, sub-banding problems normally associated
with dimeric microsatellites were minimal with the trimeric and tetrameric
microsatellites utilised.

Table 2. Allele frequency distribution for 69 individuals at locus HUMTHO1

Allele size (bp)	Frequency
191	0.22
195	0.20
199	0.11
203	0.12
207	0.34

ANALYSIS OF FIXED SURGICAL SPECIMENS

Four DNA samples were extracted from paraffin-embedded surgical tissue specimens, which were thought to have been mis-paired, using essentially the protocol of Wright and Manos (1990). Attempts were made to amplify the samples at loci ApoB, D1S80, D17S5, HUMTHO1[AATG]n and HUMFABP[AAT]n (Edwards unpublished results), broadly using the conditions described previously. No amplification products were generated at loci ApoB and D1S80, but 2 of the samples generated a single band of 304bp at locus D17S5. Failure to amplify bands within the size range of ApoB and D1S80 (381-932bp) is likely to be due to the DNA being predominantly of very low molecular weight. In contrast, all 4 samples yielded strong results from HUMTHO1 and HUMFABP (size range 191-238bp), which correlated with the D17S5 match result and confirmed that the samples had been incorrectly paired. These results may indicate that the use of microsatellites for forensic purposes may prove to be preferable to VNTRs.

REFERENCES

Boerwinkle E, Xiong W, Fourest E, Chan L (1989) Rapid typing of tandemly repeated hypervariable loci by the polymerase chain reaction: application to the apolipoprotein B 3' hypervariable region. Proc Natl Acad Sci USA 86: 212-216

Hagelberg E, Gray IC, Jeffreys AJ (1991) Identification of the skeletal remains of a murder victim by DNA analysis. Nature 352: 427-429

Horn GT, Richards B, Klinger KW (1989) Amplification of a highly polymorphic VNTR segment by the polymerase chain reaction. Nucleic Acids Research 17: 2140

Kasai K, Nakamura Y, White R (1990) Amplification of a variable number tandem repeat (VNTR) locus (pMCT118) by the polymerase chain reaction (PCR) and its application to forensic science. J Forensic Sci 5: 1196-1200

Litt M, Luty JA (1989) A hypervariable microsatellite revealed by in vitro amplification of a dinucleotide repeat within the cardiac muscle actin gene. Am J Hum Genet 44: 397-401

Mayrand PE, Robertson J, Ziegle J, Hoff LB, McBride LJ, Kronick MN Annales de Biologie Clinique (in press)

Nakamura Y, Leppert M, O'Connell P, Wolff R, Holm T, Culver M, Martin C, Fujimoto E, Hoff M, Kumlin E, White R (1987) Variable number of tandem repeats (markers) for human gene mapping. Science 235: 1616-1622

Weber JL, May PE (1989) Abundant class of human DNA polymorphisms which can be typed using the polymerase chain reaction. Am J Hum Genet 44: 388-396

Wu S, Seino S, Bell GI (1990) Human Collagen, type II, alpha 1, (COL2A1) gene: VNTR polymorphism detected by gene amplification. Nucl Acids Res 18: 3102

PCR Typing Including High Resolution Gel Electrophoresis Reveals new Alleles in the COL2A1 VNTR

E.S. Berg and B. Olaisen

Institute of Forensic Medicine
Rikshospitalet, N-0027 Oslo, Norway

INTRODUCTION

The AT-rich variable number of tandem repeat (VNTR) near the collagen type II gene (COL2A1) is a candidate to increase the discriminative power in PCR based DNA typing. The aim of the present study was to investigate the COL2A1 VNTR in Norwegian family- and population materials, and to evaluate the system for forensic purposes.

POLYMERASE CHAIN REACTION (PCR)

PCR typing of the COL2A1 VNTR have been described by Priestly et al. (1990) and Wu et al. (1990). We did not, however, achieve high sensitivity and robustness with the published PCR. The primers were therefore redesigned by aid of computer programs (Oligo[TM] and GCG software). The new PCR primers had the sequences:

    LCOL: 5'-ATCCCTGCCCCTGCTTCCTC-3'
    HCOL: 5'-CACCTGCTCTCCTCCGACCC-3'

The PCR was performed as Perkin-Elmer Cetus recommend for their AmpliTaq[TM] with 1.5 mM $MgCl_2$ and a thermo profile including an annealing temperature of $58°C$.

MATERIALS

The COL2A1 VNTR was studied in a Norwegian population material of 200 unrelated individuals and in 50 small Norwegian family groups.

NONDENATURATING POLYACRYLAMIDE GEL ELECTROPHORESIS

The electrophoresis of the PCR products was performed in a nondenaturating polyacrylamide gel (PAGel) in apparatus (V15-17) from Bethesda Research Laboratories.
Figure 1 is a picture of an ethidium bromide stained non-denaturating PAGel with COL2A1 VNTR PCR products from 13 unrelated individuals. Four of the allelic variants described by Priestly et al. (1990) are present in figure 1. We found a heterozygote frequency of 58% in our population material for this VNTR.

Advances in Forensic Haemogenetics 4
Edited by Ch. Rittner and P. M. Schneider
© Springer-Verlag Berlin Heidelberg 1992

45

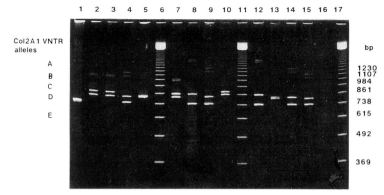

Fig. 1. Nondenaturating PAGel with COL2A1 VNTR PCR product of
13 unrelated individuals. Lane 6, 11 and 17 are molecular
weight standard. Lane 16 is the negative control

DENATURATING POLYACRYLAMIDE GEL ELECTROPHORESIS

In the nondenaturating gel system there appeared several
alleles which were difficult to classify because they migrated
slightly different from standard alleles. The higher
resolution power of the denaturating PAGel (sequencing gel)
was necessary to resolve this problem. Prior to the
electrophoresis the PCR product was labelled as described by
Ludwig et al. (1989) by addition of an endlabelled internal
primer before the last five cycles of the PCR. The internal
primer had the sequence:

ICol: 5'-TCATGAACTAGCTCTGGTGG-3'

Figure 2 is a picture of the autoradiogram of one such gel. As
compared to the nondenaturating gels, further subdivision of
some alleles may seen. The denaturating gel system has so far
revealed 16 allelic variants of this VNTR in the same
Norwegian population material and a heterozygosity of 76.4%.

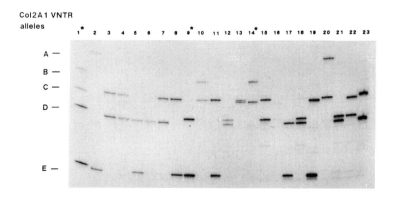

Fig. 2. Denaturating PAGel, which also includes all
individuals in figure 1. The allelic ladder in lane 1 is a
mixture of the PCR product from the individuals in lanes 9 and
14

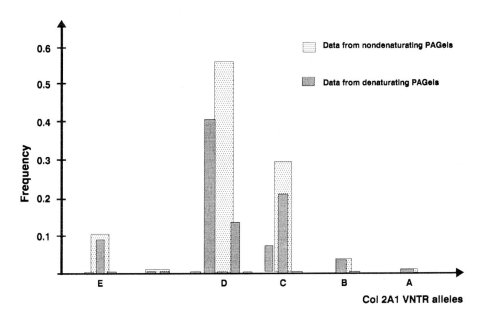

Fig. 3. This is a schematic drawing of the different allelic variants detected by the two resolution systems. In light colour bars are the alleles detected by nondenaturating PAGels. Norwegian gene frequencies are similar to those published by Priestly et al. (1990). The further subdivision of the allelic variants obtained in denaturating PAGel is represented by dark colour bars

Stoker et al. (1985) have shown that the COL2A1 VNTR is similar in construction to the Apo B VNTR. Our sequencing data support their findings. The small differences in size between the variable tandem repeat units, 31 and 34 bp, are visible only in the high resolution gels.
Sequencing of more alleles is necessary for further characterization of the Col2A1 VNTR, and should form basis for a more appropriate nomenclature.

REFERENCES

Ludwig HE, Friedl W, McCarty BJ (1990) High-resolution analysis of hypervariable region in the human apolipoprotein B gene. Am J Hum Genet 45:458-464
Priestly L, Kumar D, Sykes B (1990) Amplification of the COL2A1 3' variable region used for segregation analysis in a family with the Stickler syndrome. Hum Genet 85:525-526
Stoker NG, Cheah KSE, Griffin JR, Pope FM, Solomon E (1985) A highly polymorphic region 3' to the human Type II collagen gene. Nucleic Acid Res 13:4613-4622
Wu S, Seino S, Bell GI (1990) Human collagen, type II, alpha 1, (COL2A1) gene: VNTR polymorphism detected by gene amplification. Nucleic Acid Res 18:3102

The Usefulness of Chelating Resins for DNA Extraction from Forensic Material Prior to PCR Amplification

M.V.Lareu, M.S. Rodriguez-Calvo, F. Barros, A. Carracedo

Institute of Legal Medicine. University of Santiago de Compostela. Galicia. Spain

INTRODUCTION

DNA extraction procedures prior PCR have been simplify since Singer-Sam et al. (1989) reported the use of chelating resins which prevents the degradation of DNA allowing the DNA extraction at high temperatures. In this paper we report a comparison between different methods of extraction, including chelatin resins, boiling with water and TE and phenol-chloroform extraction prior to the amplification of HLA DQA1 and pMCT118 systems.

MATERIAL AND METHODS

Samples.- Bloodstains [Recent (up to 6 months old); old (10 years old)] and hair

DNA extraction methods

Bloodstains:

A.- Chelating resin

Pippete 1 ml of water into a sterile 1.5 ml microfuge tube. Add bloodstain. Incubate at room temperature for 15 to 30 minutes. Mix occasionally by inversion or gentle vortexing. Spin in a microcentrifuge for 2 to 3 minutes at 10.000 to 15.000 xg. Remove supernatant (all but 20 to 30 µl) and discard. Add 5% chelating resins to a final volume of 200µl. Incubate at 56°C for 15 to 30 minutes. Vortex at high speed for 5 to 10. Boil in a boiling water bath for 8 minutes. Vortex at high speed for 5 to 10 seconds. Spin in a microcentrifuge for 2 to 3 minutes at 10.000 to 15.000 xg. Add 20 µL of supernatant to the PCR mix.

B.- Conventional method with phenol-chloroform

C.- Water boiling.- Chelating resin is substituted in method A by distilled water.

D.- TE boiling.- Chelating resin is substituted in method A by TE.

Hair:

E.- Chelating resin

Use a clean scalpel to cut a 5 to 10 mm portion from the root end of the hair. Add the root portion of the hair to 200 µL of 5% chelating resin in a 1.5 mL microfuge tube. Incubate at 56 °C overnight (at least 6-8 hours). Vortex at high speed for 5 to 10 seconds. Boil in a boiling water bath for 8 minutes. Vortex at high speed for 5 to 10 seconds. Spin in a microcentrifuge for 2 to 3 minutes at 10.000 to 15.000 xg.Add 40 µL of the supernatant to the PCR mix.

F.- Conventional method with phenol-chloroform

PCR.- HLA DQA1: Primers and amplification conditions according to Cetus AmpliType protocol. Dot-blot with Aso-probes (Amplitype). pMCT-118: Primers

Advances in Forensic Haemogenetics 4
Edited by Ch. Rittner and P. M. Schneider
© Springer-Verlag Berlin Heidelberg 1992

and amplification conditions according to Budowle et al. (1990). Detection by SDS-PAGE, T= 10-15, 100 Vh, followed by silver-staining according to Barros et al. (1991).

RESULTS

Table 1.- RECENT-OLD BLOODSTAIN COMPARISON

METHOD / BLOODSTAIN (50µl)	CHELATING RESINS		PHENOL-CHLOR.	
	DQA1	pMCT-118	DQA1	pMCT-118
RECENT	+++	+++	+++	+++
OLD (10 years old)	++	++	–	–

Table 2.- MINUTE BLOODSTAINS

METHOD / BLOODSTAIN (2 years old)	CHELATING RESINS		PHENOL-CHLOR.	
	DQA1	pMCT-118	DQA1	pMCT-118
0.5 µl	++	++	–	–
1 µl	++	++	–	–
5 µl	+++	+++	–	–

Table 3.- CHELATING RESINS/WATER/TE COMPARISON

METHOD / BLOODSTAIN	CHELATING RES.		WATER		TE	
	DQA1	pMCT	DQA1	pMCT	DQA1	pMCT
0.25 cm²	++	++	+	+	–	–
0.50 cm²	++	++	+	+	–	–
1 cm²	+++	+++	+	+	–	–

Table 4.- ROOT HAIRS

METHOD / SAMPLE	CHELATING RESINS		PHENOL-CHLOROFORM	
	DQA1	pMCT-118	DQA1	pMCT-118
ROOT HAIR	++	++	–	–

CONCLUSIONS

1.- Extraction with chelating resins provided positive results in 10 years old bloodstains whereas phenol-chloroform extraction gave negative results.

2.- Extraction with chelating resins provided positive results in minute bloodstains 2 years old whereas phenol-chloroform extraction gave negative results.

3.- Chelating resins increases the PCR signal when compared with a simple water extraction (boiling). TE gives negative results.

4.- Extraction with chelating resins provided positive results in root hairs whereas phenol-chloroform extraction gave negative results.

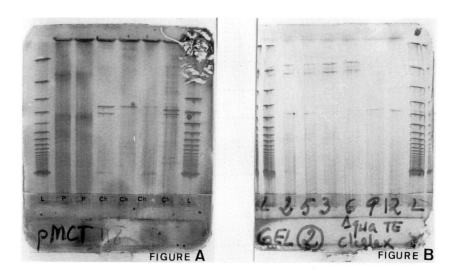

Figure A.- Comparison between chelating resin and phenol-chloroform methods in old bloodstains and hair. P= phenol-chloroform extraction, Ch= chelating resin extraction, L= 123bp DNAladder (BRL). (Hair: lanes 2,4; bloodstains: lanes 3,5,6,7).

Figure B.- Comparison between differents DNA extraction methods in old bloodstains. (Water: lanes 2,5; chelating resin: lanes 3,6; TE: lanes 9,12)

ACKNOWLEGEMENTS

This study was supported by grants from Ministerio de Educación y Ciencia (CICYT PA86-0453) and Xunta de Galicia (XUGA 84-20689)

REFERENCES

Barros F, Carracedo A, Lareu MV, Rodriguez-Calvo M (1991) Electrophoretic HLA-DQA1 DNA typing after polymerase chain reaction amplification. Electrophoresis (In press)

Budowle B, Giusti AM, Allen RC (1990) Analysis of PCR products (pMCT-118) by polyacrylamide gel electrophoresis. In: Polesky HF, Mayr WR (eds) Advances in forensic haemogenetics 3. Springer-Verlag, Berlin, pp 148-150

Singer-Sam J, Tanguay RL, Riggs AD (1989) Use of Chelex to improve the PCR signal from a small number of cells. Amplifications 3:11

The Isolation of DNA for Forensic PCR Analysis.
An Evaluation of Available Methodologies

R. Coquoz

Institut de Police Scientifique et de Criminologie, University of
Lausanne, place du Château 3, 1005 Lausanne, Switzerland

INTRODUCTION

PCR is generally considered to require less stringent sample
purification than other analytical methods such as RFLP analysis.
However, since it is intended to be used on particularly difficult
samples (small, old, degraded,...), the success of the analysis
will be highly dependent upon parameters like yield of the DNA
isolation and presence of PCR inhibitors. For this reason, an
evaluation of the merits of a few common or more recent DNA
isolation methods was undertaken.

MATERIALS/METHODS

Stains

10μl stains were prepared from blood, sperm and saliva, diluted
with NaCl 0.9% , giving stains containing from o.1 to 10μl of the
corresponding body fluid. These stains were allowed to dry and
some were submitted to other conditions, giving rise to 4 types of
stain treatment :
A) drying at room temperature for 24h
B) 5 days of direct exposure to summer sun (at 46° latitude north)
C) 1 week heating at 75°C
D) 1 week heating at 50°C in a water saturated atmosphere

DNA Extraction :

I. Chelex method (Singer-Sam et al. 1989) : add 500μl H_2O to the
stain and incubate 30 min at room temperature. Spin 2 min at 15000
g and remove the supernatant {these first 2 steps are used only
with blood and sperm stains}. Add 100μl 5% Chelex 100 (100-200
mesh, sodium form, Bio-Rad) {in the case of sperm, add also 1μl
Prot.K 10 mg/ml and 4μl DTT 1M}. Incubate 30 min at 56°C (1h. for
sperm). Vortex 5 sec. Boil for 8 min. Vortex 5 sec.

II. Methidium-Sepharose extraction (Harding et al. 1989) : to the
stain, add 190μl 10mM Tris-HCl pH 8, 10mM EDTA, 100mM NaCl, 39mM
DTT, 0.5% SDS, and 10μl prot.K 10 mg/ml. Incubate 1h. at 60°C.
Punch a hole in the tube ; spin and recover the liquid phase.Add
50μl DNA capture reagent (Gibco-BRL) and agitate for 1h. Decant

the supernatant and wash the resin twice with 10mM Tris-HCl pH
7.5, 1mM EDTA, 100mM NaCl. Add NaOH 0.2M and agitate 10 min.
Recover the eluted DNA and precipitate with ethanol. Dissolve the
DNA in 100µl H2O

III. Standard proteinase K digestion & phenol extraction

IV. Proteinase K digestion alone (Turck et al. 1990)

<u>PCR Amplification of the D1S80 Locus</u>

The efficiency of the DNA extraction was estimated by using 1/10
of the extract to amplify the locus D1S80 according to the method
of Kasai (1990) with minor modifications. The PCR products were
analysed on 2% agarose gel followed by staining with ethidium
bromide.

RESULTS

In all the situations tested, the methods (II) and (IV) were at
various degrees less efficient than the other two methods (fig.
1). Only methods (I) and (III) were retained for further testing.

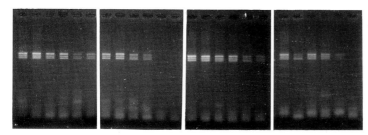

Fig. 1. Efficiency
of the DNA
extraction methods
(I) to (IV) (from
left to right)
with fresh 10, 1,
0.1µl blood stains
(in duplicate)

Of the four stain treatment conditions tested, the exposure to sun
was the most detrimental. But methods (I) and (III) had the same
efficiency in the DNA extraction of such mistreated stains (fig.
2).

```
     A          B          C          D       :stain treatment
  I   III    I   III    I   III    I   III    :extraction method
```

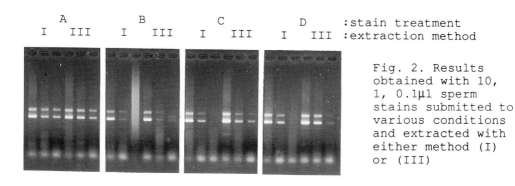

Fig. 2. Results
obtained with 10,
1, 0.1µl sperm
stains submitted to
various conditions
and extracted with
either method (I)
or (III)

This is true for most of the stain types tested, with two
exceptions (fig. 3):
- blood stains on blue denim, where only method (I) gave a result;
- saliva stains on stamps where only method (III) was effective.

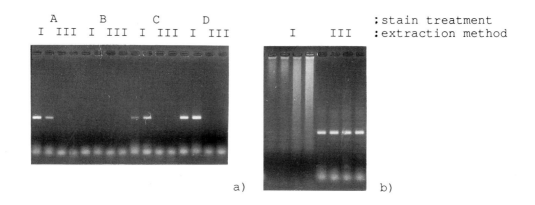

a)   b)

Fig. 3. Results obtained with a) 1µl blood stains on blue denim
submitted to various conditions and extracted with either method
(I) or (III) b) stamps pasted using 10µl saliva and extracted with
either method (I) or (III).

REFERENCES

Harding JD, Gebeyehu G, Bebee R, Simms D, Klevan L (1989) Rapid
    isolation of DNA from complex biological samples using a novel
    capture reagent - methidium-spermine-sepharose. Nucl Acids Res
    17(17):6947-6958
Kasai K, Nakamura Y, White R (1990) Amplification of a variable
    number of tandem repeats (VNTR) locus (pMCT118) by the
    polymerase chain reaction (PCR) and its application to forensic
    science. J Forens Sci 35(5):1196-1200
Singer-Sam J, Tanguay RL, Riggs AD (1989) Use of chelex to improve
    the PCR signal from a small number of cells. Amplifications 3:11
Turck A, Schall B, Maguire S, Belluscio L, Nawoschik S, McKee R,
    Grimberg J, Eisenberg A (1990) A simple and efficient non-
    organic procedure for the extraction of DNA from evidentiary
    samples. In : Advances in forensic haemogenetics, vol 3 ,
    Springer, p.26

This work was supported by a grant from the Swiss National Fund
for Scientific Research

DETECTION OF THREE DIFFERENT VNTR'S BY DNA-AMPLIFICATION

Ate Kloosterman; Rolf Vossen; Deborah Wust; Wiljo de Leeuw[*] & André Uitterlinden[*]
Dutch Forensic Science Laboratory; Volmerlaan 17; 2288 GD Rijswijk, The Netherlands. [*]Medscand Ingeny; PO Box 685; 2300 AR The Netherlands

Introduction

The Polymerase Chain Reaction (PCR) can enhance the detection of known VNTR loci, particularly in forensic situations where limited amounts of DNA are available. PCR amplification of several polymorphic VNTR regions has been described. Here, we describe the application of the DNA-amplification technique for the detection of three variable minisatellite loci: the VNTR loci D1S80 (D1S58) and D17S30 (D17S5) and the hypervariable region 3' of the apolipoprotein B gene. Polymorphic PCR-fragments were detected on ethidium-bromide stained polyacrylamide gels.
Table 1 summarizes the characteristics of the three different VNTR-loci involved in this study.

Table 1. Properties of the VNTR's in this study

VNTR	Chromosome Localization	Locus[b]	Repeat Length	% GC[a] content	Ref.
Apo B	2p24-p23		2x15[c]	4	[1,2]
MCT 118	1p	D1S80 (D1S58)	16	58	[3,4]
YNZ 22	17p	D17S30 (D17S5)	70	64	[5]

[a] : GC content of the VNTR repeat units
[b] : Human Gene Mapping Symbols
[c] : The Apo B alleles differ in length from its next neighbouring allele by 30 bp or two 15-bp repeat units.

The primer sequences for the three different VNTR loci were:

Apo B : 5'-primer: 5'-ATGGAAACGGAGAAATTATG-3' (20 mer).
3'-primer: 5'-CCTTCTCACTTGGCAAATAC-3' (20 mer). (Boerwinkle [1]).

pMCT118 : primer 1: 5'-GAAACTGGCCTCCAAACACTGCCCGCCG-3' (28 mer).
primer 2: 5'-GTCTTGTTGGAGATGCACGTGCCCCTTGC-3' (29mer).
(Kasai [4] & Budowle [3]).

pYNZ22 : primer 1: 5'-CGAAGAGTGAAGTGCACAGG-3' (20 mer)
primer 2: 5'-CACAGTCTTTATTCTTCAGCG-3' (21 mer). (Horn [5]).

MATERIALS AND METHODS

1. Isolation of total high molecular weight DNA from liquid blood samples

DNA for PCR analysis was isolated from 1 ml aliquots of blood by standard procedures. DNA concentrations were estimated by minigel electrophoresis in 1% agarose to which 1 μg/ml ethidium bromide was added. Concentration standards used were dilutions of cell-line K562 DNA (Promega).

2. Primer synthesis

Oligonucleotides were synthesized on the Gene Assembler plus (Pharmacia) and were purified by ethanol precipitation.

3. Size fractionation of DNA-amplification products in 6% polyacrylamidegels

PCR products were separated by electrophoresis on a Protean II xi Slab Cell (Biorad) using 6% polyacrylamide (29:1 Acrylamide/Bis mixture; Biorad), in 1x TAE buffer (40 mM Tris-acetate; 1 mM EDTA). Electrophoresis was performed at 200 V (35 mA) for 3-4 hours depending on the genetic system. The fragment sizes were determined by comigration of 500 ng of a 1kb-ladder (BRL) and a 123 bp ladder (BRL).
The amplification products were visualized directly after staining the gel in 1 μg/ml ethidium bromide for 0.5 hours.

Advances in Forensic Haemogenetics 4
Edited by Ch. Rittner and P. M. Schneider
© Springer-Verlag Berlin Heidelberg 1992

RESULTS

Amplification of target DNA by the Polymerase Chain Reaction (PCR)

Temperature cycling conditions and optimal reation parameters for each of the three systems are specified in table 2.

**Table 2. Optimal reaction parameters and temperature cycling conditions
for the three different VNTR-loci**

Locus	pMCT118 (D1S80)	ApoB (3' ApoB)	pYNZ22 (D17S30)
[MgCl$_2$]	1.0-1.5 mM	1.0-1.5 mM	1.0-1.5 mM
glycerol	10%	10%	10%
Optimal DNA-input	0-100 ng	5-100 ng	10-200 ng
Minimal DNA-input	<5 ng	<5 ng	<1 ng
3'& 5' primer conc.	0.45 ng	0.30ng	0.30 ng
# cycles	26	26	34
initial denaturation	4' 94°C	4' 94°C	4' 94°C
denaturation	2' 94°C	2' 94°C	2' 94°C
annealing	2' 65°C	6' 58°C	30" 55°C
extension	4' 72°C		4' 72°C
final extension	10' 72°C	10' 72°C	10' 72°C

General Conditions:
1x PCR buffer: 50 mM KCl; 10 mM Tris pH 8.30; 0.2 mg/ml acetylated BSA; 1.0/1.5 mM MgCl$_2$ dNTP's: 200 μM; Taq Polymerase: 2 Units; Final Reaction-volume: 50 μl.

a. Locus D1S80 (pMCT 118)

Data from the PCR experiments demonstrate that the MgCl$_2$concentration is a most critical parameter. High concentrations of Mg^{2+}generate additional bands and/or reduced amounts of locus specific PCR product. A Mg^{2+}concentration of 1.0 - 1.5 mM was found as an optimum. Standard amounts of primer and Taq polymerase are sufficient for locus specific amplification. It was noted that in our PCR-system some individuals show faint extra bands of high molecular weight. The sensitivity of this system allows detection of alleles of the D1S80 locus without hybridization. However especially with the appearance of shady extra bands in forensic samples it may be desirable to use a DNA-probe to confirm whether or not the fragments are derived from the D1S80 locus. After electroblotting and hybridization we observed that the extra high molecular weight bands did not hybridize with the pMCT118 probe and it may be concluded that these sequences are unrelated to the D1S80 locus.
An example of the allelic variation of the D1S80 locus is given in figure 1. Each lane represents the genomic DNA from a different individual. All alleles could be separated. The resolution obtained could distinguish alleles differing only 16 bp (i.e. one repeat) in length. A suitable marker system was obtained by preparing a cocktail of alleles from different individuals. With this allelic ladder the unknown alleles can be designated directly without measuring relative migration distances. Experiments for a population screening are in progress.

b. Locus ApoB

It was found that amplification of the AopB locus is the most robust system of the three. The system produces easy-to-identify PCR-fragments in a broad Mg^{2+}concentration range. Comparison of annealing at 58°C and extension at 72°C or annealing and extension at 58°C showed that a better amplification was obtained at an annealing & extension temperature of 58°C. This phenomenon is probably due to the very low GC content of the ApoB sequence; which causes the template to denature before complete extension occurs at the standard extension temperature of 72°C. An example of the allelic variation of the apoB locus is given in figure 2. Each lane represents the genomic DNA from a different individual. All alleles could be separated. Experiments for a population screening are in progress.

c. Locus D17S30 (pYNZ22)

Data from the PCR experiments demonstrate that here also the MgCl$_2$concentration is a most critical parameter. The major problem with amplification of the D17S30 locus is that products with fewer repeat units (short alleles) are preferentially amplified over longer alleles. The reason for this phenomenon is that Taq polymerase is more efficient on shorter fragments of this locus. In forensic VNTR-typing this problem can induce ambiguity into the typing results. In order to amplify and directly visualize long D17S30 alleles it was necessary to increase the number of amplification cycles. Optimum amplification was at 34 cycles. We also found that the addition of 10% glycerol to the PCR reaction-mix had both an advantagous effect on the stability of the Taq polymerase during thermocycling and on the sharpness of the bands in the eventual polyacrylamide electophoresis. Because of these findings 10% glycerol was added in all three PCR systems. Decreasing the input of genomic DNA also seemed to increase the efficiency of amplification of the larger alleles. A succesful approach for the suppression of ladder bands in this system was the shortening of the annealing time. Optimum annealing time was found to be 0.5 minute. An example of the allelic variation of the D17S30 locus is given in figure 3.

DISCUSSION AND CONCLUSION

A rapid and relatively simple procedure for the detection of hypervariable regions in the human genome is presented. Making use of oligonucleotide primersets from DNA flanking the minisatelite regions and thermostable Taq Polymerase reproducible and faithful amplification of the loci D1S80 and ApoB has been demonstrated. The electrophoretic separation system used (17 cm vertical 6% PAA gels) appears to be sufficient for separation of most if not all alleles of the VNTR loci analysed. For the D17S5 locus, PCR conditions have to be optimized especially so for the amplification of the longer alleles. The PCR conditions for the three VNTR systems will have to be evaluated through testing in more different biological materials and in real case work. Typing these hypervariable regions by the PCR technique is extremely sensitive. Nanogram amouts of template DNA generated detectable signals in all three systems.

A problem with the VNTR loci analysed here is the inability to determine the exact identity of the alleles. Identification of the alleles would greatly simplify the construction of a population database and the exchange of results. The marker systems used in this study (the "1-Kb"- and the "123 bp" ladder) can give only an approximation of the size of the alleles after PCR analysis. An improved marker system was obtained in the VNTR locus D1S80 by preparing a cocktail of alleles from different individuals. A problem here is the availability of individuals with rare alleles.

The VNTR loci used for PCR analysis all have a relatively low level of heterozygosity in common when compared to the most optimal VNTR loci used in Southern blot hybridization analysis. Consequently, these PCR-based DNA-identification systems have a lower discriminating power than the Southern hybridization-based systems such as multi-locus DNA-fingerprinting or locus-specific DNA-profiling. As noted by Sullivan these three VNTR loci combined have a discriminating power of 0.9997. As a result the occurence of inconclusive PCR results in identity disputes will be relatively frequent when compared to traditional methods of DNA-profiling. It is therefore essential to have several more "PCRable" VNTR loci available in order to reach a high level of discrimination power. This, however poses no severe problem in view of the relative abundance of VNTR loci in the human genome. Several other PCRable VNTR systems have been described and they can be included in the set of loci to be typed in forensic material.

Literature

[1]   Boerwinkle E, Xiong W, Fourest E, Chan L (1989).
        Rapid typing of tandemly repeated hypervariable loci by the Polymerase Chain Reaction: Application to the apolipoprotein B3 hypervariable region.
        Proc. Natl. Acad. Sci **86**: 212-216.
[2]   Ludwig EH, Friedl W & McCarthy BJ (1989).
        High-Resolution analysis of a hypervariable region in the Human Apolipoprotein B gene.
        American J. Hum. Genet. **45**: 458-464.
[3]   Budowle B, Chakraborty R, Giusty AM, Eisenberg AJ & Allen RC (1991).
        Analysis of the VNTR Locus D1S80 by the PCR followed by High-Resolution PAGE.
        Am. J. Hum. Genet. **48** : 137-144.
[4]   Kasai K, Nakamura Y & White R (1990).
        Amplification of a variable number of tandem repeats (VNTR) Locus (pMCT118) by the polymerase chain reaction (PCR) and its application to forensic science.
        Journal of Forensic Sciences **35** : 1196-1200.
[5]   Horn GT, Richards B & Klinger KW (1989).
        Amplification of a highly polymorfic VNTR segment by the Polymerase Chain Reaction. Nucleic Acids Research **17**: 2140.

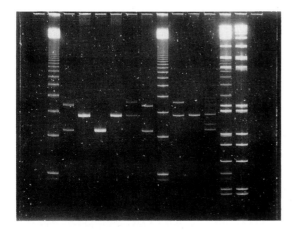

Fig. 1
Amplification of the D1S80 locus for 8 different individuals. The size standards are the 1-kb and the 123-bp ladder (BRL). An example of an allelic ladder is shown in lane 11

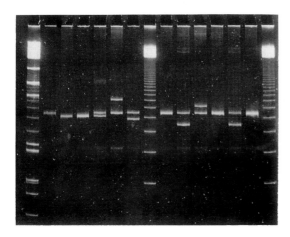

Fig. 2
Amplification of the ApoB locus for 12 different individuals. The size standards are the 1-kb and the 123-bp ladder

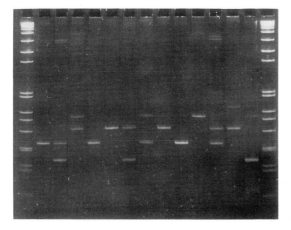

Fig. 3
Amplification of the D17S30 locus for 13 different individuals. The size standard is the 1-kb ladder

1.3 Practical Application

VALIDATION OF THE USE DNA AMPLIFICATION FOR THE ANALYSIS OF FORENSIC SAMPLES BY COMPARISON WITH TESTS USING NON-AMPLIFIED DNA POLYMORPHISMS

L. Perlee, I. Balazs

Lifecodes Corporation, Valhalla, NY, USA

SUMMARY

The utility and reliability of DNA amplification for forensic DNA samples was tested using material previously analyzed with single locus RFLP. Aliquots containing about 10 ng of DNA were amplified for two repeated sequences present in the X (DXZ1) and Y (DYZ2) chromosomes, then amplified for the polymorphic loci, DQα, D1S80, ApoB and Col2A1. The alleles identified in the amplified evidentiary DNA were compared to those obtained from the exemplars to determine whether they were the same. In all cases there was agreement for the matches and non-matches obtained by DNA amplification vs. previous testing with RFLP. However, some samples from sexual assault cases showed the presence of contaminating female DNA more readily with DNA amplification than RFLP analysis. Approximately one half of the evidentiary samples, that did not contain sufficient intact DNA for RFLP testing, produced interpretable results using AMP-FLP. Other samples could only be typed for the presence of male and/or X DNA.

INTRODUCTION

To date, the most common DNA analysis method used in forensic casework includes the analysis of single locus restriction fragment length polymorphism (RFLP). This method of identity testing has gained world wide acceptance due to its robustness and sensitivity. However, one of the main limitations of RFLP is that it will not generate results if a large fraction of the DNA sample is degraded. The use of the polymerase chain reaction (PCR) has been shown to have the potential of producing results with degraded samples (Higuchi et al.1988, Roewer et al.1991). Therefore, using PCR, it may be possible to expand the fraction of samples for which DNA profiles can be generated.

There have been numerous genetic markers, described in the literature, for the analysis of DNA polymorphisms by PCR. In general, the polymorphisms detected at these loci are the result of changes in DNA sequence (e.g. DQα), or result from variations in the number of tandem repeats, (AMP-FLP), (e.g. Col2A, ApoB). The purpose of this report is to validate the use of PCR with forensic samples by comparing the results obtained by DNA amplification with results obtained by RFLP analysis.

MATERIALS AND METHODS

<u>Processing of DNA sample</u>. DNA samples used in this study were isolated from liquid blood, semen or blood stains. The general procedure used for the analysis of samples

Advances in Forensic Haemogenetics 4
Edited by Ch. Rittner and P. M. Schneider
© Springer-Verlag Berlin Heidelberg 1992

by PCR consisted of: 1. Determine the quality and quantity, of a 5 to 10% aliquot of DNA, using a yield gel (McNally et al. 1989). Samples of degraded DNA or those containing less than 10 ng of DNA were quantitated by slot blot hybridization to Alkaline Phosphatase-conjugated probes (AP-oligo) for human and bacterial DNA, detected by chemiluminescence (Nano-Blot^{TM}, Lifecodes, Corp.). 2. Amplification of sequences from the X and Y chromosomes. 3. Amplification of polymorphic sequences. 4. Gel fractionation of amplified product.

Slot blot hybridization. A 5% aliquot of the DNA sample was denatured with NaOH and applied to a charged nylon membrane (PALL-Biodine B) that had been placed into a slot blot apparatus (BRL). Known amounts of human and bacterial DNA (0.5, 1, 2, 5, 10, 20ng) were added as controls to the remaining slots. After washing with neutralization solution and drying, the DNA was hybridized 10 min. to an AP-oligo homologous to human repeated sequences or to bacterial ribosomal genes. Filter(s) was washed and sprayed with the chemiluminescent reagent Lumi-Phos 450^{TM}(Lumigen Inc.), sealed in a plastic folder and exposed to XAR5 (Kodak) X-ray film for about 1 hour at 37°C. After developing the film, the amount of human or bacterial DNA in the sample could be estimated by comparing the intensity of the band relative to that of the control DNA.

RFLP analysis. The fractionation of PstI-digested DNA samples and the determination of a match among DNA profiles was performed by the analysis of several VNTR loci (e.g. D2S44, D4S163, D14S13, D17S79, D18S27, DXYS14).

Amplification of DNA sequences. Amplification for X, Y and AMP-FLP was done for 30 cycles. DQα was amplified for 32 cycles. The amount of human DNA used per amplification reaction was about 5 to 10ng. The primers and conditions used for the amplification of the non-polymorphic repeated sequences, DXZ1 and DYZ2, were those described by Witt & Ericson (1989). The cycling parameters used for the amplification of each sequence were optimized for maximum sensitivity and specificity and were significantly different for each locus. Therefore, the simultaneous amplification of 2 or more loci, did not have the same sensitivity as individual amplifications. The primers for DQα and D1S80 were obtained from Cetus Corp. and used under conditions recommended by the manufacture. The conditions for amplification of ApoB were 30" at 94°C, 3'at 58°C, and for Col2A1, 30" at 95°C, 1' at 55°C, 1' at 72°C. The general formats used for the detection of these polymorphisms were the reverse dot blot (i.e. Cetus Corp., for DQα) or size fractionation, by gel electrophoresis, of the different size DNA fragments (i.e. X, Y, AMP-FLP).

RESULTS AND DISCUSSION

DNA samples derived from a variety of sources were analyzed by electrophoresis in yield gels. About half of the DNA samples were extensively degraded or the amount of DNA could not be measured by EtBr staining (i.e. <10ng of high molecular weight DNA). These type of samples were quantitated by slot blot hybridization to human or bacterial DNA.

All samples were tested for their ability to generate the amplified 130 bp fragment of the DXZ1 locus and the 170 bp fragment of the DYZ2. The amplification of the

DXZ1 sequence served as an indicator to predict the ability to obtain result for the polymorphic loci. Since these DNA fragments represent repeated sequences and they are small in size, they can be detected in degraded samples containing subnanogram quantities of human DNA. Many amplified samples, negative for the polymorphic sequences, produced the DXZ1 DNA fragment. However, samples negative for DXZ1 did not yield results for the polymorphic markers. Evidentiary DNA from sexual assault cases, in which the alleles did not match the victim, were positive for DYZ2. There was good agreement between the extent of DNA degradation and the loss of amplifiable DNA fragments. As expected, the largest fragments were the first to be lost as amplification products. Since the DNA fragments for the DQα alleles are the smallest of all the polymorphic markers tested, they were the most resistant to DNA degradation. The relative sensitivity of the markers amplified was X and Y > DQα > ApoB > Col2A1 > D1S80.

The results of the RFLP analysis were compared with those obtained by PCR. There was complete agreement, in term of sample matches, in the results obtained by both procedures. About half of the evidentiary samples were partially degraded and about half of them produced results only by DNA amplification. Samples derived from sexual assault cases were processed by a differential lysis procedure that separates most of the male DNA from the female DNA. RFLP analysis of the male fraction reveals in most cases only the DNA pattern from the assailant. However, in some cases the female pattern can be visualized as a fainter pattern. Using DNA amplification, several male DNA fractions showed the pattern of DNA fragments from the victim. Many times the intensity of the contaminating female DNA was similar to that of the male DNA.

In conclusions, the result obtained by RFLP analysis and DNA amplification were consistent with each other, validating the reliability of these PCR markers for forensic application.

REFERENCES

Higuchi R, Beroldingen CH von, Sensabaugh GF, Erlich HA (1988) DNA typing from single cells. Nature 332:543-546

McNally L, Shaler MS, Baird M, Balazs I, De Forest P, Crim D, Kobilinsky L (1989) Evaluation of deoxyribonucleic acid (DNA) isolated from human bloodstains exposed to ultraviolet light, heat, humidity, and soil contamination. Journal of Forensic Science 34:1059-1069

Roewer L, Rieb O, Prokop O (1991) Hybridization and polymerase chain reaction amplification of simple repeated DNA sequences for analysis of forensic stains. Electrophoresis 12: 181-186

Witt M, Erickson RP (1989) A rapid method for detection of Y-chromosomal DNA from dried blood specimens by the polymerase chain reaction. Hum Genet 82:271-274

Investigations on the Forensic application of 4 AMPFLP systems

P. Wiegand, S. Rand, B. Brinkmann

Institut für Rechtsmedizin, Westfälische-Wilhelms-Universität,
Von-Esmarch-Str. 86, 4400 Münster, Germany

INTRODUCTION

One major problem with stain examinations is that the amount of biological material is often too small
and the extracted DNA is highly degraded due to the environmental conditions. It is therefore highly
probable that only PCR can be successfully used for DNA analysis and individualisation.
Recently 4 amplifiable fragment length polymorphisms have been under intensive investigation:
MCT118 - APOB - YNZ22 - COL2A1
These systems seem to be very powerful tools for resolving the problem of highly degraded DNA. But
before they can be established in casework, basic experience is necessary to prove the reliability of the
results.

MATERIALS AND METHODS

The investigated blood samples were obtained from paternity cases from the Münster area. DNA was
extracted from EDTA blood as previously described (Brinkmann et al. 1991).
Chelex extraction from blood stains was carried out as described by Walsh et al (1990).
The vaginal swabs were taken 1-2 days after sexual intercourse and extracted using "single lysis" or "mild
preferential lysis" (Wiegand et al. 1991 in press).
The extraction of the cigarette butts (crime case 1) was carried out using proteinase K, phenol-chloro-
form-isoamylalcohol (24:24:1) and ethanol precipitation.
PCR-amplification was performed using published conditions and primers:
MCT118 (Budowle et al. 1991)
APOB (Boerwinkle et al. 1989)
COL2A1 (Wu et al. 1990)
YNZ22 (the following conditions were used;B. Budowle, pers. com.)
Primer sequence:
5'-AAACTGCAGAGAGAAAGGTCGAAGAGTGAAGTG-3'
5'-AAAGGATCCCCCACATCCGCTCCCCAAGTT-3'

temp.: 94 / 63 / 72 °C
time : 1   1   6   min
cycl.: 27

Thermocycler: Triothermoblock (Biometra, FRG)

Amplification was carried out with 2.5 U Taq polymerase (Promega corporation, USA) in 10mmol Tris-
HCl, pH 8.3, 50 mmol KCl, 1.5 mmol $MgCl_2$, 0.1% Triton-X, 0.5 μM each primer and 200 μM each dNTP.
The total volume was 50 μl with the addition of 30 μl oil overlay.
The electrophortical separation of the amplified fragments was carried out in polyacrylamide gels (6% T,
3% C; thickness 400 μm) with piperazine diacrylamide as cross-linker (Budowle et al. 1991) using a
discontinous buffer system (Allen et al. 1989). The separation distance was 10 cm. Visualisation of the
bands was performed by silver staining (Budowle et al. 1991).

RESULTS AND DISCUSSION

The most common stain materials are bloodstains, mixtures of vaginal cells, semen and sometimes hairs.
Chelex extraction from blood stains (3 mm^2 area on cotton), which were stored at room temperature over
different time periods, clearly showed visible bands for each stain (Fig. 1).

Advances in Forensic Haemogenetics 4
Edited by Ch. Rittner and P. M. Schneider
© Springer-Verlag Berlin Heidelberg 1992

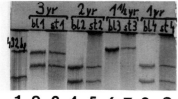

Fig. 1: Comparison between amplified blood DNA and
corresponding Chelex extracted bloodstains after
different storage time. System: MCT118
lane 1   : 123 bp ladder (Gibco-BRL, UK)
lane 2, 4, 6, 8: phenol-chloroform extracted blood
DNA
lane 3, 5, 7, 9: Chelex extracted bloodstains
(5-10 ng DNA template)

A very problematical area is the application of PCR to mixtures of cells or body fluids which are present
in different proportions and is a problem mainly encountered with secretions from sexual organs. Firstly
it is necessary to know the weakest concentration which can be detected.
If different ratios of a mixture of 2 sperm populations were amplified, the recognition of the weakest
component was possible down to a minimal concentration of 10 % (Fig. 2). But in these cases disadvantageous effects can also occur: In a 1 : 5 mixture ratio of spermatozoa from 2 individuals, the larger fragment was virtually suppressed (Fig. 3, lane 4).

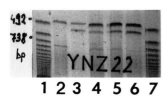

Fig. 2: Amplification of sperm mixtures from 2 individuals
in 3 different ratios in comparison to the corresponding blood DNA
lane 1,7:   123 bp ladder (Gibco-BRL, UK)
lane 2 :   blood DNA from individual 1
lane 3 :   blood DNA from individual 2
lane 4 :   semen mixture in 1:1 ratio (25:25ng template
DNA)
lane 5 :   semen mixture in 1:5 ratio (10:50ng template
DNA)
lane 6 :   semen mixture in 1:10 ratio (5 :50ng template
DNA)

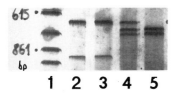

Fig. 3: Amplification of a semen mixture (1:5) from 2 individuals in comparison to the corresponding blood and
semen DNA. System: APOB
lane 1: 123 bp ladder (Gibco-BRL, UK)
lane 2: blood DNA from individual 1
lane 3: semen DNA from individual 2
lane 4: semen mixture from individual 1 and 2 (10:50ng
template DNA)
lane 5: blood DNA from individual 2

A situation which occurs frequently in practice is that in vaginal smears the concentration of vaginal cells
is much greater than the spermatozoa. If a preferential lysis (Gill et al 1985) is carried out, a considerable number of spermatozoa could be lysed in the first step and will therefore be lost. Performing single
lysis on the total extract has the disadvantage that the weak component can be suppressed. Therefore for
such cases a "mild preferential lysis" was applied. This procedure avoids excess destruction of spermatozoa in the first step and achieves a considerable reduction of female DNA. It is achieved by halving the
incubation time and incubation temperature and reduction of the amount of proteinase-K.
After single lysis were the female bands much more intensive than the male because of the unfavourable
proportions. After mild preferential lysis the vaginal proportion was distinctly reduced (Fig. 4). The
female bands became weaker but now both male bands are visible.

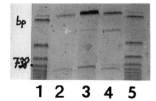

Fig. 4: Amplification of DNA fragments extracted from
vaginal swabs in comparison to the female blood
DNA. System: YNZ22
lane 1,5 : 123 bp ladder (Gibco-BRL, UK)
lane 2   : female blood DNA
lane 3   : swab extraction, single lysis
lane 4   : swab extraction, mild preferential lysis

A further application of these PCR systems is the analysis of hairs. If hair roots are available there is a good chance of obtaining interpretable results.
One hair root was extracted with Chelex and approximately 5 ng DNA were used for amplification. For both systems (APOB, COL2A1) the expected band patterns were visible (Fig. 5).

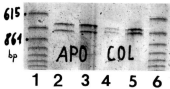

Fig. 5: Chelex extracted hair root DNA in comparison to the corresponding blood DNA using the APO B and COL2A1 systems
lane 1,6 : 123 bp ladder (Gibco-BRL, UK)
lane 2,4 : Chelex extracted hair root (5 ng template DNA)
lane 3,5 : phenol-chlorophorm extracted blood DNA

The amplification of hair shaft DNA only is much more problematical: the blood DNA pattern showed 2 bands, after amplification using 2 hair shafts only 1 of the 2 bands was visible (Fig. 6). Such results can lead to a misinterpretation.

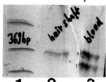

Fig. 6: Comparison between amplified hair shaft DNA and corresponding blood DNA. System: MCT118
lane 1: 123 bp ladder (Gibco-BRL, UK)
lane 2: DNA from 2 hair shafts, extracted after Higuchi (1989)
lane 3: phenol-chloroform extracted blood DNA

In cases where only a minimal amount of DNA is available, coamplification of 2 systems can be useful. Using side-to-side comparison with blood DNA the corresponding bands can be clearly distinguished (Fig. 7).

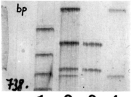

Fig. 7: Coamplification of 2 systems using blood DNA
lane 1: 123 bp ladder (Gibco-BRL, UK)
lane 2: coamplification of the systems MCT118 and YNZ22
lane 3: corresponding DNA fragments in MCT118
lane 4: corresponding DNA fragments in YNZ22

A coamplification with the COL2A1 system and the sex-specific Amelogenin system (Akane et al. 1991) was successfull possible (Fig. 8). Males have 2 bands in defined positions, females only 1 band. Because the ranges do not overlap, these systems can be successfully combined.

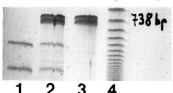

Fig. 8: Coamplification of 2 systems using blood DNA
lane 1: male specific Amelogenin bands
lane 2: coamplification of the Amelogenin and COL2A1 system
lane 3: corresponding COL2A1 bands
lane 4: 123 bp ladder (Gibco-BRL, UK)

Two casework investigations should give an example for the forensic application of the AMPFLP systems: In both cases only highly degraded DNA could be extracted.
The first case involved 2 suspects and 2-year-old cigarette butts (4 butts) were investigated. The band pattern shows that both suspects could be excluded with YNZ22 (Fig. 9) and MCT (not shown).

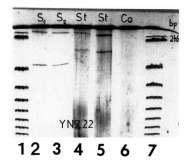

Fig. 9: Amplification of DNA fragments extracted from 2-year old cigarette butts in comparison to the band pattern of 2 excluded suspects
lane 1,7: 123 bp ladder (Gibco-BRL, UK)
lane 2 : blood DNA from suspect 1
lane 3 : blood DNA from suspect 2
lane 4 : DNA extracted from cigarette butts amplified with addition of BSA (200 μg/ml)
lane 5 : DNA extracted from cigarette butts amplified with addition of BSA (400 μg/ml)
lane 6 : negative control, no template DNA was added to the amplification

The last example is a rape case. Clear results could be obtained with 3 AMPFLP systems (Fig. 10; 1 system is shown). The swab extraction was carried out in a 1 step procedure without preferential lysis. In the stain pattern the bands corresponding to the victim and to the suspect could be clearly distinguished. Victim and suspect have 1 common band in the same position.

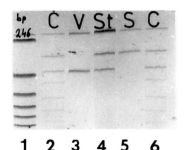

Fig. 10: Amplified DNA fragments in a rape case.
System: YNZ22
lane 1 : 123 bp ladder (Gibco-BRL, UK)
lane 2,6:   YNZ22 allele cocktail
lane 3 : victim blood DNA
lane 4 : swab extration, single lysis
lane 5 : suspect blood DNA

To summarise: The AMPFLP systems provide a very promising new generation of methods for forensic haemogenetics which can be applied to solve numerous forensic problems. However one of the prerequisites for the application is the establishment of own data bases and the performance of numerous experimental investigations by each laboratory, so that possible artefacts can be assessed and taken into consideration when interpreting results.

REFERENCES

Akane A, Shiono H, Matsubara K, Nakahori Y, Seki S, Nagafuchi S, Yamada M, Nakagome Y (1991) Sex identification of forensic specimens by polymerase chain reaction (PCR): two alternative methods. For Sci Int 49: 81-88

Allen RC, Graves G, Budowle B (1989) Polymerase chain reaction amplification products separated on rehydratable polyacrylamide gels and stained with silver. Bio Techniques 7: 736-744

Boerwinkle E, Xiong W, Fourest E, Chang L (1989) Rapid typing of tandemly repeated hypervariable loci by the polymerase chain reaction: application to the apolipoprotein B 3' hypervariable region. Proc Natl Acad Sci USA 86: 212-216

Brinkmann B, Rand S, Wiegand P (1991) Population and family data of RFLP's using selected single- and multi-locus systems. Int J Leg Med 104: 81-86

Budowle B, Chakraborty R, Giusti AM, Eisenberg AJ, Allen RC (1991) Analysis of the variable vumber of tandem repeats locus D1S80 by the polymerase chain reaction followed by high resolution polyacrylamide gel electrophoresis. Am J Hum Genet 48: 137-144

Gill P, Jeffreys AJ, Werrett DJ (1985) Forensic applications of DNA "fingerprints". Nature 318: 577-579

Higuchi R (1989) Sinple and rapid preparation of samples for PCR. In: Erlich HA (ed) PCR technology - principles and applications for DNA amplification. Stockton Press, New York London Tokyo Melbourne Hong Kong pp 31-39

Walsh PS, Metzger DA, Higuchi R (1991) Chelex 100 as a medium for simple extraction of DNA for PCR-based typing from forensic material. Biotechniques 10 (4): 506-513

Wiegand P, Schürenkamp M, Schütte U (1991 in press) DNA extraction from mixtures of body fluid using mild preferential lysis. Int J Leg Med

Wolff RK, Nakamura YR, White R (1988) Molecular characterization of a spontaneously generated new allele at a VNTR locus: no exchange of flanking DNA sequence. Genomics 3: 347-351

Wu S, Seino S, Bell GI (1990) Human collagen, type II, alpha 21, (COL2A1) gene: VNTR polymorphism detected by gene amplification, Nucleic Acids Res 18: 3102

SDS-PAGE Typing of HLA-DQA1 and pMCT118 after PCR Amplification

F. Barros, M.C. Vide*, M.V. Lareu, A. Carracedo
Dep. of Legal Medicine, University of Santiago de Compostela, Galicia

INTRODUCTION

The development of PCR for amplifying DNA sequences has raised the possibility that VNTRs and other DNA polymorphisms might be analyzed using this approach. Some methods for detecting single base changes in DNA after PCR amplification have been proposed as ribonuclease cleavage, denaturing gradient gel electrophoresis and the PCR amplification of specific alleles. These methods have rarely been used in practice because they involved complicated methodology or else , its use in forensic or clinical casework has not been proved until now. Here we propose a method for detecting DNA polymorphisms, not only in coding DNA but also in repetitive DNA (e.g. minisatellites). The method involves a DNA extraction with a chelating resin, PCR amplification, SDS-PAGE in gradient non-denaturing gels and silver staining. Its usefulness is exemplified by typing the HLA-DQA1 system and the VNTR in the position D1S80.

MATERIAL AND METHODS

DNA was extracted from 4 µl blood by a method described previously (Singer-Sam et al. 1989) using a chelating resin (Sigma, St Louis, MO). The total extraction time was 45 min. The oligonucleotides used as primers for HLA-DQA1 amplification were GH26 (5′ GTGCTGCAGGTGTAAACTTGTACCAG 3′) and GH27 (5′ CACGGATCCGGTAGCAGCGGTAGAGTTG 3′) and for pMCT118 were 5′ GAAACTGGCCTCCAAACACTGCCCGCCG 3′ and 5′ GTCTTGTTGGAGATGCACGTG-CCCCTTGC 3′. These primers amplified a 16-base pair repeating unit, the different alleles containing 15-36 repeating units. Each sample amplified contained 1-10 ng DNA, 10 mM Tris-HCl (pH 8.3), 2.5 mM MgCl$_2$, 50 mM KCl, 0.01% gelatin, 2.5 units of AmpliTaq DNA Polymerase (Cetus), 0.188 mM of each dNTP and 0.2 µm of each primer. The volume of each sample was 50 µl. The cycling reaction was done in a programmable heat block (Perkin-Elmer/Cetus) set to heat at 94°C for 1 min (denature), cool at 60°C for 30 sec (anneal), and incubate at 72°C for 30 sec (extend). After 32 repetitions, the samples were incubated an additional 7 min at 72°C. PCR amplification of pMCT118 was achieved by the method described by Budowle et al (1990) with slight modifications. Each amplified sample contained 1-10 ng DNA, 10 mM Tris-HCl (pH 8.3), 50 mM KCl, 1.5 mM MgCl$_2$, 0.01% gelatin, 2.5 units of AmpliTaq DNA Polymerase, 1 µM of each primer and 200 µM of each dNTP, for a total volume of 50 µl. The PCR was carried out for 30 cycles. Each cycle was one minute at 95°C for denaturation, one minute at 65°C for primer annealing, and eight minutes at 70°C for primer extension. Electrophoresis was carried out in PhastGels Gradient 10-15 and 8-25 (Pharmacia-LKB) using the PhastSystem. Polyacrylamide gels (5 x 5 cm) have a 13 mm stacking gel zone, at a gel concentration of 4.5% and cross-linking of 3%, and a 32 mm separation gel zone with a continuous 10-15% or 8-25% gradient with 2% cross-linking. The buffer system in the gels is of 0.112 M acetate and 0.112 M Tris, pH 6.4. The electrode buffer contained 0.20 M tricine, 0.20 M Tris and 0.55% SDS, pH 7.5. The buffer strips are made of 2% agarose (Agarose IEF, Pharmacia-LKB). Samples (1 µl of amplified product) were applied to the cathodic end of the gel. Electrophoresis was carried out at 50 V/cm, 10.0 mA and 3.0 W for a total of 50 volt-hours. Detection of the PCR amplified products was made with the silver staining method of Heukeshoven and Dernick (1988) Alternatively, normal size gels (10x20x0.4 cm) with the same discontinuous buffer system were used. A 123 bp DNA ladder (Gibco-BRL) was used as size marker. For comparison dot-blot analysis with HLA-DQα AmplyType (Cetus) was carried out using protocols provided by the manufacturer.

* Institute of Legal Medicine. Coimbra. Portugal

Advances in Forensic Haemogenetics 4
Edited by Ch. Rittner and P. M. Schneider
© Springer-Verlag Berlin Heidelberg 1992

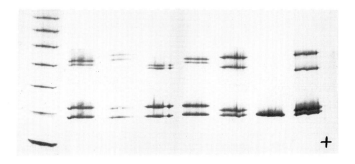

Fig.1. SDS-PAGE of PCR amplification of HLA-DQA1 locus. From left to right HLA-DQA1 genotypes 3-4; 4-4; 2-3; 1.1-4; 1.2-4; 1.1-2; 1.2-4 and 123bp ladder marker. Electrophoresis was carried out in PhastGel 10-15 for 100Vh at 15 C

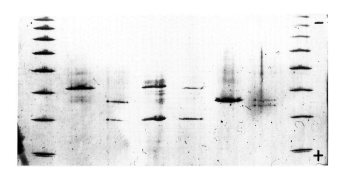

Fig. 2. SDS-PAGE of PCR amplification of locus D1S80. Electrophoresis was carried out in PhastGel 10-15 for 100Vh at 15 C. Samples are 2µl 5 years old bloodstains

RESULTS AND DISCUSSION

  Limitations of PCR dot-blot method for HLA-DQA1 typing are, first, that commercially available systems are expensive since they involved immobilized ASO probes and, second, the number of ASO probes do not permit the identification the entire variation of the system and only the more common alleles. The electrophoretic method reported overcomes such limitations, since single substitutions can be detected and enzymes or probes are not necessary. A complete correlation between the electrophoretic patterns of HLA-DQA1 phenotypes and dot-blot results was observed. HLADQA1 products differing only 4 bp substitutions such as the alleles DQA1*0201 and DQA1*0301 can be distinguished in homoduplexes and DQA1 alleles differing a single base substitution in heteroduplexes such as the subtypes DQA1*0101 and DQA1*0103 which can be distinguished in any heterozygotes with other DQA1 alleles(Fig.1). With reference to the electrophoretic method, clear separations were obtained only when discontinuous electrophoretic systems were used. The use of 0.112M acetate (leading ion) and 0.112M Tris, pH 6.4 as buffer system in the gels, and 0.20M tricine (trailing ion), 0.20M Tris and 0.55% SDS, pH 7.5 as buffer in the agarose strips (bridge) gave particularly good results. Homogeneous polyacrylamide gels provided poor resolutions. Only gradient polyacrylamide with stacking gels can be used to obtain a good result. Optimal resolution are obtained with the gradient T=10-15, with a stacking gel of T=4.5%. Tas (1990) recently proved that DNA molecules are separated readily and rapidly by gel electrophoresis with SDS in a conventional static electric field. We have here observed the same effect for small DNA molecules, HLA-DQA1 cannot be typed if SDS is not added at least in the agarose bridge buffer. Furthermore these small molecules migrated during SDS-PAGE faster than proteins of identical molecular mass, and thus, the number of volthours habitually used for conventional SDS-PAGE separation of proteins has to be considerably shortened. With SDS, DNA molecules form sharper bands and separate better, and this effect can be used for analyzing other DNA polymorphisms. The use of automatized systems for miniaturized gels such as the PhastSystem are particularly recommended, firstly because polyacrylamide gel miniaturization improves protein visualization and increases the sensitivity for detecting low abundance components, and secondly because all variables are controlled, and so results can be always reproduced and samples do not have manipulated by adding bromophenol blue since migration can be controlled by counting the number of volthours. An additional advantage of using the PhastSystem is the possibility of controlling the temperature. Temperature control is essential since the electrophoretic behaviour of heteroduplexes critically depends on it and reproducible results are obtained only when bands are separated at the same temperature. An optimal resolution is obtained between 3 and 15°C. In any case reproducible and short separations can be carried out with the proposed methodology, even when the method is applied to forensic casework. Important advantages of the proposed method for typing the HLA-DQA1 system over commercially available dot-blot systems with ASO probes are the time needed for the entire process (5h for 10h), the cost (at least ten times less) and the sensitivity (positive results were obtained with low amounts of amplified products given dot-blot negative results). The system can also be applied to the analysis of VNTRs and so pMCT 118 alleles can be easily recognized. PhastGel 10-15 and the same electrophoretic discontinuous buffer system gives the best results (Fig.2). Single tandem repeats (16 bp) can be distinguished and the method can used in forensic casework with the advantage over previously published methods, that results can be obtained in only 5 h including extraction. Heteroduplexes are not observed after pMCT118 amplification and the temperature control is not essential in this case. The factors influencing the generation of recombinants are not known and our system can be used as a model to study this fact and the electrophoretic behaviour of small DNA molecules.

ACKNOWLEDGMENTS

This study was supported by grants from Ministerio de Educación y Ciencia (CICYT PA86-0453) and Xunta de Galicia (XUGA8420689).

REFERENCES
Budowle, B., Giusti, A.M., Allen, R.C.(1990) in Advances in Forensic Science 3 (Polesky, H.F. and Mayr, W.R. Eds), pp 148-150, Springer-Verlag, Berlin-Heidelberg
Heukeshoven, J., Dernick, R. (1988) Electrophoresis 9, 28-32
Singer-Sam, J., Tanguay, R.L., Riggs, A.D. (1989) Amplifications 3, 11
Tas, S. (1990). Anal. Biochem. 188: 33-37

Gene frequencies of APOB alleles in a sample of random Italian individuals (Central and Southern Italy)

E.d'Aloja, M.Dobosz, M.Pescarmona, A.Moscetti, and V.L.Pascali

Immunohematology laboratory, Institute of Forensic Medicine, Catholic University, Rome, Italy

INTRODUCTION

The region situated downstream of the apolipoprotein B exon contains a hypervariable sequence (APO B HVR, APO B) organized in tandem repeat units. Its polymorphism was described by Boherwinkle et al (1989) using the polymerase chain reaction technique (PCR). These authors reported the existence of 12 allelomorphic fragments in Caucasians with a heterozygosity index amounting to 0.75. Since then, APOB has become a widespread marker, frequently used in forensics.
In view of the application of this polymorphism to our routine casework, we have undertaken a population survey on the distribution of its alleles in the population of Central and Southern Italy. Here we report data referring to a first share of typed samples (109 unrelated individuals) from our reference population.

MATERIALS AND METHODS

Genomic DNA was obtained by phenol-chloroform extraction. Samples of 50 to 100 Ng were amplified by a standard PCR procedure, using a couple of flanking oligonucleotide primers (Boerwinkle et al, 1989) (final ratio 0.1 fM w/v). Amplification conditions were: denaturation: 94°C, 60 sec; annealing: 58°C, 60 sec; extension: 59°C, 300 sec (overall 30 cycles; with a 600 sec extension in the final cycle). Amplified products were separated by agarose (NuSieve, FMC, 2.5% w/v) submarine electrophoresis (80 V, 6h). Phenotypes were classified with the help of a commercial MW standard ladder (123 bp, BRL). In cases of controversial allele classification, a home - made ladder formed by admixture of the commonest allele fragments was used as reference.

RESULTS AND DISCUSSION

In Table I the distribution of observed and expected APOB phenotypes is shown. APOB allele frequencies are sketched in a bar histogram in Fig.1.

Advances in Forensic Haemogenetics 4
Edited by Ch. Rittner and P. M. Schneider
© Springer-Verlag Berlin Heidelberg 1992

Individual alleles apparently originated from iteration (29 to 47 repeat) of the expected 14-16 bp long repeat unit. Eleven common alleles and 28 phenotypes were identified. We found a favorable distribution of fragments sizes in the system, which helped to achieve a safe amplification of the alleles and minimized the risks of false homozygosity. Mistyping was also avoided by the use of the self-established marker of common APOB types. As a consequence, observed and expected types were consistent with the assumption of population equilibrium (chisquare = 19.61, 11 df, $0.10 > p > 0.05$, compliance with the Hardy Weinberg rule).

The average heterozygosity of the system amounted to 0.74. APOB polymorphism is now used in our laboratory as a routine marker for solving dubious paternity cases. A trial is also under way for the introduction of this system in the analysis of criminal cases.

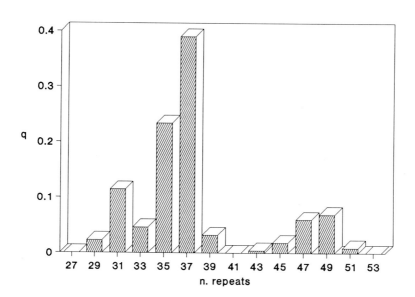

APO B

Fig. 1. APO B gene frequencies in 109 unrelated Italians

Table 1. Observed and expected APO B phenotypes

TYPE	OBS	EXP	%
31-31	4	1.43	3.67
35-35	6	5.97	5.50
37-37	18	16.57	16.51
29-47	1	0.30	0.92
31-43	1	0.11	0.92
31-47	1	1.49	0.92
31-49	1	1.72	0.92
33-49	2	0.69	1.83
35-29	3	1.17	2.75
35-31	1	5.85	0.92
35-33	3	2.34	2.75
35-39	2	1.64	1.83
35-45	1	0.94	0.92
35-47	4	3.04	3.67
35-49	7	3.51	6.42
35-51	1	0.47	0.92
39-31	2	0.80	1.83
39-33	1	0.32	0.92
37-29	1	1.95	0.92
37-31	11	9.75	10.09
37-33	4	3.90	3.67
37-35	17	19.89	15.60
37-39	2	2.73	1.83
37-45	2	1.56	1.83
37-47	6	5.07	5.50
37-49	5	5.85	4.59
37-51	1	0.78	0.92
45-47	1	0.24	0.92
sum	109	100.06	100.00

REFERENCES

Boerwinkle E, Xijong W, Fourest E, Chan L (1989) Rapid typing of tandemly repeated hypervariable loci by the Polymerse chain reaction: Application to the apolipoprotein B 3'hypervariable region. Proc Natl Acad Sci USA 86:212-216

Study of the HLA DQα polymorphism in the population of Catalonia (Spain)

M. Gené, E. Huguet, A. Carracedo, J. Mezquita

Forensic Haemogenetics Laboratory. Legal Medicine Department. School of Medicine. University of Barcelona. Av Joan XXIII s/n. 08028 Barcelona. Catalonia. Spain

INTRODUCTION

We report here the results of a survey of HLA DQα polymorfism studied by the polymerase chain reaction (PCR) in 110 samples from people living in Catalonia (North-east Spain). In agreement with others, we conclude that it is a useful marker in forensic evidence analysis and in paternity testing.

MATERIAL AND METHODS

The study was carried out with blood donor samples obtained from a Blood Bank, "Hospital Clínic", Barcelona, and from unrelated paternity cases. The HLA DQα alleles were characterized after enzymatic PCR amplification of specific DNA sequences, using allele specific oligonucleotide probes (ASO probes) and reverse dot-blot methodology (Cetus 1990). The method identifies four common types of alleles called DQα 1, 2, 3, 4, and distinguishes three genetic variants (subtypes) of allele 1 (DQα 1.1, 1.2, 1.3), defining a total of twenty-one different genotypes.

RESULTS AND DISCUSSION

Calculation of the phenotype distribution and gene frequencies indicates that there is no deviation from the Hardy-Weinberg equilibrium (Chi-square of 8.64 with 15 degrees of freedom, and p>0.75). The results of population studies are given in Table 1. The gene frequencies of the twenty-one genotypes range from less than 0.09 (allele 1.3) to 0.15 (alleles 1.1 and 1.2) except for allele 4 in wich the frequency was 0.37.

When compared with the frequencies given from Cetus and Roche Biomedical Laboratories (Cetus 1990), the distribution of some of the variants shows few differences between Catalans and other caucasians, but larger ones in relation to other ethnic groups.

We have performed the HLA DQα polymorphism in 52 paternity testing cases. 35 cases of paternity practically proved (W ≥ 99.73 %) using conventional markers were confirmed, supporting the assumed autosomal codominant way of inheritance. The percentage of exclusions (11 incompatibilities in 17 cases of

Advances in Forensic Haemogenetics 4
Edited by Ch. Rittner and P. M. Schneider
© Springer-Verlag Berlin Heidelberg 1992

non paternity 64.7%) using this method proved the theoretical a priori chance exclusion value (C.E.= 0.59) obtained from gene frequencies in our population.

Table 1. Hardy Weinberg equilibrium for the locus HLA DQα

Types	Obs.	Exp.	Dif.	X^2
1.1 - 1.1	3	2.63	0.37	0.05
1.1 - 1.2	3	5.10	-2.10	0.86
1.1 - 1.3	5	3.25	1.75	0.95
1.1 - 2	5	4.17	0.83	0.16
1.1 - 3	4	3.55	0.45	0.06
1.1 - 4	11	12.67	-1.67	0.22
1.2 - 1.2	2	2.47	-0.47	0.09
1.2 - 1.3	2	3.15	-1.15	0.42
1.2 - 2	6	4.05	1.95	0.94
1.2 - 3	4	3.45	0.55	0.09
1.2 - 4	14	12.30	1.70	0.23
1.3 - 1.3	1	1.00	-0.00	0.00
1.3 - 2	3	2.58	0.42	0.07
1.3 - 3	3	2.20	0.80	0.30
1.3 - 4	6	7.83	-1.83	0.43
2 - 2	1	1.66	-0.66	0.26
2 - 3	0	2.82	-2.82	2.82
2 - 4	11	10.06	0.94	0.09
3 - 3	2	1.20	0.80	0.53
3 - 4	8	8.57	-0.57	0.04
4 - 4	16	15.28	0.72	0.03
Total	110	109.99		8.64

HLA DQα 1.1 = 0.1545		
HLA DQα 1.2 = 0.1500		X^2 = 8.64
HLA DQα 1.3 = 0.0955		df = 15
HLA DQα 2 = 0.1227		P > 0.75
HLA DQα 3 = 0.1045		CE = 0.59
HLA DQα 4 = 0.3727		EM value = 9.55

REFERENCES

Beroldingen CH, Blake ET, Higuchi R, Sensabaugh GF, Erlich H (1989) Applications of PCR to the analysis of biological evidence. In: Erlich HA (ed) PCR technology. Principles and applications for DNA amplification, 1st edn, Stockton Press, New York, p 209

Cetus (1990) Amplitype. User guide, Cetus Corporation, Emerville

Erlich HA, Bugawan TL (1989) HLA Class II gene polymorphism: DNA typing, evolution, and relationship to Disease Susceptibility. In: Erlich HA (ed) PCR technology. Principles and applications for DNA amplification, 1st edn, Stockton Press, New York, p 193

Erlich HA, Bugawan TL (1990) HLA DNA typing. In: Innis MA, Gelfand DH, Sninsky JJ, White TJ (ed) PCR protocols, 1st edn, Academic Press, San Diego, p 261

Use of PCR for Forensic Analysis of DNA from Formaldehyde fixed and Paraffin embedded Human Tissues

B. Ludes *, M.C. Tortel **, P. Mangin *

*   Institut de Médecine Légale 11 rue Humann 67085 Strasbourg
      France
**   Centre Hospitalier Louis Pasteur 68021 Colmar – France

Some fixation methods damage DNA and avoid subsequent classical fingerprint analysis.
Previous authors (Dubeau, 1986 ; Goelz, 1985) showed that high molecular weight DNA can be yielded from paraffin embedded tissues and analysed by the RFLP technic.
The polymerase chain reaction is a powerfull tool for the analysis of the fixed tissues. DNA in treated tissue can serve as a template for amplification of the HLA DQ alpha region.
The results from our study indicate that PCR results can be achieved from two years old paraffin embedded muscle and heart blocks. This kind of fixation is used in medical studies conducted in remote regions where samples require fixation and storage for extended periods of time before analysis. The storage require fixation methods which preserve the DNA of specimens for future study.

MATERIAL AND METHODS

1)   Paraffin blocks

The skeletic muscle and heart paraffin blocks have been prepared for routine histopathologic examination of surgical resection specimen. Their ages varied from 24 to 36 months.

2)   Preparation of the samples

For the embedded samples, it was important to cut away as much of the paraffin as possible before weighing and to mince the tissue extremely finely.

The minced pieces were less than 0.5 mm in any dimension and weighed 0.30 gr. They were placed in a 1.5 ml microfuge tube. Deparaffinization of the sections was performed with a twice xylene (1 ml) extraction followed by two ethanol rinses and a centrifugation. Pellets were air dried. The pellets were suspended in 200 µl of digestion buffer (50 mM Tris, 10 mM EDTA, pH = 7.4, 1 % SDS, 10 mM NaCl, 300 µg/ml proteinase K) and incubated during 60 hours at 37°C. Fresh aliquots of proteinase K were added every 16 hours.

Advances in Forensic Haemogenetics 4
Edited by Ch. Rittner and P. M. Schneider
© Springer-Verlag Berlin Heidelberg 1992

After this step, the samples underwent under classical phenol-chloroform extraction and a yield gel was performed.

Aliquots of 2 µl of DNA were amplified in duplicate according to the amplitype™ kit method. Cycling parameters were 32 cycles, 94°C for denaturation (1 mn), 60°C for annealing (30 sec) and 72°C for elongation (30 sec) in a DNA thermal cycler (Perkin Elmer Cetus[R]). 10 ng from K 562 cell line are used as a human DNA control.

RESULTS

From each specimen 15-20 ng DNA/mg tissues were extracted. The variation in yields were partially due to different densities within the tissues and to the quantity of paraffin left which contributed to the mesured weight. Amplification products (1/20e of the reaction) were electrophoresed on a 4 % Nusieve (3:1) gel, stained with ethidium bromide and photographed under UV light. Aliquots of 20 ng were amplified and hybridized onto the nylon strip where the allele specific probes of the HLA DQ alpha region were disposed. As an example, we present the analysis of a two years old breast carcinoma biopsy fixed and paraffin embedded after contestation by the patient of the diagnostic on the base of a possible inversion of samples from different patients by the laboratory. Therefore a control of the origin of the samples was required and refered to our laboratory for DNA identification.

DISCUSSION AND CONCLUSION

In previous studies, several authors (Greer 1991) studied different fixation methods found in clinical settings. Goelz and coworkers (1985) showed that even if DNA is not completely intact, it is double stranded, cleavable with restriction endonucleases and hybridized efficiently with labeled probes.

In our study, the material was unusable for Southern blot analysis but the remaining DNA was a sufficient template for successfull amplification. Therefore, DNA from routinely fixed and embedded tissue was suitable for the analysis of the HLA DQ alpha region by PCR. These results were in agrement with the work of Greer and coll (1991) who succeded to amplify the human B-globin gene.

In our case work the donnor of the biopsy was the right patient. The routine histopathologic fixation and conservation method provided acceptable histology analysis and suitable DNA for PCR analyse. This fixation procedure might be a good method for specimen storage for extended periods of time before analysis.

REFERENCES

Goelz SE, Hamilton SR, Vogelstein B (1985) Purification of DNA from formaldehyde fixed and paraffin embedded human tissue. Biochem Biophysic Res Commun, 130:188-126

Greer CE, Lund JK, Manos MM (1991) PCR amplification from paraffin-embedded tissues : Recommandations on fixatives for long-term storage and Prospective studies. PCR methods and application, 1:46-50

Greer CE, Peterson SL, Kiviat NB, Manos MM (1991) PCR amplification from paraffin-embedded tissues : Effects of fixative and fixation time. Am J Clin Pathol, 95:117-124

Comparison of Population data using 3 AMPFLP systems

K. Skowasch, M. Schürenkamp, S. Rand
Institute of Legal Medicine, Münster, Germany

INTRODUCTION AND AIMS

The so-called AMPFLP's (amplified fragment length polymorphism) generally have fragment lengths of up to 1000 bp. With a good electrophoretic set up the alleles can be defined. The advantages are as follows: - discrete alleles are definable - amplification of alleles can be reliable carried out because the allele length is relatively small (1 kb) - amplification is also possible with highly degraded DNA.

Population data has been carried out for 3 different AMPFLP - systems in a north German population. The aims of investigation were: - to obtain allele frequencies in a German population sample - to perform family studies for preliminary information about possible new mutations - a comparison with other population studies to show whether differencies could be seen - to test the Hardy-Weinberg equilibrium.

MATERIALS AND METHODS

Blood samples were obtained from routine paternity cases whereby results from unrelated individuals (i. e. mother and putative fathers) were included in the population studies. DNA was extracted from EDTA blood as previously described (Brinkmann et al 1991). Each amplification sample contained:
100ng DNA, 2 Units taq-Polymerase (Promega), 0,5 mmol each Primer, 200 mmol each NTP, 5 μl PCR-Buffer (Promega).
The following primers were used: Apo B (Boerwinkle et al, 1989)
                        pMCT 118 (Budowle et al, 1991)
                        YNZ 22   (Budowle pers. com.)
                        5'-AAA CTG CAG AGA GAA AGG TCG AAG AGT GAA GTG-3'
                        5'-AAA GGA TCC CCC ACA TCC GCT CCC CAA GTT-3'
The electrophoretical separation of the amplified fragments was carried out in short polyacrilamide gels (8 cm, YNZ 22; Budowle et al 1991, Sambrook et al 1989) or long polyacrilamide gels (18-20cm, pMCT 118, Apo B) using a discontinuous buffer system (Allen et al 1989). Visualisation of the bands was carried out by silver staining (Budowle et al 1991). Allele determination was carried out by comparison with an allele cocktail in addition to the size marker (123Bp-Ladder).

RESULTS

I. Population data

In pMCT there are 2 fragments with a frequency of more than 20%, allele Nr. 7 has a frequency of nearly 40%. In Apo B there are two fragments with frequencies of approximately 20% can be found. YNZ 22 also has 3 fragments with frequencies between 15-25%. From the allele frequencies a mean exclusion chance for the 3 systems of 0,58 - 0,7 was calculated and the combined exclusion chance is approximately 93%. For the 3 AMP-FLP systems the value of the discrimination index ranged from 0,29 - 0,05 with a combined value of $1,6 * 10^{-3}$
As the AMPFLP systems shown here have many alleles it is possible to construct a variety of allele groups which can then be treated as one allele. Chi square tests can then carried out on these allele groups to test for Hardy-Weinberg-equilibrium. Hardy-Weinberg calculations have been carried out using a 4- allele model (pMCT 118, Apo B)or a 5-allele-model (YNZ 22). As the combined chi-square value shows that there is no significant deviation between expected und observed values the population is assumed to be in Hardy Weinberg equilibrium: For Apo B x = 12,37, p = 0,1-0,2 (df 9); for pMCT x = 5,51, p = 0,7-0,8 (df 9); for YNZ x = 4,73, p = 0,99 - 0.97 (df 4,73).
Although the repeat lengh of pMCT is assumed to be 16bp, two additional intermediate bands were found in the range of 369 - 492 bp.

Advances in Forensic Haemogenetics 4
Edited by Ch. Rittner and P. M. Schneider
© Springer-Verlag Berlin Heidelberg 1992

II. Comparison of different population studies

A comparison of different population studies using smoothed curves for convenience showed clear conformity for all systems. With Apo B a comparison of 2 European studies shows a very similar profile. A shift can be seen in the lower frequency region between repeats 27 - 29 and between repeats 45 - 49. With pMCT there are only 2 peaks with obvious differences in the peak height. Alleles 6 and 7 give a combined allele frequency of approximately 43% in the German study and 35% in the American study. With YNZ the smoothed curves show good correlation. In the German study a large peak can be seen in the range of the 2nd -4th alleles which is much smaller in the American study. The peak between 8-10 alleles is similar in both studies.

III. Family studies:

The results are in Fig. 3. In Apo B 76% were in agreement with the basic investigation, for YNZ 89% and for pMCT 118 86%. As 24% for Apo B, 11% for YNZ, 14% for pMCT of investigated families show exclusion in the basic investigations and no exclusion in PCR. There was no evidence of new mutations found.

DISCUSSION

Population studies should be carried out by each laboratory for the calculation of population specific allele frequencies. Deviations between various populations seem to be relatively small but it must be taken into consideration that the sample sizes of these studies are as yet too small for a reliable comparison. The classical method for testing if a population sample is in Hardy-Weinberg equilibrium is impractical and not statistical suitable for systems containing large numbers of alleles as suggested by Brenner and Morris (1989) for a quasi continuous distribution of alleles. No significant deviations from Hardy-Weinberg equilibrium could be found in all 3 AMPFLP systems.

This paper is an updating from Rand S, Puers C, Skowasch K, Wiegand P, Budowle B, Brinkmann B: Population genetics and forensic efficiency data of 4 AMPFLP's (in press: Int. J. Leg. Med.).

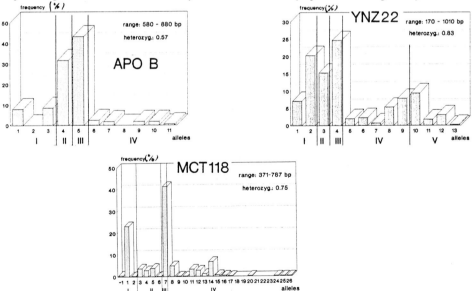

Fig. 1: Population data: Distribution of alleles in the AMPFLP systems Apo B (1a), MCT 118 (1b), YNZ 22 (1c). The nomenclature for the allele number for Apo B is as given by Ludwig et al 1989, for pMCT as given by Budowle et al 1991, for YNZ as given by Horn et al 1989. I-V indicate the groups of alleles used to estimate the Hardy Weinberg equilibrium for APO B, MCT, YNZ

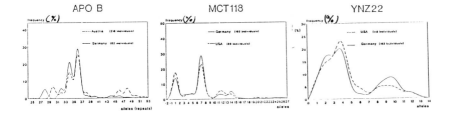

Fig. 2: Comparison of data from Münster with data from Ludwig et al 1989, for Apo B, for pMCT 118 with Budowle et al 1991, for YNZ 22 with Bataninan et al 1990

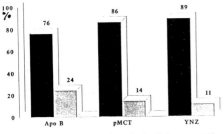

PCR and "basic investigations" in agreement
(using classical serological methods
and single locus DNA investigation)

Exclusion in "basic investigations",
non-exclusion in PCR

Fig. 3: Family studies for Apo B, pMCT 118, showing a comparison of the results from PCR and basic investigation. Family studies have been carried out for different AMPFLP systems and the results habe been compared to the "basic paternity investigation" using classical serological methods and a single-locus DNA investigation

REFERENCES

Allen RC, Graves G, Budowle B (1989): Polymerase chain reaction amplification products separated on rehydratable polyacrylamide gels and stained with silver. Biotechniques 7: 736-744

Batanian JR, Ledbetter SA, Wolff RK, Nakamura Y, White R, Dobyns WB, Ledbetter DH (1990): Rapid diagnosis of Miller-Dieker syndrome and isolated lissencephaly sequence by the polymerase chain reaction. Hum. Genet. 85: 555-559

Boerwinkle E, Xiong W, Fourest E, Chan L (Jan. 1989): Rapid typing of tandemly repeated hypervariable loci by the polymerase chain reaction: Application to the apolipoprotein B 3'hypervariable region. Pro. Natl. Acad. Sci. USA, Vol 86: 212-216

Brenner C, Moris JW: Paternity index calculation in single locus hypervariable DNA probes: Validation and other studies in: Proceedings for the International Symposium on Human Identification, Promega corporation, Madison, USA 1989

Brinkmann B, Rand S, Wiegand P (1991): Population anf family data of RFLP's using selected single- and multi-locus systems. Int. J. Leg. Med. 104: 81-86

Budowle B, Chakraborty R, Guisti AM, Eisenberg AJ, Allen RC (1989): Analysis of the VNTR-locus D1S80 by the PCR followed by high-resolution PAGE. American Journal of Human Genetics 48: 137-144 (1991)

Horn GT, Richards B, Klinger KW: Amplification of a highly polymorphic VNTR segment by the polymerase chain reaction. Nucleic Acid of Research 17: 2140

Ludwig EH, Friedl W, McCarthy BJ (1989): High resolution analysis of a hypervariable region in the human apolipoprotein B gene. Am. J. Genet. 45: 458-464

Sambrook J, Fritsch EF, Maniatis T: Molecular Cloning - a laboratory manual. 2nd edition, Cold Spring Harbor, New York 1989. Vol. 2, Chapter 14

The Amplified Fragment Length Polymorphism Study of Locus pMCT118 and Its Application in Forensic Biology

Li Boling, Ding Yan, Ni Jintang, Chen Song, Hu Lan, Ye Jian

Institute of Forensic Science, Ministry of Public Security, Beijing 100038, People's Republic of China

INTRODUCTION

DNA restriction fragment length polymorphism (RFLP) analysis has been used more and more in forensic science on individual identification and paternity test. But the RFLP analysis needs relatively large quantity of undegraded DNA ($>$300ng for mutilocus probe) and the manupulation is complicated (Jeffreys 1985, 李伯龄 1991). In actual cases, the samples to be detected usually contain too little high molecular DNA to conduct RFLP analysis. The development of in vitro DNA amplification provides a new way to solve this problem. The sequences flanked the target VNTR locus are chosen as primers, and the use of polymerase chain reaction to amplify the VNTR can result in different length DNA fragment. The polymorphism is called amplified fragment length polymorphism (Amp—FLP) (Bugoele 1991).
According to the results of Kasai (1989), we chose pMCT118 locus to analysis the Amp—FLP. The question related to forensic sciences were discussed.

MATERIALS AND METHOD

DNA extraction: The DNA extraction from blood, semen, tissue and organ were discribed elsewhere (李伯龄 1991).

Amplification of pMCT118 locus: The PCR was carried out in a final volume of 100µl or 20µl. The content were 50mM KCl, 10mM Tris—HCl, pH8. 3, 1. 5mM MgCl$_2$ 0. 01mg/ml gelatin, 200mM of each dNTP, 0. 1µM of each primer, 1—100ng sample DNA. After denatured at 95^{0}C for 5min, 2. 5U or 1. 25U of Taq DNA polymerase was added. Then overlay the mix with 50µl or 20µl of mineral oil. The PCR was carried out in Thermal Cycler (PE co. USA) with 95^{0}C for 1 min. 65^{0}C for 1 min. 70^{0}C for 3 min. as one cycle. Ten second was added after each cycle. Thirty three cycles were conducted for each PCR.

Detection of the amplified sample: 5%T, 3%C, 0. 75mm mini vertical plate polyacrylamide gel electrophoresis and silver stain was used to detect the Amp—FLP.

Advances in Forensic Haemogenetics 4
Edited by Ch. Rittner and P. M. Schneider
© Springer-Verlag Berlin Heidelberg 1992

RESULTS

Blood extracted DNA of 98 unrelated Chinese was analyxed by PCR of pMCT118 locus. The Amp—FLP results show 22 alleles, ranging from 340 to 780bp. The allele distribution frequencies range from 0. 5— 30% with a heterozygosity of 0. 79.

Two families of three generation with 5 persons and four families of two generation with 3 persons were analysed of pMCT118 locus Amp—FLP. The Amp—FLP bands of the child were inherited from either mother or father. These were consistant with the Mendelian Inheritance Law.

The pMCT118 locus Amp—FLP of sperm DNA prepared from mixed stains were compared with that of the male and female blood DNA. The results showed that the sperm DNA prepared from the mixed stain was not contaminated by the female DNA and that a genotype was the same as that of the male blood DNA. Fifty samples were conducted and none of them showed female alleles.

The result of pMCT118 locus Amp—FLP of DNA extracted from 1μl saliva has been got.

Using the method discribed above, the PCR have been conducted with DNA prepared from blood, semen, and different organs of the same person. The results are the same.

DNA from a sample, even the quantity varied more than 100 times (1ng to 100ng) or have different degrade level, can all get the same results. The sample quantity as little as 1ng DNA, 1μl blood, 0. 1μl semen or semen stain, single hair root and 1μl saliva can all get PCR results. In a study of 20 blood samples, 1μl blood was analysed and all get good results. If use 0. 1μl blood, 16 of 20 samples were positive in a percentile of 80%.

DISCUSSION

The pMCT118 locus is a VNTR with a core sequence as GNNGTCCC. The analysis of unrelated 98 Chinese shows that pMCT118 locus has 22 alleles ranging from 340 to 780 bp compared to the results of Kasai (1989) with 21 alleles ranging from 387 to 723bp when studying of 67 Japanese. There is obvious difference between the two results. There are also differences on the alleles distribution frequency of the two studies. And some results infer the repeat unit of the alleles is an 8 base sequence (will be reported elsewhere) . So the Amp—FLP result of this locus is different in different race. In 200 samples we have detected, two samples show three bands. The reason of that would be studied further.

About 60% of the 98 studied samples show one or two extra bands, some show three or four. These extra bands are stable. They do not change according to the change of DNA sample quantity. The Amp—FLP of different organs from one individual also show stability. They seemed to be individual specific. But they can not be inherited and do not interfere the analysis. In addition, samples of some individuals show a weak band on allele except ordinary bands. These may be caused by the sensitive detect method. When we use 3% agarose gel electrophoresis and ethidium bromide fluorescence to detect , the weak band can not be seen. In our analysis, we overlooked this band. If the primer concentrition was raised to 1μM, the extra bands are likely to exist according to the sample DNA quantity and the bands were visible by agarose electrophoresis detection.

REFERENCES

Bugoele B, Chakraborty R, et al. (1991) Analysis of the VNTR Locus D1S80 by the PCR followed by high—resolution PAGE. American Journal of Human Genetics. Vol. 48. pp 137— 44

Jeffreys A, J, et al. (1985)Individual spectific fingerprints of human DNA. Nature 316:76—79

Kasai R, K, et al. (1989) Amplification of VNTR locus by the polymerase chain reaction(PCR). Proceedings of an International Symposium on the Forensic Aspects of DNA Analysis, Govermental Printing Office , Washingten. D. C.

李伯龄等(1991)α一珠白蛋—3' HVR 探针 DNA 指纹图法医应用的研究,遗传(3) (in press)

DNA typing from formalin-fixed, paraffin-embedded tissues

H. Fukushima, M. Ota, K. Tanaka[*], A. Ichinose[*], K. Sato, and K. Honda

Department of Legal Medicine and[*]Department of Anesthesiology, Shinshu University School of Medicine, 3-1-1 Asahi, Matsumoto, Nagano 390, Japan

INTRODUCTION

Serologically defined individual variation has been shown to be considerable in HLA class I and class II. Recently, HLA alleles were defined using polymerase chain reaction(PCR-DNA typing). As previously reported(Ota 1991), the PCR-restriction fragment length polymorphism(PCR-RFLP) method is the most useful to define the HLA-DQA1, DQB1, DRB1 and DPB1 alleles. The advantage of this method is the use of some informative restriction enzymes, which have either a single cleavage site or alternatively no cleavage site in the amplified DNA region.

In this study, we attempted to extract DNA from old formalin-fixed, paraffin-embedded samples of tissues, such as brain, heart, lung, liver and kidney. The extracted DNA was amplified and typed using the PCR-RFLP method.

MATERIALS AND METHODS

For comparison with DNA extraction from (1)long-term, formalin-fixed and embedded samples, and (2)short-term, formalin-fixed and long-term embedded samples, brain ,heart, lung, liver and kidney tissues were fixed in phosphate buffered formaldehyde (3-5%) or unbuffered formaldehyde(3-5%) at room temperature for two months or two years. 5-μ sections were cut from blocks and deparaffinized by immersion for 30 minutes at room temperature in 1ml of xylene, spun 5 minutes in a microfuge, and decanted (Shibata 1988). This procedure was repeated. The sections were rinsed once with 100% ethanol by inverting the tube two or three times. The samples were then centrifuged and the liquid decanted. The procedure was repeated with 100% ethanol. The last rinse was decanted and the remaining ethanol evaporated under vacuum. The sections were resuspended in 300μl of digestive buffer(10mM Tris-HCl,pH8.0, 10mM EDTA, 0.1M NaCl) containing 1%SDS and proteinase K(250μg/ml). The mixture was incubated for over 5 hours at 50°C. After the solution was extracted with water-saturated phenol, TE buffer was added. The solution was concentrated on a Centricon 30 microconcentrator(Amicon)(Pääbo 1988). After addition of distilled water and a second concentration, the solution was used for the DNA template.

For PCR amplification, the reaction mixture was subjected to 30 cycles of 1 minute at 92°C, 1 minute at 62°C, and 2 minutes at 72° by automated PCR thermal cyclers. The DQA1 gene was amplified

Advances in Forensic Haemogenetics 4
Edited by Ch. Rittner and P. M. Schneider
© Springer-Verlag Berlin Heidelberg 1992

using the PCR primers GH26 and GH27 at 1 µM. After amplification, aliquots of the reaction mixtures were digested with the restriction endonucleases, ApaLI, HphI, BsaJI, FokI and MboII, for 5 hours after adding the appropriate incubation buffer. Samples of the restriction-enzyme-cleaved amplified DNAs were subjected to electrophoresis in 12% polyacrylamide gel in a minigel apparatus. Restriction fragments were detected by staining with ethidium bromide.

RESULTS AND DISCUSSION

Genetic characterization of individuals for identity testing is being performed increasingly at the DNA level. A new, technically more feasible strategy for individual identification at the DNA level is the use of PCR. The advantage of the PCR technique is that it enables the analysis of minute amounts of DNA from various sources, including impure or degraded samples (Higuchi 1988). DNA analysis from the formalin-fixed, paraffin-embedded tissues was performed by the PCR procedure with Tag DNA polymerase. This method has been applied successfully to DNA extracted from 2-year-old paraffin blocks as well as from 2-year-old formalin-fixed tissue stored at room temperature (Table 1). Although it is reported that unbuffered formalin markedly degrades DNA, our procedure shows that amplification of short specific DNA sequences is still possible.

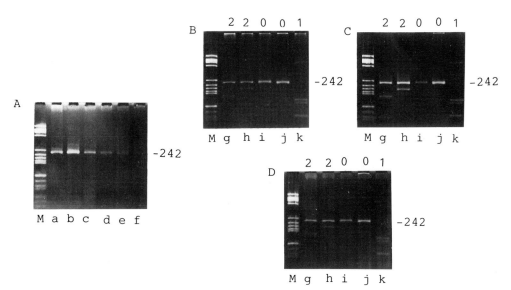

Fig. 1   PCR amplification and restriction analysis of HLA-DQA1 fragments in various organs(buffered formalin)

A:amplified DNA	B:brain	g:ApaLI	0:not cleaved
a,d:brain	C:heart	h:HphI	1:cleaved
b,e:heart	D:liver	i:BsaJI	
c,f:liver		j:FokI	
1-week-old(a,b,c)		k:MboII	
2-month-old(d,e,f)			

83

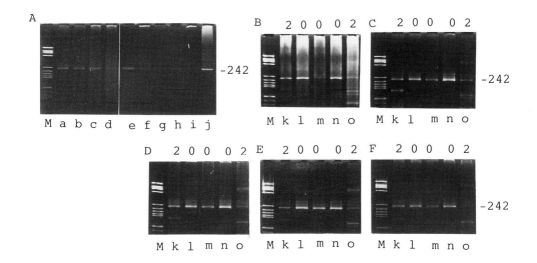

Fig. 2 PCR amplification and restriction analysis of HLA-DQA1
fragments in various organs(unbuffered formalin)
  A:amplified DNA   B:blood   k:ApaLI   0:not cleaved
    a,e:brain, b,f:heart   C:brain   l:HphI   1:cleaved
    c,g:liver, d,h:kidney   D:heart   m:BsaJI
    i:lung,   j:blood   E:liver,F:kidney   n:FokI,o:MboII
    2-year-old paraffin-embedded(a,b,c,d)
    2-year-old formalin-fixed(e,f,g,h)

Table 1.   HLA-DQA1 genotyping from tissues using PCR-RFLP

	Genotype	Restriction endonucleases				
		ApaLI	HphI	BsaJI	FokI	MboII
case I(2-month-old)	0103/0301	2	2	0	0	1
case II(2-year-old)	0102/0301	2	0	0	0	2

0: not cleaved, 1:cleaved, 2:both for heterozygote. DQA1 0101 and 0102
can be discriminated by RFLP bands (23 bp and/or 40 bp) digested with
MnlI enzyme. case I and case II: blood, brain, heart, liver, kidney, lung.

REFERENCES

Higuchi R, Beroldingen CH von, Sensabaugh GF, Erlich HA (1988)
  DNA   typing from single hairs. Nature 332:543-546
Ota M, Seki T, Nomura N, Sugimura K, Mizuki N, Fukushima H, Tsuji
  K, Inoko H (1991) Modified PCR-RFLP method for HLA-DPB1 and
  DQA1 genotyping. Tissue Antigens 38: 60-71
Pääbo S, Gifford JA, Wilson AC (1988) Mitochondrial DNA sequences
  from a 7000-year old brain. Nucl Acids Res 16:9775-9787
Shibata DK, Arnheim N, Martin WJ (1988) Detection of human
  papilloma virus in paraffin-embedded tissue using the
  polymerase chain reaction. J Exp Med 167:225-230

HLA-DQA1 and HLA-DPB1 gene polymorphisms in the Japanese populations

A. Ichinose, M. Ota[*], H. Inoko[**], K. Sato[*], K. Tanaka, K. Kiyono, K. Honda[*] and H. Fukushima[*]

Department of Anesthesiology and[*] Department of Legal Medicine Shinshu University School of Medicine, 3-1-1 Asahi Matsumoto 390.
[**]Department of Transplantation, Tokai University School of Medicine, Bohseidai, Isehara, 259-11. JAPAN

INTRODUCTION
Highly polymorphic HLA systems have greatly contributed to paternity testing and personal identification in forensic work. Recently HLA alleles in the class II region has been identified easily at the nucleotide level using PCR method. The PCR procedure involves the PCR-SSO (sequence specific oligonucleotide) method and the modified PCR-RFLP method (1). Those two methods permit precise and direct analysis of allelic variations by using less than 1 ng of DNA. The modified PCR-RFLP method provides a simpler and more rapid technique for accurate definition of the HLA-class II alleles. In this study, HLA-DQA1 and -DPB1 alleles were defined in 150 unrelated healthy Japanese individuals using the modified PCR-RFLP method. Exclusion probability (EP) was calculated from the allele frequencies of DQA1 and DPB1 obtained in this population.

MATERIAL AND METHOD
DNA samples : Genomic DNAs from 150 healthy Japanese volunteers' whole blood were isolated by phenol extraction of sodium dodecyl sulfate (SDS)-lysed and proteinase K-treated cells.

PCR amplification: Genomic DNA (1 µg) was amplified by the PCR procedure with 2.5 units of the Taq DNA polymerase (Perkin Elmer Cetus Inc.). The reaction mixture was subjected to 30 cycles of 1 min at 94 $^\circ$C, 1 min at 62 $^\circ$C, and 2 min at 72 $^\circ$C by automated PCR thermal sequencer (Iwaki Glass Inc.). The second exon of the DQA1 gene was amplified by using PCR primers, GH26 and GH27 at 1 µM and the second exon of the DPB1 gene was amplified by using the PCR primers, DPB101 and DPB201 at 1 µM (Table 1).

Digestion with restriction endonucleases and acrylamide gel electrophoresis: Restriction enzymes of ApaLI, HphI, BsaJI, FokI, MboII and MnlI were used for digestion of the amplified DQA1 gene and Bsp1286I, FokI, DdeI, BsaJI, Cfr13I, RsaI, EcoNI and AvaII were used for digestion of the amplified DPB1 gene. Samples of the restriction enzyme-cleaved amplified DNAs were subjected to electrophoresis in 12% polyacrylamide gels in a horizontal mini-gel apparatus (Mupid, Cosmo Bio Co.). Cleavage or no cleavage of amplified fragments was detected by staining with ethidium bromide.

Advances in Forensic Haemogenetics 4
Edited by Ch. Rittner and P. M. Schneider
© Springer-Verlag Berlin Heidelberg 1992

CONCLUSION
For the DQA1 alleles, 36 combinations including 8 homozygotes and 28 heterozygotes can be unequivocally determined by the modified PCR-RFLP method (1). DQA1 gene frequencies are shown in Table 2. Cleavage patterns of DQA1 genes are shown in Fig.1. DQA1*0301 was the most frequent (37.8%) allele. EP of the DQA1 genotype was 0.51. For the DPB1 alleles, 190 combinations including 19 homozygotes and 171 heterozygotes could be determined. DPB1 gene frequencies are shown in Table 3. Cleavage patterns of DPB1 gnes are shown in Fig.2. EP of the DPB1 genotype was 0.57. The HLA-DQA1 and -DPB1 polymorphisms are useful for paternity test and personal identification.

REFERENCE
1) Ota M, Seki T, Nomura N, Sugimura K, Mizuki N, Fukushima H, Tsuji K, Inoko H. (1991) Modified PCR-RFLP method for HLA-DPB1 and DQA1 genotyping. Tissue Antigens 38:60-71

Table 1. PCR primers for amplification of DQA1 and DPB1 genes

Gene	Primers	Sequences (5' to 3')
DQA1	GH26	GTGCTGCAGGTGTAAACTTGTACCAG
	GH27	CACGGATCCGGTAGCAGCGGTAGAGTTG
DPB1	DPB101	GTGAAGCTTTCCCCGCAGAGAATTAC
	DPB201	CACCTGCAGTCACTCACCTCGGCGCTG

Table 2. DQA1 gene frequency

Type	n	P.F.	G.F.
DQA1*0101	45	0.300	0.163
DQA1*0102	48	0.320	0.175
DQA1*0103	56	0.373	0.208
DQA1*0201	1	0.007	0.004
DQA1*0301	92	0.613	0.378
DQA1*0401	1	0.007	0.004
DQA1*0501	22	0.147	0.076
DQA1*0601	4	0.027	0.014

P.F.: Phenotype Frequency
G.F.: Gene Frequency
Total number examined=150

Table 3. DPB1 gene frequency

Type	n	P.F.	G.F.
DPB1*0101	0	0.000	0.000
DPB1*0201	48	0.320	0.175
DPB1*0202	14	0.093	0.048
DPB1*0301	10	0.067	0.034
DPB1*0401	14	0.093	0.048
DPB1*0402	35	0.233	0.124
DPB1*0501	83	0.553	0.331
DPB1*0601	1	0.007	0.004
DPB1*0801	0	0.000	0.000
DPB1*0901	29	0.193	0.102
DPB1*1001	0	0.000	0.000
DPB1*1101	0	0.000	0.000
DPB1*1301	4	0.027	0.014
DPB1*1401	3	0.020	0.010
DPB1*1501	0	0.000	0.000
DPB1*1601	2	0.013	0.007
DPB1*1701	0	0.000	0.000
DPB1*1801	0	0.000	0.000
DPB1*1901	0	0.000	0.000

P.F.: Phenotype Frequency
G.F.: Gene Frequency
Total number examined=150

Fig.1 Cleavage patterns of polymorphic restriction
fragments in the PCR-amplified DQA1 genes
obtained from DNAs of 12 normal individuals
after digestion with 5 restriction enzymes

Fig.2 Cleavage patterns of polymorphic restriction
fragments in the PCR-amplified DPB1 genes
obtained from DNAs of 7 normal individuals
after digestion with 9 restriction enzymes

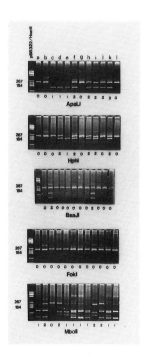

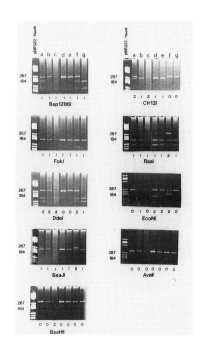

DQA1 genotype

a:DQA1*0301/0301
b:DQA1*0301/0501
c:DQA1*0101/0102
d:DQA1*0102/0103
e:DQA1*0103/0103
f:DQA1*0103/0301
g:DQA1*0301/0301
h:DQA1*0103/0301
i:DQA1*0103/0501
j:DQA1*0102/0301
k:DQA1*0103/0301
l:DQA1*0301/0301

DPB1 genotype

a:DPB1*0402/0501
b:DPB1*0201/0202
c:DPB1*0401/0501
d:DPB1*0201/0402
e:DPB1*0201/0402
f:DPB1*0501/0901
g:DPB1*0501/0501

The Study of apoB Locus Apm—FLP and Its Application in Forensic Sciences

Li Boling, Ding Yan, Ni Jintang, Chen Song, Hu Lan, Ye Jian

Institute of Forensic Science, Ministry of Public Security, Beijing 100038, People's Republic of China

INTRODUCTION

The restriction fragment length polymorphism (RELP) analysis needs a relatively large quantity of high molecular DNA, which is hard to meet in actual cases. In 1985, Saiki et al reported DNA amplification in vitro, which provided a new method to solve the problem. The technique used polymerase chain reaction (PCR) to amplify specific template DNA sequence to more than 10^8 times (Saiki 1988). This method is sensitive and suitable to the sample with minute quantity or degraded DNA.

ApoB gene, which located on the chromosome 2 of human genome, is a marker to show the probability to suffer cardiovscular diseases. In 3' end of the gene has a VNTR locus which contains an A—T rich core sequence. Using special flanked primers, the locus can be amplified. Based on the method reported by Boerwinkle (1989), we have studied blood, blood stain, semen, semen stain, mixed stain, tissue, hair and degraded DNA with PCR. Reliable result has been got.

MATERIALS AND METHOD

PCR was carried out in 100μl system. Each cycle includes denaturing at 95°C for 1 min, annealling and extension at 58°C for 6 min. Thirty five cycles as a PCR.

The results were detected with mini vertical PEAG and silver stain.

The composition of the gel is as follows:

30% acrylamide	810μl
20% bis	375μl
10x TBE	500μl
DDW	3285μl

Mix and then add 3.5μl TEMED and 35μl 10% $(NH_4)_2S_2O_8$, gel for 1 hour. Pre—electrophoresis for 10 min and then the sample was loaded. Electrophoresis was carried out under 200V for 45 min. Silver staining was carried out as follows: fix with 10% ethanol and 5% acetic acid for 15 min and stain with 12 mM Ag-NO$_3$, for 30 min, 0.25M Na$_2$CO$_3$, 0.04% HCHO stain for 10 min, stopped with 10% acetic acid. Gel was dried with drier.

Advances in Forensic Haemogenetics 4
Edited by Ch. Rittner and P. M. Schneider
© Springer-Verlag Berlin Heidelberg 1992

RESULTS

We have investigated the apoB locus Amp—FLP of 100 unrelated individuals in Beijing area. Eleven alleles have been determined. The fragments range from 600—1000bp. Gene frequences are 0.5—52.5% with a heterozygosity of 70%.

ApoB Amp — FLP of four families each contains 3 persons have been analysed. With family 3 as example:

The mother, father and the son each show two bands. The two bands of the son match either the mother or the father, which is consistant with Mendelian Law.

Compare the Amp—FLP get from semen stain with that from blood, the same results were got.

The apoB Amp—FLPs of the sperm DNA prepared from mixed stain were got and compared with that of the male and female blood DNA. The Amp—FLP of the sperm DNA prepared form mixed stain is the same as that of the male and different from that of the female.

The Amp—FLP of different organs show the same bands.

1μl blood, 0.1μl semen, 1 ng DNA and single hair root can all be detected respectively with the method described above.

We have used this time—saving technique as a prThe unexcluded sample cann' t be used to conduct DNA fingerprinting. The identification rate has been raised.

DISCCUSION

Uniformity study of different nucleate cells DNA (include kinds of tissue, blood, blood stain, semen, semen stain, hair and so on) has been done. The results show that DNA from different nucleate cells of one individual gives the same form Amp — FLP pattern. Even to the DNA easily degraded organs such as' liver, spleen, kidney, which usually get only partial fingerprints, can also get good amplified fragment same to other tissues. The sameness is the base for the application of this technique. We repeat amplification of some sample DNA which show sameness. In apoB locus Amp—FLP, some samples show extra bands. The reason need farther discussion.

Blood or blood stain separated from the substrate have been amplified directly and good results have been got. And the method was proved to be a simple and time—saving method . PCR, as a simple, time—saving preexperinment of DNA fingerprint, have rasied the identification rate of DNA fingerprint. A series of VN-TR locus Amp—FLP should be an even more prowerful tool in forensic sciences.

REFERENCES

Boerwinkle E, et al. (1989) Rapid typing of tandemly repeated hypervariable loci
   by the PCR: Application to the apolipoprotein B 3' hypervariable region. Proc. Natl. Acad.

Sci. USA 86;212—216 SaikiP. K,et al. (1985)Enzymatic amplification ofβ—globin genomic

sequences and restriction site analysis for diagnosis of scikle cell anemia. Science

230;1350

SaikiR. K,et al. (1988)Primer—directed enzymatic amplification of DNA with a thermostable

DNA polymerase. Science 239;487. Printing Office,Washington. D. C. 李伯龄等(1991)α—珠蛋白—

3' HVR 探针 DNA 指纹图法医应用的研究. 遗传(3)(in press)

Application of HLA-class II Genotyping by the Modified PCR-RFLP Method to the Forensic Science

M. Ota, H. Inoko[*], T. Seki[**], A. Ichinose, K. Honda, K. Tsuji[*] and H. Fukushima

Department of Legal Medicine and [**]Department of 2nd Internal Medicine, Shinshu University School of Medicine, 3-1-1 Asahi Matsumoto 390. [*]Department of Transplantation, Tokai University School of Medicine, Bohseidai, Isehara, 259-11. JAPAN

INTRODUCTION

The HLA class II antigens(HLA-DR, -DQ, -DP), located in the short arm of chromosome 6, show a great deal of polymorphisms. These antigens have been usually defined by serological procedures (for DR and DQ) using alloantisera or monoclonal antibody and cellular assay procedure (for Dw and DP). Definition of HLA class II antigens became possible at the DNA level using Southern blot hybridization technique with class II antigen cDNA probes. More recently, detection of nucleotide sequence polymorphisms in the HLA class II region has become feasible with the advent of polymerase chain reaction (PCR) technique. The PCR method permits precise and direct analysis of allelic variations with as little as 1 ng of genomic DNA. We earlier reported the modified PCR-RFLP methods (1-3), which were legible and easy to use in the accurate definition of HLA class II (DQA1, DQB1, DRB1 and DPB1) alleles. This method allows discrimination of 36, 91, 946 and 190 combinations, including homozygotes and heterozygotes of the DQA1(8 alleles), DQB1(13 alleles), DRB1(43 alleles) and DPB1(18 alleles) respectively. In this study, we examined the possibility of HLA-class II genotyping by the modified PCR-RFLP method for DNA samples extracted from hairs, a small volume of whole blood, fresh or old dental pulp tissues.

MATERIALS AND METHODS

1) DNA extraction and amplification: Genomic DNAs were extracted from blood, a single plucked hair with a length of 3 cm and fresh or old dental pulp tissues (300 mg) by a rapid DNA extraction technique (Fig. 1) using Centricon 30 dialysis/concentration tube (Amicon Co.).
2) Amplification: DQA1, DQB1, DPB1 and DRB1 genes were amplified by using PCR primers (1, 2, 3). After amplification, aliquots (10 μl) of the reaction mixture were digested with each objective restriction endonuclease (1, 2, 3).
3) Acrylamide gel electrophoresis: Samples of the amplified DNAs cleaved with restriction enzyme were subjected to electrophoresis in 12% polyacrylamide gel in a minigel apparatus (Mupid, Cosmo Bio Co.). Cleavage or non-cleavage of amplified fragments was detected by staining with ethidium bromide.

RESULTS

1) DQA1 and DQB1 genotyping from blood.
   DQA1 and DQB1 genes could be amplified with DNAs extracted

Advances in Forensic Haemogenetics 4
Edited by Ch. Rittner and P. M. Schneider
© Springer-Verlag Berlin Heidelberg 1992

from 250 μl of stored blood in a 1.5 ml eppendorf tube for 2 years at room temperature (Fig. 2). Their genotypes could be determined by the modified PCR-RFLP method (I: DQA1*0103/0301, DQB1*0601/0401; II: DQA1*0101=2/0301, DQB1*0501/0303).

2) DRB1 genotyping from hair.

DRB1 gene could be amplified with DNAs extracted from a single plucked hair with 3 cm length using group-specific primers. This genotype was determined by the modified PCR-RFLP method (Fig. 3 : DRB1*0803/0803).

3) DQA1 and DPB1 genotyping from dental pulp tissues.

The DQA1 genes from both fresh and old (over one year) dental pulp tissues could be amplified, but the DPB1 genes could be amplified only from fresh samples (Fig. 4. A; DQA1*0103/0301: DPB1*0402/0402, B; DQA1*0103/0301: DPB1*0202/1801, C; DQA1*0103/0301: DPB1*0501/0501, D; DQA1*0102/0103, E; DQA1* 0102/0102).

REFERENCES
1) Nomura N, Ota M, Tsuji K, Inoko H: (1991) HLA-DQB1 genotyping by a modified PCR-RFLP method combined with group-specific primers. Tissue Antigens 38:53-59
2) Ota M, Seki T, Nomura N, Sugimura K, Mizuki N, Fukushima H, Tsuji K, Inoko H: (1991) Modified PCR-RFLP method for HLA-DPB1 and -DQA1 genotyping. Tissue Antigens 38:60-71
3) Ota M, Seki T, Fukushima H, Tsuji K, Inoko H: HLA-DRB1 genotyping by modified PCR-RFLP method combined with group-specific primers. Tissue Antigens in press

Fig.1 A rapid DNA extraction technique using Centricon 30 dialysis/concentration tube

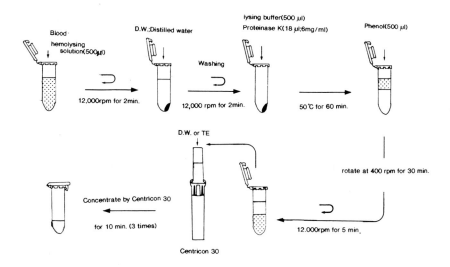

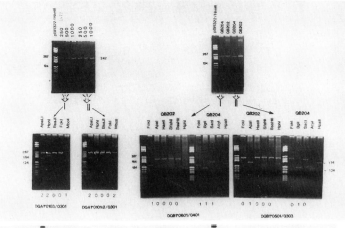

Fig. 2 Modified PCR-RFLP typing for the DQA1 and DQB1 genes using DNAs extracted from stored blood for 2 years

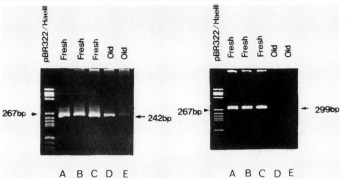

Fig.4 PCR-RFLP typing for the DQA1 and DPB1 genes using DNAs extracted from dental pulp tissues

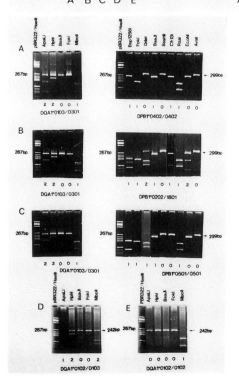

Fig.3 Modified PCR-RFLP typing for the DRB1 genes amplified by group specific primers using DNAs extracted from a single hair

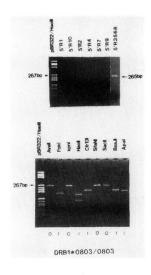

Simultaneous DNA analysis of HLA-DPB and -DQB loci from single hairs: a criminal case report

S. Pelotti, V. Mantovani*, G. Angelini°, F. Barboni* and G. Pappalardo

Institute of Legal Medicine University of Bologna, via Irnerio 49 40126 Bologna, Italy
*Tissue Typing Laboratory Malpighi Hospital, Bologna, Italy
°National Cancer Institute, Genova, Italy

INTRODUCTION

Polymorphic DNA sequences can be amplified over a millionfold with polymerase chain reaction (PCR), therefore samples can be typed even when the DNA is degraded or very small amount is available. The HLA Class II genes HLA-DR, -DQ, and -DP present a high degree of polymorphism and are suitable as genetic markers for individual forensic identification (Korman et al 1985). Higuchi et al (1988) typed for HLA-DQA single hairs by using PCR. We report a case concerning five hairs found on the hands of a murdered man. HLA-DPB polymorphism was analyzed from all the single hairs, for two simultaneously with HLA-DQB polymorphism. The typing was compared to that obtained from plucked hairs of the victim and the suspect.

MATERIALS AND METHODS

Morphological examination of evidence samples showed 5 human hairs of their natural colour, at different growth phases (one anagen with sheath, three catagen with residues of sheath, one telogen), four 6 cm and one 3 cm in lenght. The specimens were cut in the middle, where a small portion was taken, cross sectioned and typed for ABO by immunoenzymatic method with inconclusive result for individual diagnosis. Finally, the hairs were stored in glycerol until DNA extraction. Reference samples consisted of plucked hairs from both victim and suspect.
For HLA-DPB typing, DNA was obtained from the root and the proximal portion of longer shafts and from the whole shortest hair. For HLA-DQB typing, the half distal part of two specimens was separately extracted. The remaining two distal shafts were retained. DNA of reference samples was obtained from the roots.

DNA Extraction

Reference samples were rinsed in distilled water, followed by absolute ethanol. For evidence samples an additional washing with absolute ethanol preceded. The samples were digested in 0.5 ml TNE, containing 0.15 mg Proteinase K, 80 mM DTT, SDS 4%, 0.05 mg RNAse for 12 hr at 37°C and then for 24 hr at room temperature. DNA was obtained by phenol/chloroform-isoamylalcohol extraction, ethanol precipitation and finally resuspended in 30 μl TE (Maniatis et al 1982).

Advances in Forensic Haemogenetics 4
Edited by Ch. Rittner and P. M. Schneider
© Springer-Verlag Berlin Heidelberg 1992

Oligonucleotide Primers and Probes

The oligonucleotide primers DB04 (5'-CAGGTACCCGCAGAGAATTAC) and PB03 (5'-CCCTCACTCACCTCGGCG) were used to amplify a 288 base pair (bp) region of the polymorphic second exon of the DPB1 gene. Sixteen oligonucleotide probes were 32P-end-labeled and used to distinguish 19 different alleles at the HLA-DPB locus (Bugawan et al 1990). Oligonucleotides for the analysis of this region were synthesized using a cyanoethylphosphoramidite method. Two primers were employed to amplify a polymorphic fragment of the second exon of the DQB1 gene. Seven sequence-specific radiolabeled probes were chosen to distinguish eight different HLA-DQB alleles. The oligonucleotide primers and probes used are described by Molkentin et al (1991).

PCR Amplification

Due to the small amount of DNA recovered from hair samples 30 cycles of amplification were followed by additional 30 cycles, the latter performed on 1/10 of the first amplification product. DNA amplification was performed in 50 μl reactions containing 50 mM potassium chloride, 10 mM Tris-HCl pH 8.4, 1.5 mM magnesium chloride, 200 mM of each deoxyribonucleotide triphosphate, 0.01% gelatin, 5% DMSO, 50 pmoles of each primer and 1.2 units of Taq-polymerase. The PCR amplification consisted in 1 min denaturation at 96°C, 2 min annealing at 50°C for the first 30 cycles and 54°C for the latter cycles, 1.5 min polymerization at 72°C. Opportune negative and positive controls were included in every stage of analysis.

Dot Blot Hybridization

Four microliters of amplified DNA were denatured in 0.4 N NaOH, 25 mM EDTA, then spotted on a nylon membrane and ultraviolet cross-linked for 5 min. Several replicate filters were done. For DPB oligotyping, membranes were hybridized and washed as previously described (Angelini et al 1989). For DQB oligotyping, the TMAC protocol according to Molkentin et al (1991) was employed.

RESULTS AND DISCUSSION

All the samples submitted to analysis were found to amplify efficiently for HLA-DPB and -DQB genes and all PCR amplification products resulted typable with oligoprobes (Fig.1). The hair roots of the five specimens showed the same DPB type: DPB1*0401/*0901; in addition, the two shafts analyzed for DQB showed the same type: DQB1*0603/*0201. Because the victim exhibited different HLA alleles (DPB1*0401/*0201, DQB1*05/*0201) and the suspect also showed different HLA typing (DPB1*0402/*0201, DQB1*03), we were able to eliminate both of them as donors of the five hair specimens.

These results indicate that, analyzing separately the root and the shaft, it is possible to simultaneously amplify and type two

different polymorphic and independent loci from a single hair.
Actually, in our experience with PCR, the shaft of most individuals with natural hair contains enough genomic DNA to perform a
molecular typing.
The high polymorphism of HLA-DPB and -DQB loci and the relative
absence of linkage disequilibrium between them, make the simultaneous typing assay a powerful tool in the field of individual
identity.

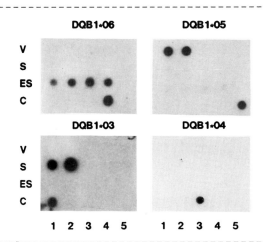

Fig. 1. Dot blot analysis of amplified DNA from the shaft of
evidence samples (ES) and from reference samples of victim (V)
and suspect (S), all in duplicate. Four oligoprobes are shown,
specific for HLA-DQB1*06, -DQB1*05, -DQB1*03 and -DQB1*04 alleles. C: positive and negative controls

REFERENCES

Angelini G, Bugawan TL, Delfino L, Erlich HA, Ferrara GB (1989)
   HLA-DP typing by DNA amplification and hybridization with
   specific oligonucleotides. Hum Immunol 26: 169-177
Bugawan TL, Begovich AB, Erlich HA (1990) Rapid HLA-DPB typing
   using enzymatically amplified DNA and nonradioactive sequence-
   specific oligonucleotide probes. Immunogenetics 32: 231-241
Higuchi R, von Beroldigen CH, Sensabaugh GF, Erlich HA (1988) DNA
   typing from single hairs. Nature 332: 543-546
Korman AJ, Boss JM, Spies T, Sorrentino R, Okada K, Strominger JL
   (1985) Genetic complexity and expression of human class II
   histocompatibility antigens. Immunol Rev 85: 45-85
Maniatis T, Fritsch EF, Sambrook J (1982) Molecular cloning: a
   laboratory manual. Cold Spring Harbor Laboratory, Cold Spring
   Harbor New York
Molkentin J, Gorski J, Baxter-Lowe LA (1991) Detection of 14 HLA-
   DQB1 alleles by oligotyping. Hum Immunol 31: 114-122

SEX DETERMINATION BY GENOMIC DOT BLOT HYBRIDIZATION AND HLA DQα TYPING BY PCR FROM FIXED TISSUES

Pötsch L., Penzes L., Prager-Eberle M., Schneider P.M., Rittner Ch.

Institute of Legal Medicine, Johannes Gutenberg-Universität, Mainz, FRG

Introduction

Recent advances in molecular biology methods have significantly increased the ability to detect genetic variation at the genomic level for forensic purposes. However, the quality requirements for blood, fresh or frozen tissue as a source of DNA are a practical limitation for typing the victim in order to conduct investigations on unsolved cases. Since paraffin embedded specimens are easily obtainable the ability to study this material would be of great value in current forensic practice.

Materials and methods

Specimen selection:

All investigations were performed using routine forensic material. The only selection criterium was the time intervall between death and autopsy which differed between 24 h and 52 hours. From autopsy cases (n = 16) blood as well as unfixed and fixed lung tissue were under investigation.

Sampling protocols:

Each lung tissue was divided into portions which were processed according the following protocols:

1) snap frozen and stored at -20°C
2) fixation in 96% ethanol
3) fixation in 4% paraformaldehyde
4) 4% buffered formaldehyde pH 7.0
5) 10% unbuffered formaldehyde.

Incubations in the fixatives were performed for 4 and 6 weeks. After these time periods samples were processed by an Autotechnicon. About 10 paraffin sections 10 μm thick were cut using a microtome. The slides were deparaffinized and rehydrated, washed 3 times by centrifugation in xylene, absolute ethanol and SSC. Unfixed and ethanol fixed lung tissue was cut using a cryostat.

DNA extraction and purification

DNA from blood, unfixed and ethanol fixed tissue was prepared using previously described methods (4). Solutions containing paraformaldehyde, 10% formaldehyde and 4% buffered formaldehyde fixed tissue were adjusted to 1% SDS, 50 mM Tris pH 8.0, and incubated at 37°C for 2 days. The preparation was centrifuged, the supernatant discarded. The pellet of lung tissue which includes large quantities of stroma was resuspended in fresh lysis mix containing: 10 mM Tris/HCl pH 7.6, 10 mM EDTA, 100 mM NaCl pH 8, 2% SDS, 40mM DDT, 1 mg/ml proteinase K. The second incubation at 42°C was stopped after 6 days. A phenol-chloroform extraction was performed and the DNA precipitated with cold ethanol. Dot hybridization could be performed with all samples at this stage. For successful PCR

Advances in Forensic Haemogenetics 4
Edited by Ch. Rittner and P. M. Schneider
© Springer-Verlag Berlin Heidelberg 1992

amplification the DNA obtained from formaldehyde and buffered formaldehyde tissue had to undergo 3 additional reextraction steps of treatment at 42°C for 24 h with the above lysis buffer followed by phenol extraction and ethanol precipitation.

Sex determination by dot hybridization

Dot hybridization on Immobilon N membranes (Millipore, Eschborn, FRG) was performed as previously described (4) with repetitive DNA probe[*] pHY 2.1, which hybridizes specifically with the long arm of the Y-chromosome (1). DNA probe was labeled by nick translation with biotin-dUTP (ENZO, Neckargemünd, FRG). Biotinylated DNA probe was visualized by a streptavidin alkaline phosphatase conjugate (Dakopatts, Hamburg, FRG) and application to a BCIP containing staining gel according to Pflug (5).

HLA DQα typing

DNA amplification was performed according to the protocol of the supplier (Ampli Type™ HLA DQα Kit, Perkin Elmer/Cetus Emeryville, USA; 40 cycles programme)

Results

Dot Hybridization

Sex was correctly classified in all cases using 50-100 ng target DNA. In some cases additional control experiments were performed: after Hae III digestion and agarose gel electrophoresis of DNA typed as male a defined fragment of 2.12 kb could be detected.

HLA-DQα-Typing

PCR and HLA DQα-typing from ethanol fixed and paraformaldehyde fixed tissue was performed without major problems and in agreement with the genotypes obtained from blood. Complete failure of DNA amplification was seen with DNA isolated from formaldehyde fixed tissues. After additional proteinase K / 2% SDS treatments the samples could be typed successfully. In one case a complete determination of the DQα genotype was nearly missed.

Discussion

When tissue specimens are processed in forensic laboratories formaldehyde fixation times are significantly different from those in clinical pathology laboratories and often vary from a few days up to several weeks. We determined the effects of various fixatives and the fixation time on DNA extractability. It seemed likely that the fixative itself and the length of fixation are important determinants of the quality and condition of DNA present in the specimen.

With crude DNA extracted from formaldehyde fixed lung tissue a PCR product could not be obtained even when the PCR was repeated several times, or more genomic DNA was added to the reaction mixture. As initial DNA denaturation is the crucial step in PCR processing we suspect the presence of formaldehyde crosslinks as a reason for PCR failure. Formylation of nucleic acids produces Schiff bases on free amino groups of the nucleotides. Exposure of nucleoproteins to formaldehyde results in the formation of crosslinks between DNA and proteins. Formaldehyde is known to react with both the imino and amino groups of the bases

---

[*] kindly provided by T. Cremer, Institut für Humangenetik, Universität Heidelberg

of DNA. It is a reagent that bridges distances of 2 Å and allows crosslinking of both histone-histone and histone-DNA regions. According to the findings of Jackson (3) for reversal of histone-DNA crosslinks the samples were adjusted to 1% SDS, 50mM Tris pH 8 at 37˚C for two days prior to DNA extraction. The observations suggest that obviously this pretreatment was not sufficient enough to cleave all crosslinks. Therefore prolonged proteinase K/2% SDS incubation is necessary in forensic case work to process human genomic DNA from formaldehyde fixed tissues in amplification experiments.

One of the effects of increasing the length of fixation was that only unspoolable DNA was obtained. To our opinion spooling of the DNA is not only a question of the samples to be kept concentrated enough during extraction procedure. Unspoolable DNA may also indicate that there are chemical alterations or changes in DNA structure. In agarose gel electrophoresis these samples showed that the mobility of DNA from fixed material was slightly slower than that of DNA from fresh tissue as reported by Goelz (2). In our study it was found that as long as DNA only partly can penetrate the gel PCR experiments should not be started. In one case heterozygosity nearly was missed. HLA DQα typing from formaldehyde tissue showed a strong 1.1 signal and a very faint signal for DQα 4. The typing result obtained from blood was 1.1,4. This phenomenon is still unclear. An explanation could be a preferential amplification of the DQα 1.1 allele due to persisting crosslinks in the DQα 4 allele region. This effect must be noticed in case work, when genomic DNA is amplified from material fixed for long time periods.

Sex always was correctly classified. No hybridization signal of the filters probed with pHY 2.1 was observed after one hour development on BCIP-staining gel of the DNA of human females. DNA probe pHY 2.1 hybridizes with about 2000 copies of DNA sequences from the distal part of the long arm on the Y chromosome and therefore should be easily visualized. There are another 100-200 copies also present in female genome which should not be detected under stringent hybridization conditions and washing procedures as shown by in situ hybridization. However, when high target concentrations (> 1 µg) for dot hybridization were used, weak signals in female DNA could be seen even after short development times. Therefore it is necessary for forensic application to determine the quantity of the extracted DNA prior to dot hybridization.

References:

1. Cooke HJ, Schmidtke J, Gosden JR (1982) Characterisation of a human Y chromosome repeated sequence and related sequences in higher primates. Chromosoma 87:491-502

2. Goelz SE, Hamilton SR, Vogelstein B (1985) Purification of DNA from formaldehyde fixed and paraffin embedded human tissue. Biochem Biophys Res Commun 130:118-126

3. Jackson V (1978) Studies on histone organization in the nucleosome using formaldehyde as a reversible cross-linking agent. Cell Vol 15:945-954

4. Maniatis T, Frisch EF and Sambrook J (1982) Molecular cloning: A laboratory manual. Cold Spring Harbor Laboratory, New York

5. Pflug W (1988) Subtyping of group specific component GC in microbloodstains and semen stains by isoelectric focusing in ultrathin immobilized pH gradient gels followed by enzyme detection. Electrophoresis 9:443-448

HLA DQα TYPING OF HUMAN FINGERNAILS

Pötsch L., Penzes L., Prager-Eberle M., Rittner Ch.

Institute of Legal Medicine, Johannes Gutenberg-Universität, Mainz, FRG

Introduction

In contrast to the extensive knowledge about protein biochemistry of keratinization, little is known about the fate of nuleic acids during these processes (1). It has been suggested that both DNA and RNA completely degenerate in the initial phase of keratinization. However, from electron microscopical studies it is known that nuclear remnants are present (1,3). From these findings and own observations one might expect that nucleic acids should still be available.

On the structure of human fingernails

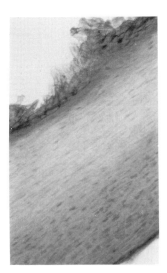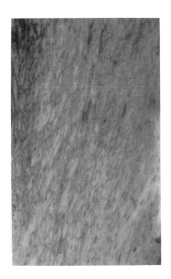

Fig 1 Sagittal section through nail clipping in x-y plane. Hematoxylin staining. For orientation see coordinates. Notice hyponychium underlying the distal edge of the nail. Microscopically closely-knit scales arranged in lamellae and different stages of keratinization can be observed

Advances in Forensic Haemogenetics 4
Edited by Ch. Rittner and P. M. Schneider
© Springer-Verlag Berlin Heidelberg 1992

Material and Methods

Fingernail clippings cut in small pieces (n=8) and sagittal sections of complete nail plates from autopsy cases (n=7) were soaked overnight in 2ml water, 0,1% NaN_3 at room temperature and filtered. For enzymatic digestion (24h, 42°C), the residues were incubated in 1ml buffer consisting of 8M urea in TEN pH 7.5 (10mM Tris/HCl, 25 mM EDTA, 25mM NaCl), 2% SDS, 2mg/ml proteinase K, 20mg/ml DTT.

From all samples the DNA was prepared by three phenol/chloroform extractions, precipitated by ethanol, centrifugated and redissolved in TE buffer.

Electrophoresis was performed in a 0,9% agarose gel at 1,5 V/cm. For HLA DQα typing, DNA amplification was performed according to the protocol of the supplier (Ampli Type™ Kit, Perkin Elmer/Cetus, Emeryville, USA; 40 cycles programme).

DNA from blood was prepared using previously described methods (2).

Results and Discussion

In this pilot study DNA was extracted from human nail clippings and nail plates. From the electropherogramms it seemed evident that always the major portion of the isolated DNA from nail was of the size in the range of 12-18kb. In addition a distinct smear of low-molecular mass nuleic acid was visible (Fig. 2).

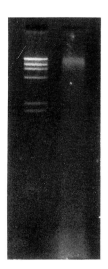

Fig. 2: Minigel, agarose 0.9%, ethidium bromide, 1,5 V/cm, 1,5 h.
Lane 1: λ-DNA/HaeIII digested
Lane 2: DNA from fingernail clipping

A rough estimation of the amount of DNA obtained from 1 nailclipping varies from 10ng to 1µg. Pretreatments and separation of the hyponychium cell layers prior to DNA extraction revealed that at least the isolated DNA did also originate from the nail plate (data not shown). Successful DNA amplification by PCR and HLA DQα typing could be performed. The results were in accordance with the genotype obtained from blood (Fig. 3). These findings demonstrate that it is possible to prepare DNA from keratinized tissue.

Comparison of the HLA DQα typing results

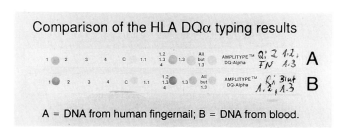

A = DNA from human fingernail; B = DNA from blood.

In principle nail keratinization seems to involve the same elements as epidermal and hair keratinization. During this process the cells flatten, their outer walls thicken and they become firmly attached to each other. Then keratinocytes undergo a dramatic transition and all the cytoplasmatic organelles including nuclei vanish.

Although our study describes preliminary experiments and must be confirmed by further investigations the persistence of high-molecular-mass DNA within cells which die in their normal differentiation may give new aspects to the process of keratinization.

References

1   Jarret A (1977) The physiology and pathophysiology of the skin. Academic Press, London

2   Maniatis T, Frisch EF and Sambrook J (1982) Molecular cloning:A laboratory manual. Cold Spring Harbor Laboratory, New York

3   Weiss L (1988) Cell and tissue biology. Urban & Schwarzberg, München

Identification of Fire Victims by Using DNA Amplification (PCR)

A. Sajantila[1,2], M. Ström[2], B. Budowle[3], P.J. Karhunen[2] and L. Peltonen[1]

[1] National Public Health Institute, Helsinki, Finland
[2] Dept. of Forensic Medicine, Univ. of Helsinki, Finland
[3] FBI Academy, FSRTC, Virginia, USA

INTRODUCTION

The most widely used approach for individualization at the DNA level is analysis of variable number of tandem repeats (VNTR) loci by restriction fragment length polymorphisms (RFLP) via southern blotting (Jeffreys 1985). Although, at present, this analysis has a major impact on identity testing, it has certain limitations. These are: (i) sufficient amount of relatively high–molecular weight (hmw) DNA is required; (ii) the RFLP–technique is comparatively laborious and time consuming; and (iii) the resolution capacity of agarose gel electrophoresis is limited.

The polymerase chain reaction (PCR) technique (Mullis 1987) offers a potential alternative to overcome the limitations of the RFLP analysis. The use of PCR can provide greater sensitivity and specificity for genotyping/phenotyping techniques. PCR obviates the need for radioisotopic detection, and it also reduces the time and laboratory work required for DNA analyses. Moreover, the PCR enables the analysis of extensively degraded samples (Bugawan 1988).

In this study the use of the PCR for genetic characterization of extensively burned fire victims was evaluated. Two different loci were analyzed using the PCR. First, the analysis of amplified fragment length polymorphisms (Amp–FLPs) at the D1S80 (pMCT118) locus (Kasai 1990). Second, a sequence polymorphism at the HLA–DQα locus (Bugawan 1988).

MATERIALS AND METHODS

Autopsy cases

The autopsy series comprised ten extensively charred fire victims. Identification by external macroscopic examination was impossible in all cases and identity could only be determined indirectly by personal effects, eyewittness statements or by forensic odontological means.

DNA extraction

Tissue specimens from the ten extensively burned fire victims were collected during autopsy and maintained at −20°C until subjected to DNA extraction. DNA extraction from each crude tissue specimen (158–1055 mg) was performed by using phenol-chloroform extraction method. DNA quality and quantity were estimated on agarose test–gels containing ethidium bromide (1 mg/ml) by direct comparison with molecular weight markers (EcoRI-HindIII digested lambda, Promega) and a dilution series of lambda DNA (Promega).

Amp–FLP analysis of the D1S80 locus

Amplification of D1S80 locus was performed using the primers described by Kasai et al (1990). The 28–mer primer was 5'-GAAACTGGCCTCCAAACACTGCCCGCCG-3'

Advances in Forensic Haemogenetics 4
Edited by Ch. Rittner and P. M. Schneider
© Springer-Verlag Berlin Heidelberg 1992

and the 29-mer primer was 5'-GTCTTGTTGGAGATGCACGTGCCCCTTGC-3'. Each reaction was composed of 100 ng of DNA in 10mM Tris-Cl, pH 8.3, 50mMKCl, 1.5mM MgC12, 0,01 % gelation, 1.0 μM of each primer, 200 μM of each dNTP and 2.5 U of Taq I polymerase (AmpliTaqTM DNA polymerase, Perkin-Elmer Cetus). The total volume of each reaction was 50 μl. The PCR cycles consisted of denaturation at 95°C for one minute, primer annealing at 65°C for one minute and primer extension at 70°C for eight minutes. A total of 25 cycles was carried out in a Perkin-Elmer Thermocycler.

The analysis of amplified D1S80 alleles was carried out on rehydratable polyacrylamide gels (4 % T, 3 % C, 400 u thick). The gels were rehydrated in 33mM tris-sulfate, pH 9.0 and 7 % glycerol for at least one hour. The trailing ion (0.14M tris-borate, pH 9.0) and bromophenol blue were contained in 2 % (w/v) agarose plugs placed on the cathodal and anodal edges of the gel. Distance between anodal and cathodal agarose plugs was 10 cm. A small volume (2.5 to 5.0 μl) of the amplification product was absorbed into 2.5 x 5.0 mm fiberglass applicator tabs (Pharmacia-LKB) and applied onto the gel surface one cm from the cathodal agarose plug. In each gel a ladder-set of known alleles was run parallel to the amplified DNA samples in every fifth lane. The electrophoretic running conditions were as previously described (Budowle 1991). The separated fragments were detected using a simple silver staining procedure also described elsewhere (Allen 1989; Budowle 1991).

HLA-DQα genotyping

HLA-DQα genotyping was performed with AmpliType™ HLA-DQα Forensic DNA Amplification and Typing Kit (Cetus Corporation, CA, USA) according to manufactures recommendations as well as the procedure published elsewhere (Bugawan 1988).

RESULTS

The qualitative evaluation of the extracted DNA from soft tissues indicated that all samples had significant degradation. The specimens from femoral muscle, psoas muscle and bone marrow yielded DNA from 500 ng/100 mg of crude tissue to greater than 6000 ng/100 mg of crude tissue. The yield of DNA extracted from post mortem blood ranged DNA from 250 ng/100 μl to 1000 ng/100 μl of blood.

All samples produced interpretable D1S80 and HLA-DQα profiles and the results were consistent in various tissues from each individual. The detected genotypes and their combined frequency in the Finnish population are shown in Table 1.

In cases no 1 and 2 a sister and a brother were burned to death in a fire at their home. Peripheral blood samples were obtained from the parents. Mendelian inheritance was demonstrated for alleles at both loci. A family perigree with genotypes is shown in Figure 1.

DISCUSSION

The identification of remains of fire victims is generally attempted by recognizing personal effects, individualizing marks (e.g. scars, tottoos, signs of known disease) and/or dental records. However, due to effects of heat and severe lacerations of the body, the identification by usual forensic means is not always possible.

The obvious limitation of RFLP analysis of DNA from post-mortem soft tissues is that the DNA can degrade rapidly. Thus, no result or minimal data may be obtained. The use of PCR based techniques may be a viable alternative for post-mortem DNA analysis in forensic cases. Virtually any defined short DNA sequence potentially can be analyzed easily and rapidly using PCR. Moreover, with PCR the amount of DNA is not as limiting a factor as it is with the RFLP methodology. Therefore, the effect of

DNA degradation will not be as pronounced with PCR compared with RFLP typing.

In the present study we have shown that PCR based analysis of D1S80 and HLA–DQα loci can be performed succesfully on DNA extracted from different soft tissue specimen from cadavers burned beyond recognition. Sufficient quantity of DNA was extracted from all tissues for PCR analysis (from 500 ng/100 mg crude tissue to grater than 6000 ng/100 mg crude tissue and 250–1000 ng/100 μl blood). On crude tissue specimen (femoral of psoas muscle and bone marrow) we found no remarkable difference between the samples and DNA yield, but post–mortem blood yielded less DNA than crude tissue in each case. DNA from all tissues was typeable and the results were consistent from tissue to tissue in each body studied. A parentage test was performed on the DNA from two victims where identity was confirmed by traditional means. The DNA data also suggests that the victims were the children of the parents. The consistency of D1S80 and HLA–DQα types in the different tissues and the Mendelian inheritance of alleles in the family study provide support that results from PCR based typing methods are reliable.

In addition to the ability to type DNA from soft tissues of charred human remains, Amp–FLP and HLA–DQα dot blot technologies enable resolution of discrete alleles. Analytical systems that provide correct genotyping and minimal measurement error permit evaluation of the goodness of fit of genotype distributions of the particular locus. The D1S80 and HLA–DQα loci satisfy the assumption of Hardy–Weinberg equilibrium (Sajantila et al., submitted; Sajantilaet al., in press). Thus, the actual allelic frequencies can be used to predict genotype frequencies.

In conclusion, PCR based techniques can provide a means for typing DNA derived from soft tissues of fire victims. The technology is simple and can provide data in an expeditious manner. When relatives are available, this approach may be useful for potential identification of human remains. We currently are performing additional validation studies involving PCR typing methodologies and investigating additional genetic markers that may prove useful for individualization.

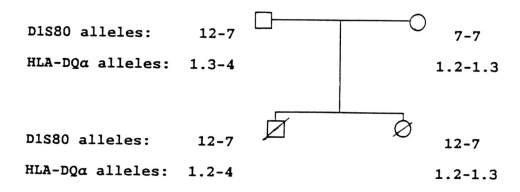

D1S80 alleles:	12–7		7–7
HLA–DQα alleles:	1.3–4		1.2–1.3
D1S80 alleles:	12–7		12–7
HLA–DQα alleles:	1.2–4		1.2–1.3

Figure 1. A pedigree of the paternity test performed in cases 1 and 2. The D1S80 and HLA–DQα alleles and the Mendelian inheritance are shown

Table 1.

Summary of the genotypes detected with Amp–FLP of D1S80 locus and HLA–DQα locus. Combined genotype frequencies are calculated from the genotype frequencies obtained in a Finnish population sample

case no.	genotype		combined genotype frequency
	D1S80	HLA–DQα	(D1S80 and HLA–DQα)
1	12–7	1.2,1.3	5.8×10^{-4}
2	12–7	1.2,4	2.4×10^{-3}
3	19–1	1.1,2	3.0×10^{-4}
4	7–7	1.1,2	3.3×10^{-3}
5	11–7	1.1,4	1.6×10^{-3}
6	11–4	1.1,4	5.4×10^{-4}
7	7–1	1.2,3	1.4×10^{-2}
8	19–1	3,4	$1.3 \times 10-3$
9	11–1	1.1,2	1.7×10^{-3}
10	7–7	1.1,1.2	7.7×10^{-3}

References

Allen RC, Graves G, Budowle B (1989) Polymerase chain reaction amplification products separated on rehydratable polyacrylamide gels stained with silver. BioTechniques 7: 736–744

Budowle B, Chakraborty R, Giusti AM, Eisenberg AJ, Allen RC (1991) Analysis of the variable number of tandem repeats locus D1S80 by the polymerase chain reaction followed by high resolution polyacrylamide gel electrophoresis. Am J Hum Genet 48:137–144

Bugawan TL, Saiki RK, Levenson CH, Watson RM, Erlich HA (1988) The use of non-radioactive ologonucleotide probes to analyze enzymatically amplified DNA for prenatal diagnosis and forensic HLA typing. Biotechnology 6:943–947

Jeffreys AJ, Wilson V, Thein SL (1985) Individual–specific fingerprints of human DNA. Nature 316:76–79

Kasai K, Nakamura Y, White R (1990) Amplification of a variable number of tandem repeats (VNTR) locus (pMCT118) by the polymerase chain reaction (PCR) and its application to forensic science. J Forensic Sci 35:1196–1200

Mullis KB, Faloona FA (1987) Specific synthesis of DNA in vitro via a polymerasecatalyzed chain reaction. In: Wu R, Grossman L, Moldave K (eds.) Methods in enzymogy, Vol. 155, Academic press, New York, pp 335–350

Sajantila A, Ström M, Budowle B, Ehnholm C, Peltonen L (1991) The distribution of the HLA–DQα alleles and genotypes in the Finnish population as determined by the use of DNA amplification and allele specific oligonucleotides. Int J Legal Med 104:181–184

Sajantila A, Budowle B, Ström M, Johnsson V, Lukka M, Peltonen L, Ehnholm C. Amplification of alleles at the D1S80 locus by the polymerase chain reaction: comparison of a Finnish and a North American Caucasian population sample, and forensic case–work evaluation, submitted

POLYMERASE CHAIN REACTION: TYPING OF DNA ISOLATED FROM VARIOUS FORMS OF BIOLOGICAL EVIDENCE

J. Schnee, S. Aab

Landeskriminalamt Baden-Württemberg, 7000 Stuttgart 50, Germany

SUMMARY

The polymerase chain reaction (PCR) is a promising technique for forensic case work because it allows the analysis of very small stains. One of the best characterized marker systems for PCR is the apo B 3' length polymorphism. We show here typing results from various forms of biological evidence and demonstrate the application of the PCR-technique in forensic case work.

INTRODUCTION

After the introduction of the RFLP analysis into forensic science the possibilities of analysing various forms of biological evidence have further been extended by the PCR. Several PCR typing systems based on length or sequence polymorphisms have been described. One of the most polymorphic systems is the apo B 3' length polymorphism on chromosome 2 about 500 bp 3' to the last codon of the apolipoprotein B gene (Knott 1986, Boerwinkle 1989). It consists of a variable number of tandem repeats, each 14-16 bp long. In Germany 14 alleles from 580 to 910 bp have been found with frequencies ranging from about 0.2 % to 37 %.
We chose the apo B polymorphism as the first PCR typing system for our case work. Some examples of DNA analysis from various stains are shown here.

MATERIAL AND METHODS

The DNA was isolated with standard methods using phenol/chloroform extraction. Mixtures of vaginal secretion and semen were separated by differential cell lysis prior to extraction. Once resuspended in TE buffer the DNA was divided into 2 or 3 aliquots containing different amounts of DNA. Each sample was amplified in a final volume of 50 ul containing 40 pmol of each primer (5' TGG AAA CGG AGA AAT TAT GGA GG 3', 5' CCT TCT CAC TTG GCA AAT ACA ATT 3'), 0.2 mM dNTPs, 2 U Taq-Polymerase and the reaction buffer (10 mM Tris/HCl pH 8.4, 2.5 mM MgCl , 50 mM KCl). After an initial denaturation step of 2 min, 27 cycles with the following steps were carried out: denaturation 90 sec at 94° C, annealing of the primers 90 sec at 61° C, chain extension 120 sec at 72° C. Electrophoresis of the amplified products was performed on 2 % agarose gels at 4 V/cm for 6-7 hours.

Advances in Forensic Haemogenetics 4
Edited by Ch. Rittner and P. M. Schneider
© Springer-Verlag Berlin Heidelberg 1992

RESULTS

We have analysed DNA from rape cases, i.e. DNA derived from sperm and/or vaginal secretion, as well as bloodstains or hair roots from murder cases or robberies. While sperm usually did not cause problems, DNA from vaginal secretion sometimes failed to amplify. We do not know whether this might be due to inhibitors or to large amounts of degraded DNA but we observed that amplifying DNA in several different dilutions steps (e.g. 1:1 and 1:10 or 1:1, 1:5 and 1:25) and/or adding BSA to the amplification mix (see Pflug et al., poster) usually leads to better results. When there were enough cells, DNA isolated from hair roots normally amplified well though the amount of amplified product did not always correlate with the number of cells estimated microscopically.

An example for PCR analysis in a rape case is demonstrated in Fig. 1. Suspect B reveals the same alleles as the stain (sperm) whereas the pattern of the victim is different. The frequency of the allele combination of the stain was in this case 0.197. This is the most common genotype in Germany. All other genotypes have frequencies of less than 0.129.

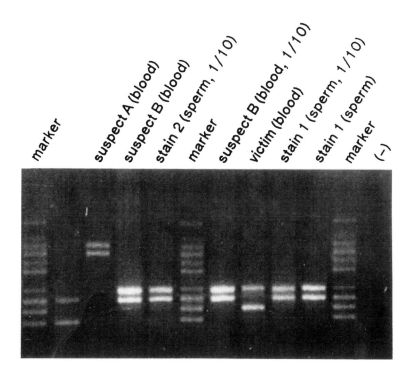

Fig. 1: apo B typing results of a rape case
(-): negative control, containing all ingredients of the amplification mix except for a DNA template,
the marker is a mixture of 10 different alleles from several individuals

DISCUSSION

The apo B 3' length polymorphism provides several advantages: it is one of the most polymorphic loci suitable for PCR, it is well characterized, the alleles are short and can therefore be amplified easily. As they differ in length blotting and hybridization is not necessary.

To get optimal results in case work we find it useful to proceed in the following manner: first we usually amplify two or three different dilutions of the DNA isolated from a stain or from blood because we observed that when one amplification was not successful a higher or lower amount of DNA often amplified well. Before running the main gel we first control the success of the amplification reaction with an aliquot (usually 1/5 of the volume). This allows us to chose the best amplification of the stain and place it between or next to the DNA of the suspect and the victim. Instead of a bacterial or viral size marker we place a ladder of 8-10 different known alleles at least every fifth slot so that determination of the unknown alleles is very easy. For frequency calculation of the allele combination we use our own statistical data which comprise about 340 German individuals up to now and which correspond well to data from other ethnic groups.

Compared to RFLP analysis typing of amplified fragment length polymorphisms is very rapid. If there are a lot of suspects which cannot be excluded by conventional methods their number can be decreased by PCR before performing RFLP analysis. Therefore, typing by PCR is also a good screening method to save time and money.

REFERENCES

Boerwinkle E, Xiong W, Fourest E, Chan L (1989) Rapid typing of tandemly repeated hypervariable loci by the polymerase chain reaction: Application to the apolipoprotein B 3'hypervariable region. Proc Natl Acad Sci USA 86: 212-216

Knott TJ, Wallis SC, Pease RJ, Powell LM, Scott J (1986) A hypervariable region 3' to the human apolipoprotein B gene. Nucleic Acids Res 14: 9215-9216

ANALYSIS OF D1S80 (pMCT 118) LOCUS POLYMORPHISM IN AN ITALIAN POPULATION SAMPLE BY THE POLYMERASE CHAIN REACTION

Tagliabracci A., Giorgetti R., Agostini A., Cingolani M., Ferrara S.D.

Istituto di Medicina Legale dell'Università di Ancona, Policlinico, I-60020 Torrette, Italy

INTRODUCTION

The D1S80 locus, identified by the probe pMCT118, is suitable for forensic haemogenetic purposes because of its wide polymorphism, the high rate of heterozygosity and the easiness and speed of the analysis method (Nakamura et al. 1988; Kasai et al.1990; Budowle et al. 1991).
Further studies are necessary to increase the number of observations, to check geographic distribution and possible genetic variations among various populations, and to make a data-base for practical application in paternity testing and individual identification. For these reasons and because of the lack of data on Italians, we studied a suitable sample of subjects living in Ancona (Central Italy).

MATERIALS AND METHODS

Whole blood collected from125 unrelated healthy subjects was stored in EDTA microcentrifuge tubes at -70° C until use.
The DNA extraction was performed by the phenol-isoamyl method described by Budowle and Baechtel (1990).
Amplification was carried out in a DNA Amplifier (Violet) with 30 cycles consisting of 1 min at 95° C for denaturation, 80 sec at 65° C for primer annealing and 7 min at 70° C for extension. The reaction mix was made up as recommended by Perkin Elmer Cetus with minor modifications in a final volume of 50 microliters. The amount of DNA sample we used was 0.2 micrograms. The amplification was performed using the primers described by Kasai et al. (2):
1) 5'GAAACTGGGCTCCAAACACTGCCCGCCG3'
2) 5'GTCTTGTTGGAGATGCACGTGCCCCTTGC3'
Electrophoresis of 10 microliters of the amplified product with 2 microliters of loading buffer (0.25 % bromophenol blue, 0.25 % xylene cyanol FF, 30% glycerol in water) was achieved on 8% polyacrylamide gel (90 min at 150 V), visualizing the bands with ethidium bromide under UV light at 300 nm. (Fig. 1).
The gel image, recorded by a video camera, was fed into a computer (Macintosh IIx) using a digitizing card (Color Capture). After image processing and enhancement, the size of alleles was calculated by comparing the band mobilities with those of a marker (PGEM-Promega) using the local reciprocal method of Elder and Southern (1983).

Advances in Forensic Haemogenetics 4
Edited by Ch. Rittner and P. M. Schneider
© Springer-Verlag Berlin Heidelberg 1992

RESULTS AND DISCUSSION

In our study we have found fourteen alleles ranging in size from ≈ 385 to ≈ 600 bp.
Allele distribution is represented in Fig. 2. The most frequent was the 467 bp allele, which corresponds to the 20 repeats in the classification of Kasai et al. The other most frequent alleles were the 21, 22 and 16 repeats. Compared with previous works we have a remarkably different distribution of the alleles and the lack of those of bigger size.
The observed heterozygosity was 79.2 %. The number of observed homozygotes was greater than expected, perhaps due to a less efficient amplification for the largest alleles. Alleles differing by only one repeat occasionally appeared as homozygotes, but they were conveniently separated after rerunning in more concentrated gel. When the attribution between similar alleles was in doubt, we reran the samples in neighboring lanes.
Finally, extra bands were occasionally present, but they have not caused any difficulties in typing the MCT region because they were located in a far position, near 2kb.

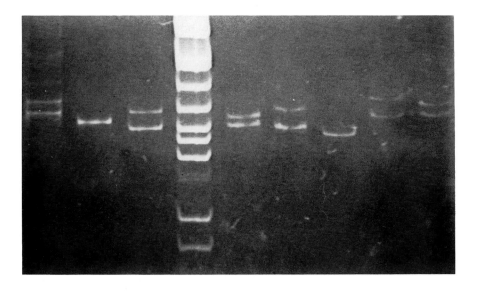

FIGURE 1. Ethidium-bromide stained polyacrylamide gel observed under UV at 300 nm after electrophoresis of 10 microliters of PCR-amplified products of D1S80 locus. From left to right: lane 1: 22/26; lane 2: 20/20; lane 3: 18/22; lane 4: pGEM Marker; lane 5: 19/21; lane 6: 18/23; lane 7: 16/16; lane 8: 21/27; lane 9: 21/24

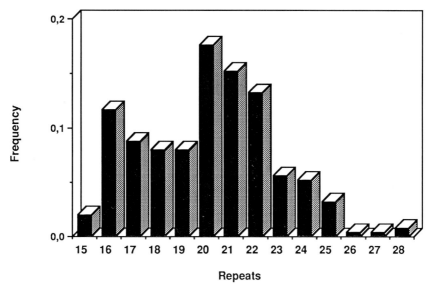

FIGURE 2. Distribution of MCT118 alleles among 125 unrelated Italians

REFERENCES

Budowle B, Baechtel FS (1990) Modifications to improve the effectiveness of restriction fragment length polymorphism typing. Appl Theor Electrophoresis, 1:181-187

Budowle B, Chakraborty R, Giusti AM, Eisenberg AJ, Allen RC (1991) Analysis of the VNTR Locus D1S80 by the PCR Followed by High-Resolution PAGE. Am J Hum Genet, 48: 137-144

Elder JK, Southern EM (1983) Measurement of DNA Length by Gel Electrophoresis II: Comparison of Methods for Relating Mobility to Fragment Length. Anal Biochem, 128: 227-231

Kasai K, Nakamura Y, White R (1990) Amplification of Variable Number of Tandem Repeats (VNTR) Locus (pMCT118) by the Polymerase Chain Reaction (PCR) and Its Application to Forensic Science. J For Sci, 35:1196-1200

Nakamura Y, Carlson M, Krapcho K, White R (1988) Isolation and Mapping of a Polymorphic DNA Sequence (pMCT118) on Chromosome 1p (D1S80). Nucleic Acids Res, 16:9364

Sex determination in bloodstains and single hairs

K. Tanaka[*], H. Fukushima, M. Ota, A. Ichinose[*], K. Sato,
K. Honda, and S. Kiyono[*]

Department of Legal Medicine, [*]Department of Anesthesiology and
Resuscitology, Shinshu University School of Medicine, 3-1-1 Asahi,
Matsumoto, Nagano 390, Japan

INTRODUCTION

Several methods for sex determination of human DNA have been
developed, focusing on detection of the Y-specific chromosomal
sequences(Gosden 1984; Fukushima 1988; Nagai 1991). The major
component is a repeated sequence family characterised by the presence
of Hae III sites spaced at 3.5kb. Various DNA extraction methods and
DNA analysis were studied, with the aim of performing sex determination of minute human materials (McCabe 1987)
    As we reported earlier, DNA was extracted from 10 μl one-year-old
dried blood spots on paper, digested with restriction enzyme, then
subjected to electrophoresis, transfer and hybridization. The human
male Y-specific probe was hybridized with Y-specific 3.5kb repetitive-
DNA.
    The polymerase chain reaction(PCR) is an extremely useful method for
primer-directed enzymatic amplification of Y-specific chromosomal
sequences(Witt 1989). In order to compare with DNA microextraction
methods for the PCR template, we have prepared many DNA samples from
bloodstains and hairs using various methods, such as Method I (phenol-
Centricon 30), Method II(phenol-ethanol precipitation), Method III
(Tween 20-treatment) and Method IV(boiling).

MATERIALS AND METHODS

    Bloodstain materials were prepared by aliquoting known quantities of
blood onto Whatman 3MM filter paper. DNA was extracted by the four
methods described below.
Method I: In general, bloodstains were cut into pieces. These samples
(bloodstains or hairs) were rinsed with cell lysis buffer (0.32M
sucrose, 1% Triton X-100, 5mM $MgCl_2$, 10mM Tris-HCl, pH7.5). Samples
were resuspended in digestive buffer(10mM Tris-HCl, pH8.0, 10mM EDTA,
0.1M NaCl) containing 1%SDS and proteinase K(20μg/ml). The mixture
was incubated for over 3 hours at 50°C. After the solution was
extracted with water-saturated phenol, TE buffer was added. The
solution was concentrated on a Centricon 30 microconcentrator(Amicon).
After addition of distilled water and a second concentration, the
solution was used for the DNA templates.
Method II:After rinsing with cell lysis buffer and centrifigation,
bloodstains(hairs) were incubated in digestive buffer. DNA was
purified by one phenol/chloroform extraction and one ethanol
precipitation.
Method III : After treatment with cell lysis buffer, samples were
suspended in another digestive buffer(50 mM Tris-HCl,pH8.5, 1mM EDTA
and 0.5% Tween 20) containing Proteinase K. The samples were
incubated for over 3 hours at 50°C, then subjected to centrifugation.
These solutions were again incubated at 95°C for 10 minutes to
inactivate the protease. The supernatant was used for PCR after
centrifugation.

Advances in Forensic Haemogenetics 4
Edited by Ch. Rittner and P. M. Schneider
© Springer-Verlag Berlin Heidelberg 1992

Method IV : Bloodstains were rehydrated in 3 ml of 0.85% NaCl for 2 hours. After centrifugation, the filter piceces were washed with 0.85% NaCl again and the elutant was spun down. The pellet was resuspended in 50μl of sterile water and boiled for 10 min. The solution was used as a template.

PCR was carried out at 94°, 55° and 72° for 30 cycles using two pairs of primers(Y1,Y2 and X1,X2)(Witt 1989). Each product was analyzed on 12% polyacrylamide gel in a minigel apparatus.

RESULTS AND DISCUSSION

The 170-bp amplification product was detected in male DNA from 0.5-1μl of three-year-old bloodstains extracted by either the phenol-Centricon-30 method or phenol-ethanol precipitation method. Although the same patterns of PCR product were obtained for 1μl of 6-month-old male bloodstain extracted by Tween 20 -treatment, amplified DNA was not detected in one-year-old or older bloodstains. In contrast, a relatively large amount of bloodstain was required for sex determination of DNA extracted by the boiling method. Amplified results were obtained from DNA of hair roots or the hair shaft(2-3cm) extracted by both the phenol-Centricon-30 and Tween 20-treatment methods.

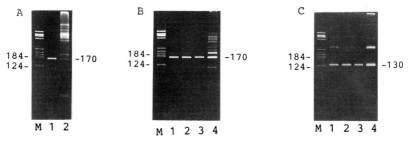

Fig.1 Effect of the Mg^{++} concentration and the amount of template DNA
A:Y-specific band(170bp)   B:Y-specific band(170bp)
     M: pBR-322/Hae III   C:X-specific band(130bp)
     1: 1.5mM MgCl$_2$
     2: 2.5mM MgCl$_2$ 1: 1ng DNA   2: 10ng DNA
                                         3: 50ng DNA   4: 100ng DNA

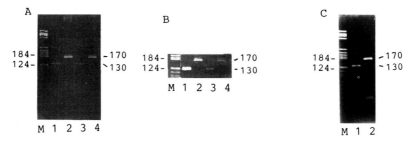

Fig.2   PCR analysis of DNA extracted from male bloodstains.
A(Method I):   B(Method III):   C(Method IV):
     Y1,Y2 primers(2,4)   Y1,Y2 primers(2,4)   Y1,Y2 primers(2)
     X1,X2 primers(1,3)   X1,X2 primers(1,3)   X1,X2 primers(1)
     1,2:0.5μl bloodstains   1,2:1μl bloodstains   1,2:50μl
     3,4:5μl bloodstains   3,4:5μl bloodstains   bloodstains

These results indicate that this PCR method may be very useful in neonatal screening for some genetic diseases and in forensic research for the analysis of biological evidence.

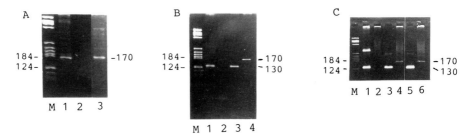

Fig.3   PCR analysis of DNA extracted from male hair shafts
A(Method I):   B(Method II):   C(Method III):
  Y1,Y2 primers(1,2,3)   Y1,Y2: primers(2,4)   Y1,Y2 primers(2,4,6)
  1:hair bulb   X1,X2: primers(1,3)   X1,X2 primers(1,3,5)
  2:1 cm   1,2:2 cm   1,2:1 cm, 3,4:2 cm
  3:2 cm   3,4:5 cm   5,6:5 cm

REFERENCES

Fukushima H, Hasekura H, Nagai K (1988) Identification of male blood-stains by dot hybridization of human Y chromosome-specific deoxy-ribonucleic acid(DNA) probe. J Forensic Sci 33: 621-627
Gosden JR, Gosden CM, Christie S, Cooke HJ, Morsman JM, Rodeck CH (1984) The use of Y-chromosome-specific DNA probes for fetal sex-determination in first trimester prenatal diagnosis. Hum Genet 66:347-351
McCabe ERB, Huang SZ, Seltzer WK, Law ML (1987) DNA microextraction from dried blood spots on filter paper blotters: potential appli-cations to newborn screening. Hum Genet 75:213-216
Nagai K, Yanagisawa I, Hayashi K (1991) The cloning of size-hetero-geneous, Y-specific repetitive DNAs and their clinical application. Mol Cell Biochem 100:71-78
Witt M, Erickson RP (1989) A rapid method for detection of Y-chromo-somal DNA from dried blood specimens by the polymerase chain reaction. Hum Genet 82:271-274

Analysis of forensic stains via PCR amplification of polymorphic simple (gata)$_n$ repeats

L.Roewer, J.Arnemann[1] and J.T.Epplen[2]

Institut für Gerichtliche Medizin, Humboldt-Universität, Hannoversche Str.6, O-1o4o Berlin, FRG

INTRODUCTION

Simple repeat sequences which are variable in length serve as highly informative, polymorphic markers in the modern forensic investigation. The typing procedures include multilocus- and single locus probing as well as -nowadays- polymerase chain reaction analysis. Mono-, di-, tri- and tetranucleotide repeats (or "microsatellites") vary extensively in motif numbers and hence in length. After PCR amplification one can demonstrate polymorphic bands in a high resolution polyacrylamide gel. Each allele can be easily sized by comparison with base for base sequenced marker DNAs. More than 150 such microsatellite polymorphisms are described till now (Reis, submitted for publication). In general simple repeats are highly informative given that the number of repeated motifs is higher than 10 (Weber 1990). Because of the high polymorphism information content (PIC) and their technically easy handling simple repeat polymorphisms represent profitable systems for forensic investigations. Under the appropriate precautions PCR can be performed on minute amounts of DNA -even when it is strongly degraded (Roewer et al. 1991, Hagelberg et al.1991). In this report the forensic application of 3 novel tetranucleotide polymorphisms located autosomally and on the Y chromosome is briefly reviewed.

METHODOLOGY AND RESULTS

We have identified several (gata)$_n$ simple repeats on cosmid clones 27 and 48 originating from the human chromosomes 12 and the Y. The corresponding plasmid clones 27H39, 4804A and 4815 were chosen for further subcloning and sequence analysis.

---

[1]National Institute for Medical Research, Mill Hill London,UK

[2]Molekulare Humangenetik der Ruhr-Universität, Universitätsstr. 150, W-4630 Bochum, FRG

Advances in Forensic Haemogenetics 4
Edited by Ch. Rittner and P. M. Schneider
© Springer-Verlag Berlin Heidelberg 1992

Flanking oligonucleotide primers for identified $(gata)_n$
stretches at 3 different loci were synthesized. The respective
sequences were PCR amplified for 30 cycles in 25 μl volumes by
the method recommended by Perkin Elmer Cetus. The denaturation
temperature was 94°C for 30 sec, primer annealing at 51°C for
30 sec and elongation for 90 sec at 72°C. The conditions are
equal for all 3 loci, so that a multilocus PCR is applicable.
After LMP gel purification and labeling in a kinase reaction
the fragments were separated in a 4% denaturing polyacrylamide
gel and exposed to an X-ray film (Roewer et al.1991). In an
initial population study (30 caucasians) at each locus a number
of different alleles were detected due to variations in the
number of gata units. The alleles differ from each other by
distinctly 4 base pair repeat units. The alleles are transmitted
regularly from father to sons (Y chromosomal locus 27H39LR)
and in families (chromosome 12 loci 4804LR and 4815LR)(Fig.1).
The heterozygosity rate of the diallelic loci 4804LR and 4815LR
is comparable to other single locus systems. Using the observed
allele frequencies we calculated the PIC values (according to
Botstein et al.1980)(Table 1). The loci are well suitable for
forensic investigations because of the shortness of the alleles
(132-248 bps), the multilocus PCR approach and the sensitivity.
We were able to clarify disputed family relationships by typing
of 4 hair roots of each person. The Y chromosomal locus 27H39LR
could be used for extremely rapid and sensitive "sexing of
stains". Meanwhile the presented $(gata)_n$ simple repeat loci
have been used for actual case work in order to exclude a man
on the basis of sperm DNA from suspicion of murder. The amount
of extracted DNA from a sperm stain was too low and the DNA was
strongly degraded so it was impossible to compare the DNAs by
multilocus- or single locus hybridization. We could unequivocally
exclude the suspect from causing the stain in all 3 analyzed
loci (for details see Roewer and Epplen, submitted for publication)

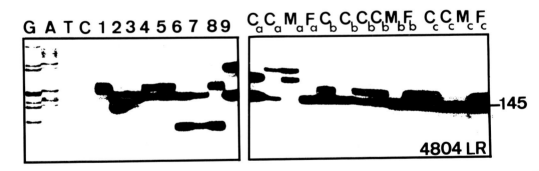

Fig.1. Variability of the simple repeat locus 4804LR as revealed
by denaturing polyacrylamide gel electrophoresis. 1-9: unrelated
individuals; F: father, M: mother, C: child of family a,b or c.
Molecular weight marker (sequenced standard DNA) is shown on the
left; the length of one allele, in bp, is depicted on the right

Table 1. Characteristics of autosomal and Y chromosomal,
hypervariable simple repeat loci (see also Roewer et al.,
submitted for publication)

DNA locus (chromosome)	heterozygosity rate (individ.)	PIC	allele frequency (base pair)	pattern of inheritance
4804LR (12)	66.7% (30)	0.61	A(132) 10% B(140) 1.7% C(144) 55% D(148) 20% E(152) 8.3% F(156) 5.0%	codominant (5 fam., 22 meioses)
4815LR (12)	86.2% (29)	0.80	A(222) 3.5% B(226) 1.7% C(230) 6.9% D(234)29.3% E(238)19.0% F(242)20.7% G(246) 8.6% H(250)1o.3%	codomonant (5 fam., 20 meioses)
27H39LR (Y)	-	0.65	A(186) 13% B(190) 47% C(194) 23% D(198) 17%	Y chromos. inherited (4 fathers, 4 sons)

ACKNOWLEDGEMENTS

This work has been supported by the DFG and the VW Stiftung.

REFERENCES

Botstein D, White RL, Skolnick M, Davis RW (1980) Construction
of a genetic linkage map in man using restriction fragment length
polymorphisms. Am J Hum Genet 32: 314-331
Hagelberg E, Gray IC, Jeffreys AJ (1991) Identification of the
skeletal remains of a murder victim by DNA analysis. Nature
352: 427-429
Roewer L, Arnemann J, Epplen JT (submitted) Simple repeat
sequences on the human Y chromosome are equally polymorphic
as their autosomal counterparts. Hum Genet
Roewer L, Epplen JT (submitted) Rapid and sensitive typing of
forensic stains by PCR amplification of polymorphic simple
(gata)n repeats.For Sci Internatl
Roewer L, Rieß O, Prokop O (1991) Hybridization an PCR amplification
of simple repeated DNA sequences for the analysis of forensic
stains. Electrophoresis 12: 181-186

Species identification by polymerase chain reaction and direct sequencing

S. Tsuchida, F. Umenishi, and S. Ikemoto

Department of Legal Medicine and Human Genetics, Jichi Medical School,
Tochigi 329-04, Japan

INTRODUCTION

Blood stain gives many informations on forensic science. Human identification of blood stains is essential for forensic practice. Immunological and biochemical methods have been used for the identification of human blood stains. However, it is difficult to determine the species of blood stains except human. In this study, we present the method for human identification by Polymerase chain reaction(PCR) and direct sequencing. This method is useful for not only human identification but also the determination of the species of forensic samples.

MATERIALS AND METHODS

Human and animal blood stains were prepared with 10 µl of whole blood on filter paper. Dried blood specimens were stored at room temperature. DNA samples were extracted from whole blood and blood stains. Oligonucleotide primers were designated based on a common conserved sequence in a region of cytochrome b of mitochondrial DNAs which were already published. Used primers were L14839: 5'-CCATCCAACATCTCAGGCATGATGA-3' and H15155:5'-TGTGGCCCCTCAGAATGATATTTG-3'. The L or H in the primer name refers to the light or heavy strand, respectively, and number identifies the base at the 3' end according to the numbering of the published sequence in human. A region of cytochrome b in mitochondrial DNA was amplified by PCR using DNA samples and primers. PCR products were separated and purified by agarose gel electrophoresis. Subsequently, single-stranded DNA was generated by an asymmetric PCR and its nucleotide sequences were determined by the dideoxy-chain termination method. DNA sequences were compared for the identification of the sample species.

RESULTS AND DISCUSSION

The fragments of cytochrome b were amplified by PCR using the DNA samples extracted from whole blood of human and several animals and primers based on a common region of cytochrome b in mitochondrial DNA. DNA sequence of 155 nucleotides in the amplified fragment of cytochrome b region was compared among human and five animal species as shown in Figure 1. The amplified DNA fragments from human and several animals showed the characteristic DNA sequences on each species. The DNA sequences from two Japanese were differed from the published data of a complete human mitochondrial DNA sequence by Anderson et al(1981). A mutation which was a transition from G to A was observed at the position of 15043 which referred to the light strand of the published sequence. However, the change did not affect amino acid sequence. Partly DNA sequences of cytochrome b in cow and mouse accorded with those in published data perfectly. There are moderate differences in the DNA sequences of PCR products among species. The mean number and frequency of the

Advances in Forensic Haemogenetics 4
Edited by Ch. Rittner and P. M. Schneider
© Springer-Verlag Berlin Heidelberg 1992

difference in nucleotides were 39.7 and 25.6%, respectively. The number and frequency of common nucleotides in 155 nucleotides of cytochrome b were 82 and 52.9%, respectively.

Using DNA samples extracted from blood stains, the fragments of cytochrome b region were also amplified by PCR in human and several animal species. The DNA sequences of amplified fragments were also determined by direct sequencing. The determined DNA sequences were in accordance with those using whole blood samples. From the blood stain of cow, only 49 nucleotides(15059-15107 region which refers to the strand of the published sequence of human) were sequenced clearly. However, the difference of nucleotides was enough to distinguish the species of blood stain from other species. The analysis of DNA sequence in the region of cytochrome b in mitochondrial DNA by PCR and direct sequencing are useful method for not only making distinction between human and animals but also the determination of the species of blood stains.

```
              14980                                    15019
Human*        CATCCGCTACCTTCACGCCAATGGCGCCTCAATATTCTTT
Human**       CATCCGCTACCTTCACGCCAATGGCGCCTCAATATTCTTT
Horse         TATCCACCATCTCCATGCTAACGGAGCGTCCATATTCTTC
Cow           CATCCGATACATACACGCAAACGGAGCTTCAATGTTTTTT
Pig           TATTCGCTATCTACATGCAAACGGAGCATCCATATTCTTT
Rabbit        CTATCGATATCTCCATGCCAATGGAGCATCGATATTTTTT
Mouse         AATCCGATATATACACGCAAACGGAGCCTCAATATTTTTT

              15020                                    15059
Human*        ATCTGCCTCTTCCTACACATCGGGCGAGGCCTATATTACG
Human**       ATCTGCCTCTTCCTACACATCGGACGAGGCCTATATTACG
Horse         ATCTGCCTCTTTATTCACGTAGGACAAGGCCTTTACTACA
Cow           ATCTGCTTATATATGCACGTAGGACGAGGCCTTATATTACG
Pig           ATTTGCCTATTCATCCACGTAGGCCGAGGTCTATACTACG
Rabbit        ATTTGCCTCTATATACACGTAGGCCATGGAATCTATTATG
Mouse         ATTTGCTTATTCCTTCATGTCGGACGAGGCTTATATTATG

              15060                                    15099
Human*        GATCATTTCTCTACTCAGAAACCTGAAACATCGGCATTAT
Human**       GATCATTTCTCTACTCAGAAACCTGAAACATCGGCATTAT
Horse         GCTCCTACACCTTCCTAGAAACATGAAATATTGGGATTCT
Cow           GGTCTTACACTTTTCTAGAAACATGAAATATTGGAGTAAT
Pig           GATCCTATATATTCCTAGAAACATGAAACATTGGAGTAGT
Rabbit        GCTCATATACATATCTAGAAACCTGAAACATCGGCATTAT
Mouse         GATCATATACATTTATAGAAACCTGAAACATTGGAGTACT

              15100                                  15134
Human*        CCTCCTGCTTGCAACTATAGCAACAGCCTTCATAG
Human**       CCTCCTGCTTGCAACTATAGCAACAGCCTTCATAG
Horse         CCTATTTCTTCCAGTAATAGCTACAGCATTCATGG
Cow           CCTTCTGCTCACAGTAATAGCCACAGCATTTATAG
Pig           CCTACTATTTACCGTTATAGCAACAGCCTTCATAG
Rabbit        TCTATTATTCTAAGAAATAGCAACAGCATTCATAG
Mouse         TCTACTGTTCGCAGTCATAGCCACAGCATTTATAG
```

Fig. 1   Comparison of partial DNA sequences in cytochrome b among human and five animal species

*: The sequences from the published data of a complete mtDNA sequence for one individual by Anderson et al(1981).

**: Two Japanese mtDNA sequences

Table 1   The number and frequencies(%) of different nucleotides in the 155 nucleotide of cytochrome b region (14980-15134)* among human and five animals

	Human[b]	Horse	Cow	Pig	Rabbit	Mouse
Human[a]	1 (0.65)	46 (29.7)	45 (29.0)	39 (25.2)	44 (28.4)	41 (26.5)
Human[b]		45 (29.0)	44 (28.4)	39 (25.2)	44 (28.4)	40 (25.8)
Horse			39 (25.2)	34 (21.9)	43 (27.7)	46 (29.7)
Cow				35 (22.6)	44 (28.4)	25 (16.1)
Pig					40 (25.8)	33 (21.3)
Rabbit						41 (26.5)

*: The number shows the nucleotide position which refers to the light strand of the published sequence by Anderson et al(1981).
a: The sequences from the published data of a complete mtDNA sequence by Anderson et al (1981).
b: Japanese mtDNA sequence

REFERENCES

Anderson S, Bankier AT, Barrell BG, de Bruijn MHL, Coulson AR, Drouin J, Eperon IC, Nierlich D., Roe BA, Sanger F, Schreier PH, Smith AJH, Staden R, Young IG (1981) Sequence and organization of the human mitochondrial genome. Nature 290:457-465

Anderson S, De Bruijn MHL, Coulson AR, Eperon IC, Sanger F, Young IG (1982) Complete sequence of bovine mitochondrial DNA Conserved features of the mammalian mitochondrial genome. J Mol Biol 156:683-717

Bibb MJ, Van Etten RA, Wright CT, Walberg MW, Clayton DA, (1981) Sequence and gene organization of mouse mitochondrial DNA. Cell 26:169-180

Gadaleta G, Pepe G, De Candia G, Quagliariello C, Sbisa E, Saccone C (1989) The complete nucleotide sequence of the Rattus norvegicus mitochondrial genome: Cryptic signals revealed by comparative analysis between vertebrates. J Mol Evol 28:497-516

2 DNA (RFLP, VNTR) Systems

2.1 General

PATERNITY INVESTIGATIONS BASED ON DNA-ANALYSIS ONLY

W. Bär and A. Kratzer, Institute of Legal Medicine, University of Zürich, Zürichbergstrasse 8, CH-8028 Zürich, Switzerland

1. Introduction

Innumerable investigations have shown that conventional blood group typing is a powerful and reliable means to solve cases of disputed paternity in simple trio cases as well as in some of the more complicated deficiency cases. The benefit of the introduction of additional systems and of the sophistication of methods, e.g. isoelectric focusing was a constant increase of the so-called positive proof of fatherhood, but the chance to find a case not already showing exclusions in other systems remained extremely small. Inherently, the plethora of methods and systems also increased almost unnoticed the chance of error. Furthermore, the training time of new technical staff considerably lengthened. The appearance of the highly polymorphic DNA systems (Jeffreys et al., 1985, Smith et al., 1990) quickly unsecured a typing system that seemed to be well established forever. Bär (1988) compared the results and the practical handling of the so-called multi-locus probes in paternity investigations as well as in stain analysis. Many reasons, e.g. the poor statistical evaluation of the results of multi-locus probes and the delicate working conditions of low stringency showed that in the hands of ordinary technical staff the work with single locus probes gives more reproducible results. Furthermore, well known and accepted statistical approaches like the one of Essen-Möller or the calculation of a paternity index are possible. The easiness of the statistical combination of DNA results with those of conventional techniques is an additional strong argument for the use of single locus probes, not unimportant in difficult cases of severe deficiency(Bär and Hummel, 1991). Based on the results of many supplementary expertises in paternity cases showing low values of probabilities , single exclusions and opposite homozygosities after conventional blood grouping, we decided in March of 1991 to completely abandon the conventional systems and to exclusively use DNA single locus probes.

2. Material and Methods

DNA analysis is independently performed by two technicians which extract high-molecular DNA from 300 µl EDTA-blood. After restriction with Hinf I band separation is done on 4 gels of 1% (2 per technician). Electrophoresis is performed over the weekend (running time 60 hrs !). Probes MS43a, MS31 and g3, yNH24 respectively are applied. Labelling is done according to Feinberg and Vogelstein (1986) using P32. Hybridization condition are of high stringency. One of the two blots per technician is cross-hybridized. Exclusions are extracted and hybridized a third time. Band length is measured with a Biolmage Visage System from Millipore. In theory, after two and a half week the report to the parties can be established. However, in praxis the mean handling time per case is longer, 33 days for cases of non-exclusion and 39 days for cases of exclusion.

3. Interpretation
3.1. Non-Exclusions

The interpretation of a match is based on a visual side-by-side comparison by two staff members. In cases of shifts, the analysis is repeated from the beginning. The visual match is backed-up by the computerized band length measurement. A match window of 2.5 % proposed by others (Gill, pers. communication) was found to be too large and too rigid taking into account that the standard deviation positively correlates with the band length. Looking at the real size of the observed band length differences based on the measurements of visually matched bands in cases of non-exclusions for the two probes MS43a and yNH24 the following observations can be reported. Probing with MS43A, of 115 pairs of mother-child and 96 child -putativfather duos about 45 % showed no difference in band length at all. The highest difference observed was 1.7 %. There was no significant difference between the samples of Mother-Child and Child-Father comparisons. If a window of 1.1 % was chosen, more than 95 % of the cases were included. Therefore our visual matches fulfilled in fact much more rigid criteria than those proposed (fig. 1). Probing with yNH24, of 109 pairs of mother-child and 90 child -putativfather duos about 50 % of the cases showed no difference in band length at all. The highest difference observed was 1.8 % of the band length. There was no significant difference between the distribution of the Mother-Child and Child-Father comparisons. If a window of 1 % was chosen, about 98 % of the cases were included. Therefore our visual matches fulfilled in fact much more rigid criteria than those proposed (fig. 2).

3.2. Band Frequency Estimation and Biostatistical Evaluation

Frequency distributions for a Swiss population sample larger than 200 unrelated persons were established for the four probes. Fixed bin sizes for yNH24 was 150 bp, for the others probes 200 bp. These bin sizes of 200 bp and 150 bp respectively which correspond to 2.5% of the mean band length for MS43A and 4.4 % for yNH24, are largely conservative taking into account the above mentioned visual match criteria which actually respect a window of about 1%. In each case of non-exclusion, the biostatistical evaluation is done according to Essen-Möller (1938), a method widely used by paternity labo-

Advances in Forensic Haemogenetics 4
Edited by Ch. Rittner and P. M. Schneider
© Springer-Verlag Berlin Heidelberg 1992

ratories and well-known by the judges. In cases of deficiency, a more common algorithm, e.g. the one of Ihm and Hummel (1975) is used. The attribution of a band frequency follows a modified fixed bin approach. The minimum band frequency employed is always 1 %. The "real" band frequencies are chosen according to band size, but in cases where the band value is close to a bin border with the adjacent bin showing a higher frequency, this higher frequency is finally used for the calculation (conservative). The use of Caucasian databases of others, e.g. Cellmark had no influence on the final decisions. The correlation of pairwise plotted W-values based on Swiss or Cellmark databases was 100 % (fig. 3). The posteriori calculation of a hypothetical mean band frequency when applying 4 probes gave values of 4.6 % , respectively 4.4 % per band for the two databases. It can therefore be concluded that a mean band frequency of 5%, proposed by us 3 years ago when databases were not yet available, would have been conservative. The general use of a mean band frequency of 10 % in cases with Non-Caucasians is again proposed.

3.3. Exclusions

24 exclusions out of 118 cases were observed corresponding to 20% of our cases which is equal to the mean value found when using conventional blood group typing. In three quarters of the cases, exclusions were seen in all 4 SL-systems and in one quarter of the cases only a single matching situation was observed. Cases of exclusions with 2 matching situations were not observed. However, cases with only one exclusion were seen in 3 instances. These latter cases cannot be solved without extension of the investigation. Either conventional markers or additional DNA single locus probes can be used to either exclude or confirm an underlying situation of a non-excluded first order relative or the occurrence of a recombination (mutation). It is worth emphasizing that when using 4 single locus probes the exclusion chance for a brother is only 1: 256 if the parents are heterozygous in the 4 systems. The extension of the investigation on only a few systems may therefore not necessarily show additional exclusions which would prove the exclusion.

3.4. Biostatistical Handling of Mutations

According to a proposition of Hummel (pers. communication), in all cases of single exclusions a biostatistical evaluation of the probability of a mutation should and can be made. The general formula of the calculation of a EM-value is: $EM_{mut}=\log c/u+10$, where c is the frequency of the "mutant" band and u is the mutation rate of the DNA system under consideration. The extension of the investigation on additional systems is usually mandatory. The integration of the EM_{mut}-value in the general formula of Essen-Möller is easily possible. Despite of the biostatistical proof of the mutation, it is necessary to report to the parties the possibility of a non-excluded first order relative.

4. Summary

DNA analysis based on 4 highly polymorphic marker systems proves to be an very powerful means to solve cases of disputed paternity and can completely replace conventional blood group techniques. The gain of evidence is very remarkable for the so-called positive proof of paternity. Despite the absence of discrete alleles the evaluation of the results can be done applying well-known methods. Visual matching is in fact even stricter than window matching since the visual match window respects a size of about 1% which is half of that proposed (2.5%). Computerized band size determination facilitates routine case work. Application of band frequencies from databases of different Caucasian population samples gives identical biostatistical results using 4 DNA probes (MS43A, MS31, g3, yNH24). Single exclusions must be further evaluated by extending the investigation on additional marker systems. The probability of a mutation can be calculated by a Bayesian approach and its value can be integrated in the W-value of Essen-Möller or the PI. However, the possibility of a non-excluded first order relative must be kept in mind.

5. References

Bär W (1988) DNA-Polymorphismen: Ihre Bedeutung in der Forensik. Habilitationsschrift. Med. Fakultät, Universität Zürich

Bär W and Hummel K (1991) DNA-Fingerprinting: Its Application in Forensic Case Work. DNA Fingerprinting: Approaches and Applications. Burke T, Dolf G, Jeffreys AJ & Wolff R (eds.) Birkhäuser Verlag Basel/Switzerland, 349-355

Essen-Möller E (1938) Die Beweiskraft der Ähnlichkeit im Vaterschaftsnachweis. Theoretische Grundlagen. Mitteil Anthopol Gesell Wien 68:9-53

Feinberg AP and Vogelstein B (1983) A Technique for radiolabeling DNA restriction endonuclease fragments to high specific activity. Anal Biochem 132:6-13

Ihm P and Hummel K (1975) Ein Verfahren zur Ermittlung der Vaterschaftswahrscheinlichkeit aus Blutgruppenbefunden unter beliebiger Einbeziehung von Verwandten. Z Immun Forsch 149:405- 416

Jeffreys A, Brookfield JFY, Semeonoff R (1985) Positive identification of an immigration test-case using human DNA fingerprints. Nature 317: 818-819

Smith JC, Anwar R, Riley J, Jenner D, Markham AF, Jeffreys AJ (1990) Highly polymorphic minisatellite sequences: allele frequencies and mutation rates for five locus-specific probes in a Caucasian population. J Forensic Sci Soc 30:19-32

Visual Match-MS43A: Distribution of Bandlength Differences in %
of the Bandlength in 115 Mother-Child and 96 Child-Putativfather
Duos

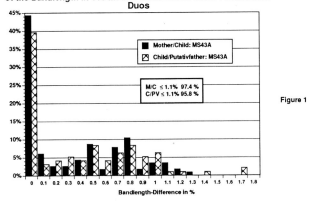

Figure 1

Visual Match-yNH24: Distribution of Bandlength Differences in %
of the Bandlength in 109 Mother-Child and 90 Child-Putativfather
Duos

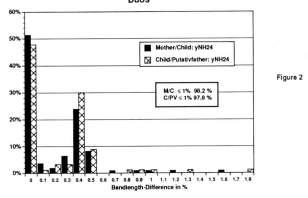

Figure 2

Simple Regression of W-Values in 60 Paternity Cases
based on Cellmark and Swiss Databases
(MS43A, MS31, g3 and yNH24)

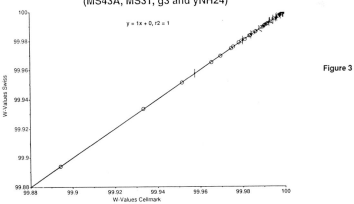

Figure 3

Achievement of Interlaboratory Uniformity - A Summary of Work Carried out by the EDNAP Group

P GILL[a], S WOODROFFE[a], W BÄR[b], B BRINKMANN[c], A CARRACEDO[d], B ERIKSEN[e], S JONES[f], A D KLOOSTERMAN[g], B LUDES[h], B MEVAG[i], V L PASCALI[j], M RUDLER[k], H SCHMITTER[l], P M SCHNEIDER[m] and J A THOMSON[n]

[a]Home Office Central Research and Support Establishment, Aldermaston (UK), [b]Institute of Legal Medicine, University of Zurich (Switzerland), [c]Institute of Legal Medicine, University of Münster (FRG), [d]Department of Legal Medicine, University de Santiago de Compostela (Spain), [e]Institute of Forensic Genetics, Copenhagen (Denmark), [f]Metropolitan Police Forensic Science Laboratory, London (UK), [g]Forensic Science Laboratory, Rijswik (The Netherlands), [h]Institute of Legal Medicine, University of Strasbourg (France), [i]Institute of Forensic Medicine, University of Oslo (Norway), [j]Institute of Legal Medicine, Catholic University, Rome (Italy), [k]Laboratoire de Police Scientifie de Paris, Ministere de L' Interier (France), [l]Bundeskriminalamt, Wiesbaden (FRG), [m]Institute of Legal Medicine, University of Mainz (FRG), [n]Department of Haematology, London Hospital Medical College (UK).

INTRODUCTION

This paper describes a collaborative exercise intended to demonstrate whether uniformity of DNA profiles results could be achieved between different European laboratories. It was shown that this goal would be obtained provided that a common protocol was followed (specifically the use of a common electrophoretic buffer is the most important parameter).

Generally lower molecular weight loci (with lower molecular weight fragments) such as YNH24 perform better than higher molecular weight loci such as MS43a. The results of the exercise are discussed in relation to the objectives of the European DNA profiling group (EDNAP).

THE WORK OF THE EDNAP GROUP

In 1989 the EDNAP group began a series of experiments to determine whether standardisation of DNA profiling systems was possible. The first series of experiments was reported by Schneider et al. (1991). Each laboratory analysed a series of samples using its own protocols (the only standardisation was use of HinfI as the restriction enzyme, and use of a common ladder marker). It was demonstrated that the sizes of fragments determined by different laboratories were within a match window of 10%. Although it was possible to compare directly results between laboratories using this wide window, interpretation and allocation of statistical significance was more difficult when such large differences were obtained between laboratories.

The second series of experiments described in this paper was carried out in order to determine whether comparable results could be obtained if different laboratories used the same protocol. Clearly, it was not possible to standardise completely because different equipment was in use. However, it was possible to standardise on electrophoretic buffer and make of agarose. Also each laboratory was supplied with a full protocol and samples of DNA; equipment was not standardised.

Advances in Forensic Haemogenetics 4
Edited by Ch. Rittner and P. M. Schneider
© Springer-Verlag Berlin Heidelberg 1992

A comparison of the within and between laboratory measurement error has been evaluated.

MATERIALS AND METHODS

DNA was bulk extracted by one laboratory (Central Research and Support Establishment CRSE) from 3 different blood samples. Half was then restricted by this laboratory with 30x excess HinfI before distribution and the other half was supplied to laboratories unrestricted so that the effect of different restriction methods could be compared. In addition, HinfI restricted K562 (genomic control; Promega) and Amersham lambda ladder was supplied to each laboratory. Each laboratory was supplied with a full protocol to follow. Probes YNH24 and MS43a were used.

RESULTS AND DISCUSSION

The differences between fragment sizes from each half of the gel were low (< 0.5%kB); it is very unlikely that different restriction buffers or different manufacturers HinfI restriction enzyme contribute to the effect.

Evett et al. (1990) introduced a method of analysis which enabled a large number of comparisons to be carried out from a relatively small database. The principle of the test involves comparison of each pair of band measurements with every other pair in the database referring to a match guideline. Part of the datafile of sample A (YNH24) is as follows:-

Identifier (laboratory)	Band Weights (bp)	
	1	2
1	4564	2724
2	4584	2735
3	4633	2776

If a match guideline is set at 2% then sample 1, band 1 and sample 2, band 1 would be deemed a match provided that each was within the range of ±1% of the mean band weight (xb) of the two fragments, ie. xb = (4564 + 4584)/2 and the match window is therefore xb ± (1/100)*xb. Of course it would also be a requirement for the second band in both samples to be within the guideline before a match was declared.

In this exercise datafiles were produced, (one for YNH24 and the other for MS43a). In each datafile there were up to 22 observations (from 11 laboratories). A match criterion was set between 2-8%. If a comparison of fragments from samples 1 and 2 was within the match criterion then a match was recorded. Sample 1 was then compared with sample 3 and so on to the end of the file. If every sample was compared in this way there was a total of n*(n-1)/2 comparisons, ie. up to 231 in this example. This process effectively simulates what would happen if a large number of casework samples were analysed in different laboratories and then compared with each other. The Home Office Forensic Science Service uses a match guideline of 2.8% for the reasons explained by Gill et al. (1991). Using this guideline approximately 97.9% of samples probed with YNH24 match between gels and between 6 different UK laboratories all using the same protocol. Use of the European protocol produced results which were comparable to (or perhaps better) than those detailed by Evett et al, (1989) and Gill et al, (1991) because a 2.8% guideline resulted in >99% matches for all YNH24 samples tested. In general, use of a 2.8% window with MS43a data was not as definitive. This was to be expected because the variation in measurement error increased with molecular weight (Gill et al, 1990).

This was a useful but simple exercise which laboratories wishing to compare results can follow. It requires only basic computing expertise to write the necessary program.

So far only the quality of the match has been considered in this paper (ie. the numerator of a Bayesian likelihood ratio). Evett et al, (1991) has examined the combined effects of the numerator, denominator (ie. band frequency) and correlation coefficient and concludes that with YNH24 and MS43a using the current EDNAP protocol, between laboratory comparisons of the same DNA sample would result in a likelihood ratio >100, with 50% of matches resulting in a likelihood ratio >10^5.

CONCLUSION

Once a protocol has been established, and agreed, then laboratories need a method to monitor the results which they achieve using an agreed quality control system which incorporates universal ladder markers and genomic controls for sizing purposes. This will enable confident interpretation between laboratories, since each autoradiograph effectively contains a universal control which can be independently checked. It would be necessary for the size of the control to fall within designated limits before inclusion into a database. Provided these simple rules are followed there would be no reason why laboratories could not exchange information and combine databases, although the latter would be dependent upon considerations relating to population structure.

The achievement of uniformity and quality control methods are currently the subject of active discussion within EDNAP and within the international DNA commission of the Forensic Haemogenetics Society.

REFERENCES

Evett IW, Werrett DJ, Pinchin R and Gill R (1990) Bayesian analysis of single locus DNA profiles. Proceedings for the International Symposium on Human Identification, 1989, 77-101
Evett IW, Scranage J and Pinchin R (1991) Efficient retrieval from DNA databases: a paper for EDNAP based on the second collaborative experiment. Submitted to Forens. Sci. Int
Gill P, Evett IW, Woodroffe S, Lygo JE, Millican E and Webster M (1991) Databases, quality control and interpretation of DNA profiling in the Home Office Forensic Science Service. Electrophoresis
Gill P, Sullivan K and Werrett DJ (1990) The analysis of hypervariable DNA profiles: problems associated with the objective determination of the probability of a match. Hum. Genet. 85: 75-79
Schneider PM, Fimmers R, Woodroffe S, Werrett DJ, Bär W, Brinkmann B, Eriksen B, Jones S, Kloosterman AD, Mevag B, Pascali VL, Rittner C, Schmitter H, Thomson HA and Gill P (1991) Report of a European collaborative exercise comparing DNA typing results using a single locus VNTR probe. Forensic Sci. Int., 49: 1-15

Cloning and Characterisation of Novel Single Locus Probes for Forensic
Purposes

C.P. Kimpton, R. Hopgood, S.K. Watson, P. Gill and K Sullivan

Central Research and Support Establishment, The Forensic Science Service,
Aldermaston, Reading, Berkshire, RG7 4PN, UK

INTRODUCTION

From the analysis of multi-locus probes (Jeffreys et al, 1986; Fowler
et al, 1988) it has previously been demonstrated that there are numerous
hypervariable loci in the human genome. Many hypervariable loci have been
fortuitously identified (Wyman and White, 1980; Bell et al, 1982; Higgs et al,
1981; Capon et al, 1983). A cloning strategy, used specifically to isolate
hypervariable DNA was developed by Wong et al (1986, 1987) who used lambda
libraries of human DNA; the insert consisting of size selected high molecular
weight (5-15kB) DNA fragments. This procedure enriched the library for
tandemly repeated minisatellites. Recently, Armour et al (1990) introduced
a more successful and simpler method for cloning hypervariable DNA by
constructing Charomid libraries (Saito and Stark, 1986). Charomids are
cosmid derived vectors which do not have the same size constraints of lambda
vectors, hence the cloning of rather unstable minisatellite fragments, which
tend to lose repeats, is much improved.

Libraries of size selected DNA (4-9kB) have been constructed in Charomid
9-36. A new hypervariable locus (B6.7) has been isolated by screening the
library with the multilocus probe 3'HVR alpha globin (Fowler et al, 1988)
under low stringency conditions.

CHAROMID CLONING AND CHARACTERISATION OF PROBES

A charomid library was prepared from human genomic DNA pooled from 20
unrelated individuals. DNA was fully digested with SauIIIa and the 6-9kB
fragments were purified by electrodialysis. DNA from this fraction was
ligated into the BamHI site of Charomid 9-36, packaged using Gigapack Gold
(Stratagene) and transfected into E. coli NM554 cells (recA mcrA, mcrB).
Charomid clones were selected on Luria Bertoni agar (LUA) containing
ampicillin (50µg/ml), grown overnight, and replica plated onto Hybond N
filters (Amersham). The DNA on the filters was subjected to denaturation
and microwave fixation.

Probe 3'HVR alpha globin was labelled with ^{32}P by random oligonucleotide
priming (Fienberg et al, 1984). Filters were incubated overnight at 61°C
in hybridisation solution (Church and Gilbert, 1984) containing 0.5ng/ml
of labelled probe, without competitor DNA. Filters were washed under low
stringency conditions in 1xSSC, 0.1% SDS at 61°C, prior to autoradiography
using Amersham-MP film. Colonies which showed signals were picked, replated
at low density and re-screened with 3'HVR. Positive colonies were picked
and overnight minipreps were grown in Luria Bertoni (LB) medium containing
ampicillin (50µg/ml). Charomid DNA was extracted from the overnight culture
by the alkaline lysis method (Sambrook et al, 1989), its concentration
established by fluorometry (Labarca and Paigen, 1980) and then restricted
with SauIIIa (10u/µg DNA) for 4-5 hours. Electrophoresis of the restricted
DNA was carried out in 0.8% agarose (Seakem GTG) gels. Insert bands were
sized against a lambda HindIII digest and a 1kb DNA ladder (Gibco BRL).
Bands sized between 2 and 9kb were recovered by electrodialysis, phenol/
chloroform extracted and ethanol precipitated twice.

Advances in Forensic Haemogenetics 4
Edited by Ch. Rittner and P. M. Schneider
© Springer-Verlag Berlin Heidelberg 1992

Probes were characterised by hybridising the radiolabelled insert DNA against Southern blots of HinfI restricted human genomic DNA prepared from the blood of a panel of random individuals. Blots were washed twice under high stringency conditions in 0.1xSSC, 0.1% SDS at 65°C and autoradiographs prepared as described previously.

The clones carrying positive insert fragments were categorised according to their hybridisation pattern:

NUMBER OF CLONES

Satellite*	2
Monomorphic	0
Polymorphic	13 (Some are characterised in Table 1)

* These clones generated a largely monomorphic ladder of hybridising DNA fragments presumed to be derived from large segments of satellite DNA.

TABLE 1. Characterisation of polymorphic clones detected by 3'HVR

Clone No.	No. of Repeat Isolates	No. of Alleles Observed	Allele Size Range (kb)	No. of People Studied	Heterozygosity
1	2	17	1.5 - 8	11	73%
4	0	16	2 - 10	11	73%
8	2	2	4.8 - 5	23	23%
10	0	7	4 - 9	17	53%
17	1	32	1 - 12	28	88%
7[a]	1	24	2 - 20	7	
19[b]	0	16	3 - 15	5	

[a] Complex pattern observed with between 3-6 bands per individual.
[b] Complex pattern observed with between 2 bands per individual.

Clone 17 (B6.7) was employed to rescreen charomid libraries resulting in the detection of approximately 600 positively hybridising clones (2% of all library clones - 4 fold more than detected by 3'HVR). Furthermore, 95% of all clones detected by 3'HVR were also hybridisation positive with clone 17. Polymorphic clones were characterised further (Table 2).

TABLE 2. Characterisation of polymorphic clones detected by clone 17

Clone No.	No. of Repeat Isolates	No. of Alleles Observed	Allele Size Range (kb)	No. of People Studied	Heterozygosity
17/9	2	18	2 - 10	21	91%
17/26	1	13	1 - 4.5	12	77%
17/45	0	9	3.5 - 6.5	10	67%
17/23[a]	0	2	4.8 - 5	23	23%

[a] Repeat isolate of 3'HVR Clone 8.

CHARACTERISATION OF PROBE B6.7

A population study was carried out using DNA from 24 unrelated white Caucasians. These results revealed at least 29 different alleles and a heterozygosity of 88%. The allele sizes in this population ranged from 1-15kb.

B6.7 shows approximately 70% homology with a sequence found in the rabbit C repeat (Cheng et al, 1984). The C family serves as a template for RNA transcription by RNA polymerase III (Fritsch et al, 1980), and shares structural properties with human Alu repeats, although their sequences are quite different. B6.7 shows no structural homology with either rabbit C or Alu repeats. There is close homology with the 3'HVR alpha-globin sequence and with the core sequence proposed by Jarman et al (1986).

COMPARISON OF B6.7 SEQUENCE WITH 3'HVR ALPHA-GLOBIN

```
TCTCTATAGGACATGAGGGTGGACAGTGAGGGGGG B6.7
        |||| | ||| |||||
     CGACACGGGGGGAAACAG          3'HVR Alpha-globin
        | |||| |||||
        GNGGGGN-ACAG            Core Sequence (Jarman et al, 1986)
```

The new probes described are the subject of patent applications. Probe B6.7 has been deposited with the Centre for Applied Microbiology and Research, Public Health Laboratory Service, Porton Down, Salisbury, Wiltshire, Deposit reference C91031501. Requests for probes should be sent to P Gill (CRSE).

REFERENCES

Armour JAL, Povey S, Jeremiah S and Jeffreys AJ (1990) Genomics 8: 501-512
Bell GI, Selby MJ and Rutter WJ (1982) Nature 295, 31: 31-35
Cheng JF, Printz R, Callaghan T, Shuey D and Hardison RC (1984) J. Mol. Biol. 176: 1-20
Church GM and Gilbert W (1984) Proc. Natl. Acad. Sci. USA 81: 1991-1995
Feinberg AP and Vogelstein B (1984) Anal. Biochem. 137: 266-267
Fowler SJ, Gill PD, Werrett DJ and Higgs DR (1988) Hum. Genet. 79: 142-146
Fritsch E, Shen CKJ, Lawn R and Maniatis T (1980) Cold Spring Harbor Symp. Quant. Biol. 44: 761-775
Higgs DR, Goodbourn SEY, Wainscoat JS, Clegg JB and Weatherall DJ (1981) Nucleic Acids Res. 9: 4213-4214
Jarman AP, Nicholls RD, Weatherall DJ, Clegg JB and Higgs DR (1986) EMBO J. 5: 1857-1863
Labarca C and Paigen K (1980) Anal. Biochem. 102: 344-352
Saito I and Stark GR (1986) Proc. Natl. Acad. Sci. USA 83: 8664-8668
Sambrook J, Maniatis T and Fritsch EF (1989) Molecular Cloning: A Laboratory Manual (Cold Spring Harbor Laboratory, Cold Spring Harbor, NY)
Wong Z, Wilson V, Jeffreys AJ and Thein SL (1986) Nucleic Acids Res. 14: 4605-4616
Wong Z, Wilson V, Patel I, Povey S and Jeffreys AJ (1987) Ann. Hum. Genet. 51: 269-288
Wyman A and White R (1980) Proc. Natl. Acad. Sci. USA 77: 6754-6758

2.2 Methodology

THE USE OF A CHEMILUMINESCENT DETECTION SYSTEM FOR PATERNITY AND FORENSIC TESTING. VERIFICATION OF THE RELIABILITY OF THE OLIGONUCLEOTIDE-PROBES USED FOR GENETIC ANALYSIS

J. Neuweiler, J. Venturini, I. Balazs, S. Kornher, D. Hintz, J. Victor

Lifecodes Corporation, Valhalla, NY, USA

SUMMARY

Several VNTR loci, that had been characterized by the use of P^{32}-labeled recombinant DNA fragments or oligonucleotides to the consensus sequence, were analyzed using oligonucleotide-Alkaline Phosphatase conjugates and a chemiluminescent detection method. The loci tested were D2S44, D4S163, D12S11, D14S13, D17S79, D18S27, DXYS14 and DNF24. Individuals, already typed using P^{32}-labeled probes, were used in this study. Pst I or Hae III-digested DNA from approximately 200 to 400 individuals, covering the full size range of alleles, were examined for each locus. The results obtained for these loci show that, with the exception of D2S44, all the alleles were recognized with the AP-oligos. D2S44 contained a subset of alleles that could only be detected by hybridization to recombinant DNA fragments. In forensic applications, results obtained using DNA recovered from evidentiary material show that most probes detect 10 ng of genomic DNA after an overnight exposure. This indicates that the sensitivity of this detection system is equal or better to that obtained with P^{32}-labeled probes.

INTRODUCTION

The use of oligonucleotides, conjugated with alkaline phosphatase (AP-oligo), and a chemiluminescent detection system provides a convenient and sensitive assay for the detection of DNA polymorphisms routinely used for identity testing (Baum et al. 1990). The detection of a polymorphism relies on the hybridization of oligonucleotides homologous to the variable number of repeats present at these loci. The size of an AP-oligo, used as a hybridization probe, varies up to 30 bases, while the size of the consensus sequences can vary from 14 to 72 bp. Thus, while some of the AP-oligos include up to 2 full copies of the consensus sequence others contain only a subset. Therefore, the purpose of this study was to test whether an AP-oligo can identify all the different size DNA fragments (alleles) of a locus.

MATERIALS AND METHODS

Isolation of DNA from samples of peripheral blood or blood stains was performed as described by Balazs et al. 1989 or Grimberg et al. 1989. DNA from semen stains was

Advances in Forensic Haemogenetics 4
Edited by Ch. Rittner and P. M. Schneider
© Springer-Verlag Berlin Heidelberg 1992

prepared by the procedure described by Giusti et al. 1986. DNA samples were digested with 10 fold excess of Hae III, Hinf I or Pst I according to manufacture recommendations. Fractionation of DNA fragments and transfer to nylon membrane has been described (Balazs et al. 1988).

Hybridization to AP-oligos to DNA-membranes was performed using the Quick-Light^{TM} hybridization kit (Lifecodes Corp.). Briefly, membranes were placed in a plastic container, pre-hybridized for 10 min, hybridized for 10 min to the AP-oligo and washed 4 times for 10 min. each. All of these incubations were done at 55°C with agitation. Membranes were treated with a blocking solution, rinsed with buffer at room temperature, sprayed with Lumi-Phos 480^{TM} (Lumigen Inc.), sealed in a plastic folder and exposed to XAR5 (Kodak) X-ray film for 1-6 hours at 37°C or overnight, at room temperature.

RESULTS AND DISCUSSION

<u>Specificity and sensitivity of AP-oligos.</u> DNA samples covering the full size range of alleles for a locus were selected from databases that had been developed using P^{32}-labeled probes. These samples were hybridized to AP-oligos and the patterns generated by these 2 types of probes were compared. For most of the loci examined, there was complete concordance between the patterns generated by both type of probes. The only exception was the oligonucleotide homologous to the consensus sequence for D2S44. This sequence does not anneal to a subset of alleles in approximately 4% of North American Black and 1% of North American Caucasian population. Although this does not pose a problem for establishing sample identity, it can result in false parental exclusion.

The temperature of the hybridization and washing steps (55°C) were found, in general, to produce minimal or undetectable cross-hybridization to DNA fragments from other loci. The AP-oligos used to detect D14S13 in Pst I and Hae III digested DNA identified, in addition to the main locus, several weaker polymorphic and monomorphic bands that did not permit easy interpretation of results. Increased stringency of hybridization or washing resulted in a loss in sensitivity without significant gain in specificity.

The sensitivity of the AP-probes was measured by hybridizing each probe to a membrane containing a serial dilution of Pst I or Hae III-digested genomic DNA, ranging from 500 to 5 ng/lane. The sensitivity of some of the AP-oligos was sufficient to detect as little as 10ng of genomic DNA after an overnight exposure.

<u>Analysis of paternity cases.</u> Each of the AP-oligos used in paternity testing, using Pst I-digested DNA, were hybridized to 400 - 500 paternity cases that had previously been typed using P^{32}-labeled probes. The most striking effect seen from the results was the increased sharpness of the bands with AP-oligos (Fig.1) as compared with P^{32}-probes (Fig.2). This resulted in easier visualization of closely spaced DNA fragments with concomitant increase in resolution.

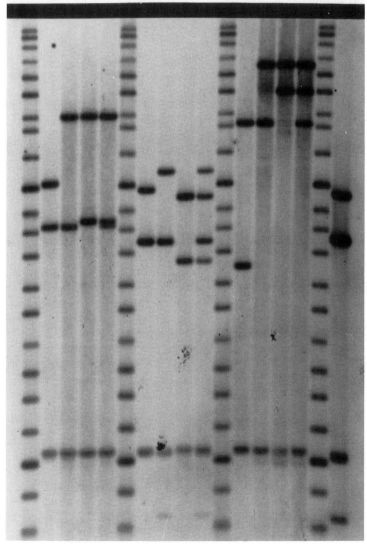

PATERNITY   PST I   LUMIGRAPH
CHEMILUMINESCENT LABELED D4S163
18 HRS EXPOSURE

PATERNITY   PST I   AUTORADIOGRAPH
³²P-LABELED D4S163   18 HR EXPOSURE

The main advantages of the AP-probes are their convenience of use, speed, and safety. This methodology, when used in conjunction with fast and simple non-organic procedures for the isolation of DNA from blood and restriction enzyme digestion (Grimberg et al.1989), can produce samples that can be loaded into gels in under 8 hrs. By using the appropriate gel concentration, electrophoresis can be performed for 16 to 20 hrs, without sacrificing resolution. After DNA transfer to a nylon membrane (3 to 6 hrs), samples are ready for hybridization. As described in Materials and Methods, the entire process, from pre-hybridization to the point of exposing to film, takes 2 to 3 hrs. Paternity cases, prepared with 0.5 to 1 μg of DNA, produced sizable results in about 2 hrs of exposure at 37 °C. Therefore, the total time required to perform an entire paternity test can be less than 2 days.

Analysis of forensic cases. DNA samples were prepared from a variety of blood and semen stains. DNA was digested with Pst I or Hae III, fractionated by gel electrophoresis, transferred to nylon membrane (neutral or charged) and hybridized to AP-oligos. Membranes were repeatedly stripped and rehybridized up to 8 times with only small decrease in sensitivity. In addition, membranes that had been previously hybridized to P^{32}-labeled probes, and stripped, produced results comparable to new membranes. Finally, the results obtained by this non-isotopic detection system were the same as those obtained with P^{32}-labeled probes in terms of sensitivity and the final conclusions that could be drawn from them.

REFERENCES

Balazs I, Baird M, Clyne M, Meade E (1989) Human population genetic studies of five hypervariable DNA loci. Am J Human Genet 44:182-190

Baum HJ, Fitz-Charles H, McKee R (1990) A non-isotopic DNA detection system with the sensitivity of P^{32}: Applications for paternity and forensic identifications. in Advances in Forensic Haemogenetics 3:37-39

Giusti A, Baird M, Pasquale S, Balazs I, Glassberg J (1986) Application of deoxyribonucleic acid (DNA) polymorphisms to the analysis of DNA recovered from sperm. J Forensic Sciences 31:409-417

Grimberg J, Nawoschik S, Belluscio l, McKee R, Turck A, Eisenberg A (1989) A simple and efficient non-organic procedure for the isolation of genomic DNA from blood. Nucleic Acid Res 17:8390

A Multi-locus Probe for Human DNA Fingerprinting Based on *chi*-like Sequences

Nasreen Z. Ehtesham* and Seyed E. Hasnain#

National Institute of Immunology, New Delhi 110067, India

INTRODUCTION

DNA fingerprinting probes based on Jeffreys minisatellite core or those exhibiting similarities with this G-rich core consensus (GGGCAGGAXG), such as the $(GTG)_5$ simple repeat (Schafer et-al 1988) or random G-rich oligodeoxynucleotides (Vergnaud 1990) presumably corresponding to VNTRs, share a degree of homology with the bacterial recombinator activator signal (*chi*), which is believed to serve as foci for recombination (Jarman and Wells 1988, Murray et-al 1988).

A synthetic oligodeoxyribonucleotide containing *chi*-like sequences was designed on the assumption that hypervariability is partly due to the presence of molecular signals which promote recombination. The utility of this probe in DNA fingerprinting is described.

RESULTS AND DISCUSSION

We designed an oligo, O-*chi*-1 (Ehtesham et-al 1991) containing novel *chi* homologues (GGAGGAGG). Our *chi* was based on sequences naturally implicated in recombination, leading to genetic variability (Table 1). A sequence resembling *chi* is also found in immunoglobulin gene rearrangements, glycine-rich plant stress proteins etc. O-*chi*-1 was chemically synthesized on the basis of the assumption that hypervariabilty is partly generated due to recombination events wherein these *chi*-like sequences are involved. A probe comprising of *chi*-like sequences when used for DNA fingerprinting should, therefore, generate individual specific fingerprints.

Human DNA was digested with different restriction enzymes, Southern transferred and probed with the 33 base long radiolabeled O-*chi*-1. Individual-specific DNA fingerprints were obtained even under extremely high stringency of hybridization and washing (6x SSC/0.2 % SDS, 65°C, 4 h). The number of bands per individual varied from 11-18, between 4-25 kb range, with an average number of 15.1 bands. Band sharing frequency data were obtained by a comparison of DNA.

---

* Present address: Plant Molecular Biology Group, International Centre for Genetic Engineering and Biotechnology, New Delhi, 110067, India; # Corresponding author

Advances in Forensic Haemogenetics 4
Edited by Ch. Rittner and P. M. Schneider
© Springer-Verlag Berlin Heidelberg 1992

Table 1. Sequences implicated in naturally occurring processes

	Sequence	Reference
O-*chi*-1	(GGAGGAGG)[*]	
E. coli chi	(GCTGGTGG)	
Minisatellite consensus	(GGGCAGGAXG)	Jeffreys et-al 1985.
Myoglobin *chi* homologue	(GCAGGAGG)	Krowczynska et-al 1990.
Mouse MHC recombination hotspot	(GGAGGTAG)	Steinmetz et-al 1986.
Homologous recombination hotspot	(AGAGGTGG)	Wahls et-al 1990.
Hamster *aprt* insertion/deletion locus	(CCAGGAGG)	Meuth et-al 1987.
Breakpoints of oncogene *bcl2* translocations	(GCAGGAGG)	Krowczynska et-al 1990.

[*]bases identical to *chi* are underlined

band patterns of unrelated individuals and parent-child combinations. The banding pattern in two individuals was compared by using the statistical calculation $D = 2N_{AB}/(N_A + N_B)$ where N_A and N_B are the number of bands in individual A and B, and N_{AB} is the number of common bands between individuals A and B (Schacker et-al 1990, Wetton et-al 1987). The band sharing frequency (D) data are presented in Table 2. Compilation of similar calculations from DNA fingerprints of a number of other individuals gives the band sharing frequency value for O-*chi*-1 to be 14.2 ± 2.7 % for unrelated individuals and 55.4 % for parent offsprings. The probability that all the bands in one individual

Table 2. D value calculations for O-*chi*-1, based on DNA fingerprints of nine different individuals[#]

	MG	AB	BN	KS	SH	EH	NH	ND
AB	.167							
BN	.190	.286						
KS	.083	.167	.190					
SH	.071	.000	.080	.071				
EH	.071	.072	.160	.143	.563			
NH	.000	.000	.000	.000	.303	.545		
ND	.067	.067	.074	.015	.177	.235	.171	
AD	.067	.067	.074	.015	.177	.235	.171	1.00

[#]Note the D values for parent-offsprings (SH/NH *vs* EH), distant degree cousins (SH *vs* NH), and homozygotic twins (AD *vs* ND)

will be common to another unrelated individual was $14.2^{15} = 1.9 \times 10^{-13}$. This value compares very well with the reported values (9×10^{-6} to 2×10^{-8}, depending upon the restriction enzyme used) for simple repeats (Schafer et-al 1988) or with that of 2×10^{-22} for a combination of the extensively used 33.15 and 33.6 minisatellite probes (Jeffreys and Morton 1987). It is significant to mention that the probability for O-*chi*-1 could further go up if fingerprinting is carried out on DNA digested with different restriction enzymes.

A closer look at Table 2 further reveals that the parents (SH and NH) of the individual (EH) also shared DNA bands between themselves - a consequence of inbreeding phenomenon fairly prevalant in certain social/caste systems in India.. This family was deliberately selected for this analysis in order to determine if O-*chi*-1 probe could also detect varying degrees of relationships between individuals. A further application of this probe in determining twin zygosity is also illustrated in Table 2. Genomic DNA was isolated from a pair of twins who presented an unusual clinical case. These twins were connected to the same placenta but by two separate umbilical chords. In usual homozygotic twins the umbilical chord is shared, whereas in heterozygotes there are two different placentae. Fingerprinting of these twins besides solving the clinical riddle, also indicated the utility of O-chi-1 in determining zygosity. A large number of exactly identical DNA bands were obtained for the twins, thus indicating their homozygotic nature. It is therefore, apparent that this probe can be also used to estimate the degree of relatedness besides paternity testing and zygosity determination.

ACKNOWLEDGEMENT

We thank Dr. Om Singh for biostatistical analyses. NZE was a Fellow of the Talwar Research Foundation, New Delhi, India.

REFERENCES

Ehtesham NZ, Das A and Hasnain SE (1991) A novel probe for human DNA fingerprinting based on chi-like sequences. Gene 00:000 (In Press)

Jarman AP and Wells RA (1988) Hypervairable minisatellites: recombinators or innocent bystanders? Trends Genet 5:367-371

Jeffreys AJ and Morton DB (1987) DNA fingerprints of dogs and cats. Anim Genet 18:1

Jeffreys AJ, Wilson V and Thein SL (1985) Individual specific fingerprint of human DNA. Nature 316:76-79

Krowczynska AM, Rudders RA and Krontiris TG (1990) The human minisatellite consensus at breakpoints of oncogene translocations. Nuc Acids Res 18:1121-1127

Meuth M, Nalban-tolfu J, Pheaar D and Miles C (1987) Molecular basis of genome rearrangements at the hamster aprt locus: In: Banbury Report 28: Mammalian Cell Mutagenesis, Cold Spring Harbor Laboratory, 183-191

Murray MJ, Haldeman BA, Grant FJ and O'Hara PJ (1988) Probing the human genome with minisatellite like sequences from the human coagulation factor VIII gene. Nuc Acids Res 16: 4166

Schafer R, Zischler H and Epplen JT (CAC)5, a very informative oligonucleotide probe for DNA fingerprinting. Nuc Acids Res 16: 5196

Schacker V, Schneider PM, Holtkamp B, Bohnke E, Fimmers R, Sonnenborn HH and Rittner C (1990) Isolation of the minisatellite probe MZ 1.3 and its application to DNA fingerprinting analysis. Forensic Sci Internatl 44:209-224

Steinmetz M, Stephan D and Lindahl KF (1986) Gene organization and recombinational hotspots in the murine major histocompatibility complex. Cell 44:895-904

Vergnaud G (1989) Polymers of short oligonucleotides detect polymorphic loci in the human genome. Nuc Acids Res 17:7623-7630

Wahls WP, Wallace LJ and Moore PD (1990) Hypervariable minisatellite DNA is a hotspot for homologous recombination in human cells. Cell 60:95-103

Wetton JH, Carter RE, Parkin DT and Walters D (1987) Demographic studies of a wild house sparrow population by DNA fingerprinting. Nature 327:147-149

THE EFFECTS OF USING DIFFERENT MOLECULAR WEIGHT MARKERS IN DNA PROFILING

M.J.Greenhalgh

Metropolitan Police Forensic Science Laboratory,
109 Lambeth Rd, London. SE1 7LP.
United Kingdom

INTRODUCTION

In forensic single locus probe analysis DNA molecular weight markers are used as a series of controls of known size. This enables bands in the profile of a blood or stain extract to be measured. By reference to a database an estimate of their rarity can then be obtained. The ability to store profiles in a numerical form is also useful as it enables comparisons to be made between crimes and suspects from different laboratories.

In order that a laboratory may use frequency data or crime intelligence data from another source it is essential that the protocols are comparable. Much of the work of the European DNA Profiling Group (EDNAP) has been directed to this end and the results of trials have shown that where common protocols are used results are directly comparable.

In this study the effects of using four different commercially available size markers are investigated.

EXPERIMENTAL

The four markers used in this study were:	catalogue No.
1) Amersham DNA analysis marker.	SJ5000
2) BRL-Life technology DNA analysis system.	4401SA
3) Promega wide range DNA marker.	DB1391
4) BRL 1KB ladder.	5615SA

The BRL 1KB ladder is not suitable for sizing bands in our system as it only extends to 12 KB and using the probes MS1,MS31 and MS43A with the restriction enzyme Hinf1, bands of a greater size are frequently encountered. It is included in this study to show the differences found when marker DNA from a different species is used.

COMPARISON OF THE AMERSHAM AND BRL-LIFE TECHNOLOGY MARKERS

Both of these marker systems are based on λ virus DNA. Our data collection had been prepared using the Amersham system and we were primarily interested in seeing if this could be used with the BRL markers.

An experiment was performed in which a gel was prepared with several samples of each marker. The band weights of each type of marker were measured using the other as control (table 1) and the logarithm of each band weight was plotted against distance migrated (Fig. 1).

As can be seen in Fig.1 the migration distances of the fragments from both marker systems are very similar. The values obtained for the band sizes of the Amersham marker using the BRL marker as standard are also close to the known sizes.

In a further study semen samples from 2 individuals were repeatedly profiled using both

Advances in Forensic Haemogenetics 4
Edited by Ch. Rittner and P. M. Schneider
© Springer-Verlag Berlin Heidelberg 1992

Table 1.   Amersham   DNA marker measured using the BRL-Life Technology
            system (all values in kilobase)

KNOWN VALUE	MEASURED VALUE	% DIFFERENCE
22.01	*	
19.32	*	
13.29	13.36	-0.5
9.69	9.78	-0.9
7.74	7.76	-0.3
6.22	6.24	-0.3
4.25	4.27	-0.5
3.47	3.45	0.6
2.69	2.69	0
2.39	2.38	0.4
1.88	1.90	-1.1
1.48	1.49	-0.7

* out of normal calibration range.

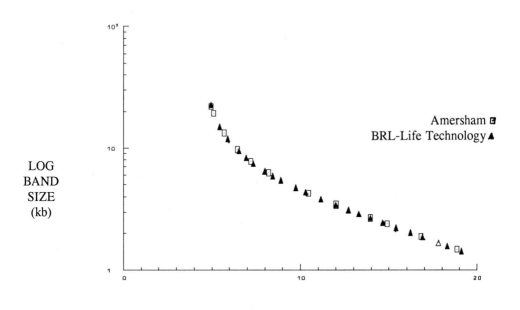

MIGRATION DISTANCE (cm)

Fig 1. Amersham and BRL-Life Technology markers
       log of fragment size vs migration distance

marker systems. A total of 12 bands were obtained ranging in size from 1.7 kb to 13.5 kb. The largest difference between values obtained using the different systems was less than 1.4%.(1 SD of the measurement at this point was 1.1%). There is no overall trend to the differences ie. the Amersham values are not always larger or smaller than those from BRL.

COMPARISON OF AMERSHAM MARKER AND PROMEGA MARKER

A similar set of experiments has been performed with the Promega wide range marker and the results (not shown here) indicate that comparable band sizes can be obtained using this system.

COMPARISON OF AMERSHAM MARKER AND BRL 1KB LADDER.

Table 2.   BRL 1KB ladder measured using Amersham DNA size marker (all values in kilobase)

KNOWN VALUE	MEASURED VALUE	%DIFFERENCE
12.22	12.72	-4.1
11.20	11.51	-2.8
10.18	10.45	-2.7
9.16	9.35	-2.1
8.14	8.28	-1.7
7.13	7.21	-1.1
6.11	6.15	-0.7
5.09	5.10	-0.2
4.07	4.09	-0.5
3.05	3.09	-1.3
2.04	2.02	1.0
1.64	1.62	1.2

The results in table 2. show considerable differences in the mobility of the BRL 1kb ladder which is derived from yeast DNA. This may be due to the different GC content of eucaryotic DNA.

DISCUSSION

The differences between the band sizes obtained using the Amersham and BRL-Life technology markers are small and it is reasonable to exchange information gathered from protocols using either of these systems. It is also likely that the Promega wide range marker is compatible. All of these systems are largely based on λ DNA fragments (some ΦX174 fragments are present in the Promega marker) and hence it is not surprising that the mobility of the fragments is very similar.

With suitable validation it may be possible to change marker systems as long as the DNA originates from the same species.

It is important to remember that forensic scientists are using a λ virus standard to measure the molecular weight of human DNA and therefore the values that we obtain are relative and not absolute.

Influence of Agarose Concentration and Electric Field Strength on the Separation of DNA-Fragments During Electrophoresis

B.L.Guo[*], M.Prinz, M.Staak

Institute of Forensic Medicine, University of Cologne,
Melatengürtel 60-62, 5000 Köln 30, FRG

Introduction

Gel electrophoretic separation of DNA fragments has been used extensively in forensic DNA typing. DNAs mobility in gels depends upon fragment length and some other features(Fisher and Dingman 1971). But the mechanism of gel electrophoresis is not well understood. The migration of the DNA molecules through the pores of the matrix must play an important role in molecular weight separations, since the electrophoretic mobility of DNA in free solution is independent of molecular weight(Olivera et al. 1964). The most successful theory of electrophoresis is the reptation theory of deGennes(1971) and Doi & Edwards(1978). The reptation theory describes the migration of polymers in the presence of fixed obstacles. The DNA fragment move along its axis through a "tube" in a neutral gel under the influence of an electric field(Lumpkin et al. 1985). The apparent mobility of DNA fragments (0.5-12kb) decreases with decreasing electric field strength and with increasing gel concentration(Nancy 1985). Separation capacity for DNA fragments is the distance between two fragments in gel electrophoresis.

Materials and Methods

The sample DNA used for the electrophoresis experiments was the standard marker Lambda Hind III(Boehringer), which contained DNA fragments of 0.564, 2.027, 2.322, 4.361, 6.557, 9.416 and 23.13kb. The loading mass of DNA was 1.2µg per well. The agarose used for all studies was Ultrapure Agarose (Gibco BRL, electroendosmosis=0.10-0.15). All gels were cast and run in Tris-borate buffer(TBE: 0.089M boric acid, 0.089M Tris-base, and 0.002M EDTA, pH8.0). The agarose was dissolved by boiling on a magnet hot plat, lost water was replaced by distilled water. After pouring, the gels were allowed to solidify for 40 min, after which the comb was removed, the gels were flooded with buffer in electrophoresis chamber(GNA-200, Pharmacia) and were allowed to stand for 20 min. Six gels with different agarose concentrations were poured on the same gel supporter. Then the DNA samples were applied and electrophoresis was started. In a preliminary investigation we have found that DNA fragments migrate with a constant velocity when the other conditions (agarose concentration, electric field strength, etc.) are constant. All electrophoresis were run at 20°C(regulated with Desaga Frigostat, Desaga). The electric field was supplied and controlled with 2197 Power Supply(LKB Bromma). After the electrophoresis the gels were stained with ethidium bromide(5µg/ml) for 15 min, and then were photographed under UV

---

[*] DAAD fellow, Institute of Forensic Science, Ministry of Justice of VR China, Guangfu Road(west) 1347, Shanghai, VR China.

Advances in Forensic Haemogenetics 4
Edited by Ch. Rittner and P. M. Schneider
© Springer-Verlag Berlin Heidelberg 1992

light. The migration distances(S, mm) of the DNA fragments were measured and the velocity was calculated as follows:

$$v=S/t \qquad\qquad (Eq.1)$$

Here t was the electrophoresis time(hours). The migration distance of the 0.564 kilobase fragment(velocity was v_1, mm/h) was converted to 180 mm. The relative migration distance(S_r, mm) of a DNA fragment (velocity was v, mm/h) was calculated with the following Equation:

$$S_r=180xv/v_1 \qquad\qquad (Eq.2)$$

Results and Discussion

1. *Separation capacity of gels with different agarose concentration.* The relationship between log(kb) and the relative migration distance of the DNA fragments in gels with different agarose concen-trations(1.6%, 1.4%, 1.2%, 1.0%, 0.8% and 0.6%) for 4V/cm electric field streng is illustrated in Figure I. The smaller ones of the DNA fragments over 4.361kb show a rapid reduction of the relative migration distance with increasing agarose concentra-tion. This causes a decrease of the distance (separation capacity) between these fragments. The longer ones of the fragments between 0.564-2.027kb also show a rapid reduction of the relative migration distance, so that the distances(separation capacity) between these fragments increase with increasing agarose concentration. For the fragment length range from 2.027 and 4.361kb there is no differnce of the separation capacity between 1% and 0.8%

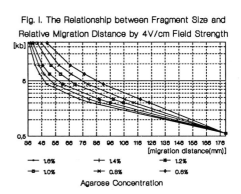

Fig. I. The Relationship between Fragment Size and Relative Migration Distance by 4V/cm Field Strength

Agarose Concentration

agarose gels. This is an important result for forensic DNA-typing, considering the rehybridisation of blots with polymorphic probes revealing different allele size distributions(e.g. MS43/Hinf I 3.5-16kb and YNH24/Hinf I 2.1-5.5kb). Since 1% agarose gels show a decreased separation capacity for fragments longer than 4.361kb and smaller fragments are equally well separated in 0.8% gels, an agarose concentration of 0.8% should be used.

2. *Separation capacity of different electric field strength.* Figure II shows the relationship between the log(kb) and the relative migration distance of DNA fragments in 1.0% agarose concentration for different electric field strength. The relative migration distances of the longer fragments increase more rapidly with increasing electric field strength than those of the smaller ones. Therefore the distances between the fragments(especially the fragments longer than 4.361kb) are reduced with increasing electric field strength. This reduction is particularly evident from 2V/cm to 4V/cm. For the fragments between 0.564kb and 2.027kb the relative migration distance does not increase as rapidly as

for the fragments between 2.027kb and 23.13kb with increasing electric field strength. The migration of long fragments(over 2kb) through agarose gels is more dependent upon the field strength than on molecular weight. This is probably caused by the field-induced distortion (Lumpkin et al. 1985)of the long fragments by high electric field strength. According to our investigation, 4V/cm electric field strength can be employed for the separation of DNA frag-

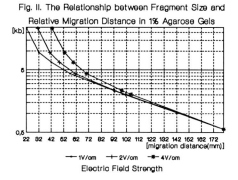

Fig. II. The Relationship between Fragment Size and Relative Migration Distance in 1% Agarose Gels

ments smaller than 2kb, without much loss of separation capacity. Moreover, only about 1/4 of the electrophoresis time for 1V/cm is needed. But since for fragments longer than 2kb the separation capacity of high voltage electric fields is much lower, a low electric field strength(e.g. 1V/cm) should be used.

Summary

The migration distances of DNA fragments undergoing gel electro-phoresis were compared, in order to study the separation capacity of gels with different agarose concentrations and of different electric field strength for given DNA fragments. High electric field strengths have lower separation capacity for DNA fragments over 2kb. A rapid separation of DNA fragments with high voltage electric field strength is not to recommend. To the separation of DNA fragments under 2kb electric field strength has scarcely influence. For DNA fragments of 4-23kb a low agarose concentration has a higher separation capacity. The fragments between 2 and 0.5kb can be separated better in gels with higher agarose concentration. Since the fragment length range from 2-4kb is equally well separated in 0.8% and 1% agarose gels, 0.8% agarose concentration is suggested for forensic DNA-typing of Hinf I digests.

References:

Fisher, M.P., Dingman, C.W.(1971) Role of Molecular conformation in the Electrophoretic Properties of Polynucleotides in Agarose-Acrylamide Composite Gels. Biochemistry 10: 1895-1899
Olivera,B.M., Baine,P., Davidson,N.(1964) Electrophoresis of the Nucleic Acid. Biopolymers 2: 245-257
deGennes, P.-G.(1971) Reptation of a Polymer Chain in the Presence of Fixed Obstacles. J.Chem.Phys. 55: 572-579
Doi, M., Edwards, S.(1978) Dynamics of Concentrated Polymer Systems J. Chem. Soc., Farad. Trans. II 74: 1789-1801
Lumpkin, O. J., Dejardin, P. & Zimm, B. H.(1985) Theory of Gel Electrophoresis of DNA. Biopolymers 24: 1573-1593
Nancy, C.S.(1985) Effect of the Electric Field on the Apparent Mobilty of Large DNA Fragments in Agarose Gels. Biopolymers 24: 2243-2255

Size Calculations of Restriction Fragments: Comparison Between Two Laboratories

L. Henke[1], P.H. van Eede[2], J. Henke[1], and G.G. de Lange[2]

[1]Institut f. Blutgruppenforschung, Otto-Hahn-Str. 39, D-4000 Düsseldorf 13, Germany
[2]Central Laboratory of the Netherlands Red Cross Blood Transfusion Service and Laboratory for Experimental and Clinical Immunology, University of Amsterdam, 1066 CX Amsterdam, The Netherlands

Material and Methods

DNA samples from 45 unrelated Caucasians were digested with Hinfl and after Southern blotting hybridized with probes MS1, MS31, MS43a, and G3. Altogether 334 restriction fragments were observed ranging from 1.6 to 29 kb.

The fragment sizes were calculated in Amsterdam by a computer aided system (TANGO) by using a digitizing tablet, and in Düsseldorf manually by using a semilogarithmic plotted curve. The following size markers were used: in Amsterdam the Lambda EcoRI/HindIII (Promega) und Lambda HindIII (BRL) and in Düsseldorf the Analytical Marker DNA Wide Range (Promega) (van Eede et al.,1991).

The results obtained in both laboratories were analysed by calculating the bias estimated by mean differences followed by the calculation of the estimated limits of agreement (Finney, 1978). The intralaboratory differences of repeated measurements of various samples were compared with the interlaboratory results.

For checking the influence of different marker systems on the estimation of fragment sizes, 60 fragments were calculated with both marker systems on the same filters.

Results

Intra-laboratory comparisons reveal a good reproducibility of fragment size measurements in each laboratory. In the range from 1.6 kb to 12 kb the standard deviation of the measurements is approximately 0.2 kb in one laboratory while the interlaboratory measurements show an increased standard deviation to approximately 0.35 kb for the same range.
Over the whole range from 1.6 to 30 kb the mean standard deviation is 0.7 kb (Fig. 1).

The data of interlaboratory comparison are shown in table 1.

Table 1: Differences (kb $size_{Düs}$ - kb $size_{Ams}$) and standard deviation in different fragment size ranges

Fragment size	1.6 - 3,9	4.0 - 5.9	6.0 - 7.9	8.0 - 9.9	10.0 - 11.9	12.0 - 30
Number of comparisons	44	87	108	64	31	18
Mean differences (kb)	0.091	-0.052	0.091	0.177	0.235	-1.92
Standard deviation	0.218	0.137	0.218	0.289	0.584	2.13

Advances in Forensic Haemogenetics 4
Edited by Ch. Rittner and P. M. Schneider
© Springer-Verlag Berlin Heidelberg 1992

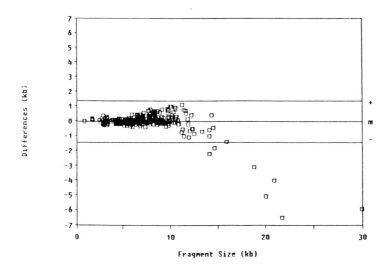

Fig. 1 Differences (kb size $_{Düs}$ - kb size $_{Ams}$) in fragment size of the same DNA samples processed in Amsterdam and Düsseldorf. Number of samples n = 352; m = mean difference; + = mean difference + $a_{0.05}$* standard deviation; - = mean difference - $a_{0.05}$* standard deviation

The influence of the different marker systems were analysed by calculating 60 fragments in the range of 3.8 kb to 20 kb with both marker systems (fig. 2). It was shown that the fragment size calculated with the Lambda markers were seemingly larger than the fragment size calculated using the Analytical Marker DNA Wide Range. The mean difference appeared to be -0.17 kb and a standard deviation of 0.10 kb. The mean diffferences increased with the fragment size.

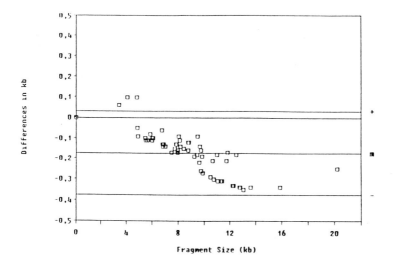

Fig. 2 Differences (kb size$_{Analytical Marker DNA}$ - kb size$_{Lambda Markers}$) in fragment size of the same fragments by using different markers. Number of samples n = 60; m = mean difference; + = mean difference + $a_{0.05}$* standard deviation; - = mean difference - $a_{0.05}$* standard deviation

Conclusions

Below a fragment size of 8 kb the results of the two laboratories appeared to be comparable. Fragments larger than 8 kb showed seemingly larger size in Amsterdam than in Düsseldorf.

This difference appeared to be at least partly due to the use of different marker systems. For pooling of data and for comparison of fragment sizes obtained in different laboratories it will be necessary to come to consenses about the marker systems.

References

Van Eede PH, Henke L, Fimmers R, Henke J and de Lange GG (1991) Size calculation of restriction enzyme *HaeIII*-generated fragments detected by probe YNH24 by comparison of data from two laboratories: The generation of fragment-size frequencies. For Sci Int 49:21-31

Finney DJ (1978) Statistical methods in biological assay, 3rd edn., Charles Griffin and Company Ltd., pp 316-348

MATCHING CRITERIA FOR PATERNITY TESTING WITH VNTR SYSTEMS

Niels Morling & Hanna E. Hansen

Institute of Forensic Genetics, University of Copenhagen,
11 Frederik Den Femtes Vej, DK-2100 Copenhagen Ø, Denmark

ABSTRACT

The variability in duplicate testings and in mother/child comparisons of RFLP VNTR data for paternity testing was analyzed. *Hinf*I digested DNA was separated by electrophoresis in agarose gels and hybridized with radiolabelled probes detecting the VNTR-systems D7S22 (g3), D5S43 (MS8), D7S21 (MS31), D12S11 (MS43), and D2S44 (YNH24). The band positions on autoradiographs were measured with a ruler with 0.5 mm resolution. Initial analyses demonstrated that, when the samples which should be compared were investigated on the same gel, the absolute difference in migration distance was the parameter with the lowest variability. Comparisons of 445 duplicate investigations on the same gel of DNA from 108 individuals showed no differences exceeding 1.25 mm. This matching criterion was used for the comparisons of 1,012 differences in 215 mother-child pairs. All mother-child differences were less than 1.25 mm except for an assumed mutation in D7S21 (MS31), and this matching criterion has been chosen for the evaluation of Danish paternity cases. The allele distributions of the five VNTR systems in 530 unrelated Danes are presented.

INTRODUCTION

We wanted to establish simple exclusion/inclusion (matching) criteria for paternity testing by means of analysis of the Restriction Fragment Length Polymorphism (RFLP) of Variable Numbers of Tandem Repeats (VNTR) regions with the single locus probe DNA technique. It was important for us (i) that the DNA investigations in paternity cases were performed with the technique which we presently use for DNA investigations in crime cases, i.e. the technique agread upon by the European DNA Profiling (EDNAP) Group, and (ii) that the background for the matching criteria and their documentation could be understood intuitively. Here, we present our matching criteria and the allele distributions of the VNTR systems investigated in Danes.

MATERIAL AND METHODS

Individuals: Blood samples were obtained in families and paternity cases from 215 mother/child pairs, 42 men who had been excluded from paternity with conventional tests, and from further 273 unrelated, random Danes.
Isolation and digestion of DNA: Genomic DNA was isolated with phenol or 6 M NaCl. The DNA was digested with the restriction enzyme *Hinf*I according to the manufacturer's specifications.
Electrophoresis: Separation of the DNA fragments was performed by electrophoresis in 0.7 % agarose gels (20 cm x 20 cm). The DNA samples from the mother, child, and

Advances in Forensic Haemogenetics 4
Edited by Ch. Rittner and P. M. Schneider
© Springer-Verlag Berlin Heidelberg 1992

the putative father(s) in a case were investigated on the same gel. At least three lanes with Amersham ^{35}S molecular weight ladder were included on each gel. The gels were run over night until the 2.39 kb band of the ladder had migrated 14.0 cm.

Hybridization: After Southern blotting, hybridization with ^{32}P radiolabelled probes was performed as sequential reprobing on the membrane. The probes detected the VNTR-systems D7S22 (g3), D5S43 (MS8), D7S21 (MS31), D12S11 (MS43) (Wong et al 1987), and D2S44 (YNH24) (Wyman & White 1980). Autoradiography was performed on X-ray films.

Band sizing: The migrations of the bands were measured with a ruler with 0.5 mm resolution, and the kilobase values were calculated by local, hyperbolic approximation (Elder & Southern 1987).

Normalized migration length: Initial investigations demonstrated that the absolute difference in migration distance was the parameter with the lowest variability. Although the variability expressed in per cent of the kb-values was almost constant for low kb-values, the variability increased with increasing kilobase values above 6 - 8 kb. When the gels were run under standardized conditions, the kb-values could be transformed into normalized migration length (NML) values:

$$NML = \frac{800}{3.8 + KB^{1.5}} + 33.75$$

The NML-value can conceptually be understood as the migration in mm on a standard (or average) gel. The NML-values fitted the normal distribution.

Calculation of upper and lower limits of matching windows: The actual kb-value of a non-maternal band of the child matching a band in the putative father was transformed into an NML-value (NML_0), and the upper (NML_U) and lower (NML_L) values of the window were defined as $NML_U = NML_0 - 1.25$ mm and $NML_L = NML_0 + 1.25$ mm. The NML_U and NML_L values were retransformed into upper (KB_U) and lower (KB_L) kb-values of the window.

Calculation of allele frequencies in matching windows: The number of alleles in the matching window ($KB_L - KB_U$) in 530 random, unrelated Danes was counted and this number was divided by the total number of alleles investigated.

RESULTS AND DISCUSSION

Variability when DNA from a person was tested twice on the same gel: DNA was isolated with (i) phenol and (ii) 6 M NaCl from the same blood sample from 108 unrelated individuals. The two DNA preparations from each person were investigated on the same gel and hybridized with five probes giving 445 bands for the analysis. No migration differences (D) exceeded 1.25 mm. The frequencies of the differences were: D = 0.0 mm: 80.4 %, D = 0.5 mm: 18.7 %, D = 1.0 mm: 0.9 %, D = 1.5 mm: 0.0 %.

Preliminary matching criteria: Based on these results, preliminary matching criteria in paternity testing were established. Thus, the hypothesis of paternity was not rejected if the migration difference between the non-maternal band in the child and the nearest band in the putative father was less that 1.25 mm in electrophoresis on the same gel.

Test of the validity of the matching criteria: The differences between the migrations of the bands identical by descent in the mothers and their children were analyzed in 215 mother/child pairs investigated with five probes giving 1,012 bands (fig. 1). All differences were less than 1.25 mm, except for a mutation in D7S21 (MS31). The migration differences between the non-maternal band of the child and the nearest band of the putative father were analyzed in 42 cases (210 bands) with a man who had been excluded as father by investigations with well established, conventional systems. In 17.2 % of the cases, the migration differences were less than 1.25 mm, but the majority of the differences (68.6 %) were above 2.5 mm (fig. 1). Although the matching criteria has not yet been tested critically on a larger group of father/child pairs, we have no reason to believe that the matching criteria cannot be used for father/child comparisons.

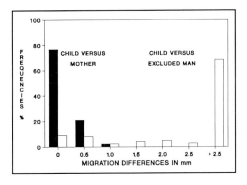

Fig. 1. Migration differences between mother/child pairs and excluded man/child pairs

Allele distributions of the VNTR systems in Danes: Figure 2 shows the allele distributions of D7S22 (g3), D5S43 (MS8), D7S21 (MS31), D12S11 (MS43), and D2S44 (YNH24) in 530 random, unrelated Danes. The frequencies were calculated in consecutive matching windows (i.e. 2.50 NML mm intervals, cf. above). The allele distribution of D7S22 (g3) was based on the analysis of 248 maternal alleles in mother/child pairs because a number of bands representing D7S22 alleles were lost for the analysis due to the size of the fragments or due to weak hybridizations with the g3 probe.

Paternity Index: Based on the estimates of the population frequencies in Danes of the paternal VNTR alleles in the child, the Paternity Index in a Danish paternity case may be calculated as previously described (Henningsen 1983).

REFERENCES

Elder JK, Southern JM (1987) Computer-aided analysis of one dimensional restriction fragment gels. In: Bishop MJ, Rawlings CJ (eds) Nucleic Acid and Protein Sequence Analysis - A Practical Approach. IRL, Oxford, pp 165-72

Henningsen K (1983) Paternity Case Analysis. In: Walker RH (ed) Inclusion Probabilities in Parentage Testing. American Association of Blood Banks, Arlington, pp 501-3

Wong Z, Wilson V, Patel I, Povey S, Jeffreys AJ (1987) Characterization of a panel of highly variable minisatellites cloned from human DNA. Ann Hum Genet 51: 269-88

Wyman AR, White R (1980) A highly polymorphic locus in human DNA. Proc Natl Acad Sci USA 77: 6754-8

152

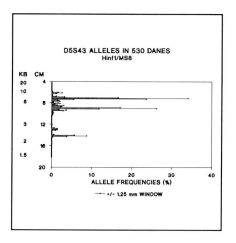

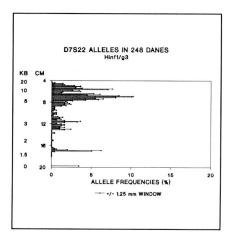

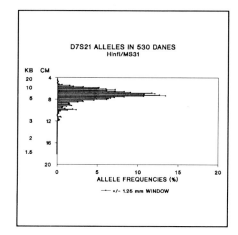

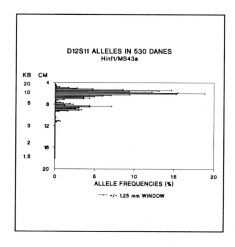

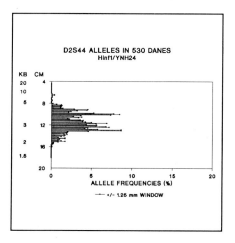

Fig. 2. Allele distribution of D5S43 (MS8), D7S22 (g3), D7S21 (MS31), D12S11 (MS43), and D2S44 (YNH24) in Danes

Computer-Aided Fragment Size Determination of Single Locus DNA Probes

M. Muche

Institut für Blutgruppenserologie und Genetik, Holsteinischer
Kamp 67, D-2000 Hamburg 76, Germany

INTRODUCTION

In recent years, several computer systems have been developed
for fragment size determination of DNA blots. As manual
evaluation is rather time-consuming, cumbersome and involves the
risk of errors in measuring, calculation or transfer of data, it
is obvious that a computer system can do much of the routine
work.

Fragment sizes of single locus DNA probes are obtained using
molecular weight markers with a known ladder of fragments. These
fragments of known size are compared to the observed bands. As
the migration distance of the standard size marker bands is not
linear to its size, a function has to be generated, resulting in
a relation between migration distance [cm] and fragment size
[kb].

REQUIREMENTS FOR A COMPUTER-AIDED SYSTEM

When DNA typing was first carried out in our laboratory, the
blots were evaluated using a manual direct method. With an
increasing work load it became difficult to obtain fragment size
values from individually drawn graphs. The first approach to
that problem we took late last year was to replace the optical
determination of fragment length by computerized calculation.
All manually measured data was entered into a computer program
that generated a function that could be used to calculate
fragment sizes. It soon became obvious that some kind of a
device should be introduced to make it easier to obtain
centimetre values from the blot but even this rather fragmental
approach proved to save a remarkable amount of time.

As an input device we decided for a digitizer. I would like to
outline why this has turned out to be a way to succesfully
shorten the procedure and to enhance the quality of evaluation:

The following questions can be applied on any system that is to
be used for DNA fragment size determination:

(1) To what degree is manual influence required?
(2) How reliable is the system? (Keyword: repeatable results)
(3) Is a closed circuit of data provided?
(4) Is the system easy to use even if the user has little or no
computer knowledge?

Advances in Forensic Haemogenetics 4
Edited by Ch. Rittner and P. M. Schneider
© Springer-Verlag Berlin Heidelberg 1992

(5) How efficient is a system?
(6) What hardware at what cost is required?

Manual influence should be limited to what is unavoidable: The
aim of any sample testing is to obtain results that are not
influenced by the measuring itself. This seems to be rather
difficult and it will be impossible to install a system that
analyzes without any human decisions, but this influence should
be restricted to clearly defined situations: We thought it
tolerable that bands are marked with a mouse-like stylus on a
pad, as certain decisions are to be made that a computer can
hardly perform: E. g. which position of a band should be used
for calculation, whether some dark dot is a band or just a
bubble.

Using an optical recognition system, such as a video camera and
corresponding software, has the same limitiations in this
respect: There will always be cases where manual corrections or
even complete manual marking is required (as for weak or broad
bands). Solely manual evaluation suffers the lack of guidance:
There is no plausibility check and there always exists the risk
of misreading the ruler.

Repeatability is an important factor. Any two fragment size
determinations of a certain sample should always result in the
same value. Although a low deviation is tolerable (and will not
be avoidable) this also is an indicator for the quality of
evaluation. Whether or not one can obtain identical results is a
question of trying: We have had a closer look at the measured
migration distances of the last 40 evaluations and found
differences between first and second value of between 0 and 0.08
cm, resulting in fragment size differences of up to 8 bp in the
range of up to 6 kb with exceptional high deviation in the range
of above 9 kb of up to 50 bp. Compared with the exactness that
is achievable with manual methods this seems to be completely
satisfactory. Very similar results were obtained in another
laboratory that uses this system.

Every computer installation should offer what is here described
as a *closed circuit*: Any data that is entered into the computer
should be used for every application it is needed for: In this
case the obtained data can be used for printing of a work sheet
for intra-laboratory use, a blot list containing results, lists
of all DNA samples examined and the calculation of probabilities
in cases of disputed paternity. It should strictly be avoided
that any bit of information has to be retyped or transferred
manually to another program, as this allows errors to occur and
drastically reduces the efficiency of the system.

Emphasis is also put on the aspect that the single steps that
have to be done in order to perform a blot analysis follow a
natural order. This is essential, so that the system can be *used
easily* also by those who do not have any experience in dealing
with computer programs or are not acquainted with the system.

The *efficiency* of the system largely depends on the following
three aspects: Time needed for setting-up of hardware devices
(e. g. adjustment of contrast for video systems or definiton of
X and Y zero positions), duration of evaluation itself and the

degree to which advanced functions are incorporated in the system (such as population statistics, calculation of probabilities or ready-to-use printouts of phenotype or case lists).

The last aspect which is not included for scientific reasons may nevertheless prove to be important for a number of laboratories that plan to introduce a computer-aided evaluation method: *Cost*. As the digitizer seems to offer a reasonable ratio between power and price (compared to some optical recognition system), it is recommenendable even for laboratories that have a limited amount of examinations but want to maintain a high standard of accuracy.

These six aims were used as a kind of guide line in developing and installing a system that is now in use in three laboratories throughout Germany, of which a brief description is given:

PROGRAM CHARACTERISTICS

The program presented here may be used for any single locus DNA system. The probes that are to be taken in calculation can be chosen by the user. However, a set of six Collaborative Research probes is included in the package. In addition, ten different size markers can be used also allowing different size markers on one blot. The definition of a size marker includes all known fragment sizes making it easy just to click the band.

Calculation of fragment sizes is carried out using the next to marker lanes for which a result can be obtained. This result is saved for future use. Up to six results per probe may be stored for each sample. Each size determination can be confirmed or corrected by a second independent measuring. It is recommended that this second measuring is carried out by another person. A protocol listing differences is printed on demand.

Once results have been obtained these can be used for creation of a population data base or for the calculation of probabilites. A wide range of different hardcopies of data is also available.

Chemiluminescent detection of single locus and multilocus hybridization patterns

M. Prinz, C. Loch, M. Staak

Institute for Forensic Medicine, University of Cologne, Melatenguertel 60-62, D-5000 Köln 30, FRG

INTRODUCTION

The chemiluminescent detection of alkaline phosphatase accelerates the time required for DNA-typing, since the signals emitted during the dephosphorylation of 3-(2'-spiroadamantane)-4-methoxy-4-(3''-phosphoryloxy)phenyl-1,2-dioxetane (AMPPD) can be visible after less than one hour.

The rate of light emission is proportional to the enzyme activity, and that means proportional to the amount of membrane bound alkaline phosphatase. Southern blot detection of low amounts of DNA therefore requires a much longer period of film exposure (compare Giles et al. 1990). Working with digoxigenin labeled probes which require blocking and antibody binding steps, these prolonged exposure times of 18 hours and more can cause severe problems with unspecific background.

We compared several modifications of the alkaline phosphatase detection with AMPPD and their effect on unspecific background and sensitivity. Working with multilocus probes, we compared the quality of the band pattern after chemiluminescent detection with the colorimetric detection.

METHODS

Up to four DNA-dilution series were run on the same gels. After Southern blotting and hybridization the membranes (Hybond N, Amersham) were divided and treated according to each modification. The single locus DNA probe used in this study was digoxigenin labeled YNH24 purchased from Promega corporation. As a multilocus probe bacteriophage M13 was labeled using the "Nonradioactive DNA Labeling and Detection Kit" from Boehringer Mannheim. The X-ray film was Agfa Curix RP1 NIF 100. Further details are given in the descriptions of the photos.

RESULTS

The influence of hybridization solutions both with and without formamide was tested for different detection protocols. In each case, after two hours of exposure, the blots hybridized with a 50% formamide solution gave more intensive signals (figure 1, A). After overnight exposure the formamide membranes showed substantial unspecific background (figure 1 C).

Advances in Forensic Haemogenetics 4
Edited by Ch. Rittner and P. M. Schneider
© Springer-Verlag Berlin Heidelberg 1992

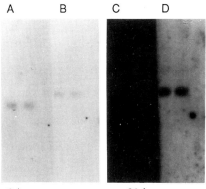

A   B   C   D

2 h exposure   20 h exposure

Fig 1. Effect of formamide in the
hybridization solution. YNH24
signals of 5µg DNA after 2 and 20
hours exposure to X-ray film.
Probe concentration was 2ng/ml.
Here detection was performed
using maleate buffer, 1% blocking
in the antibody dilution and
0.235mM AMPPD in tris-buffer
pH9.5
A: hybridization solution 50%
formamide and 5% Boehringer
blocking reagent
B: no formamide and 0.5% blocking

According to ALLEFS et al. (1990) and the updated manufacturers
instructions by Boehringer Mannheim, unspecific background can be
reduced by diluting the anti-digoxigenin/alkaline phosphatase
conjugate in a buffer containing Boehringer blocking reagent. We
tested this to see if it would not impair the sensitivity of the
detection assay. DNA-dilution series from 1µg to 10ng DNA were
blotted and treated as described in figure 2 A,B. The background
is reduced for the antibody/blocking procedure, while the
sensitivity is the same. In both cases the 3.0kb fragment could
be detected among 25ng DNA. With a DNA content of a human diploid
cell of 6.2pg and with the value of 1pg corresponding to
0.965×10^9 bp (Lewin 1987) the heterozygote single copy 3.0kb band
in the 25ng track represents a 0.012pg target sequence. For the
smaller 1.5kb fragment this amount of target sequence is contained in 50ng (lane 7). The hybridization pattern for the smaller
fragment corresponds to this detection limit.

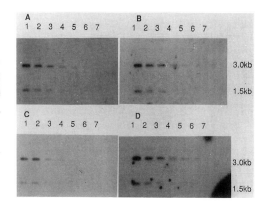

A
1 2 3 4 5 6 7   B
1 2 3 4 5 6 7

3.0kb

1.5kb

C
1 2 3 4 5 6 7   D
1 2 3 4 5 6 7

3.0kb

1.5kb

Fig 2. Influence of different detection buffers.
Probe concentration of YNH24
was 4ng/ml. A: digoxigenin
antibody conjugate was
diluted in maleate buffer
(0.1M maleic acid, 0.15M
NaCl, pH 7.5 adjusted with
NaOH)
B: antibody conjugate
diluted in maleate buffer
containing 1% blocking
reagent
A and B: AMPPD diluted to
0.235mM in tris-buffer pH9.5
(0.1M TrisHCl, 0.1M NaCl,
0.05M $MgCl_2$), film exposure
20h
C: antibody-conjugate diluted in maleate buffer 1% blocking,
AMPPD diluted in carbonate buffer pH 9.5 (0.05M $NaHCO_4$/Na_2CO_4,
0.001M $MgCl_2$), 20 h exposure
D: as C after 72h exposure

Comparing the alkaline buffers for the dilution of AMPPD, e.g. as the pH 9.5 carbonate buffer used by Tropix Inc. to the pH 9.5 tris-buffer used by Boehringer Mannheim, the carbonate buffer showed a much lower rate of background but also a decreased, or at least slower light emmission rate (figure 2 C). In comparing blots B and C of figure 2 it is noticeable that after the 20h exposure to X-ray film the signal intensity and sensitivity of the assay using tris-buffer is higher. Only after prolonged exposure times can the carbonate assay reach the same sensitivity (figure 2 D).

To test the influence of enhancer molecules DNA-dilution series were incubated for 5 minutes in AMPPD diluted in carbonate buffer, AMPPD diluted in carbonate buffer 10% EMERALD enhancer, and in LUMIPHOS 530 reagent which contains AMPPD, cethyltrime-thylammoniumbromide and aminofluorescein (Carlson et al. 1990). The addition of EMERALD enhancer produced dark background, where as there was no difference in background between the AMPPD solution and the Lumiphos 530 reagent. Using Lumiphos 530 the sensitivity was increased.

Prolonging the incubation of the membrane with AMPPD substrate from 5 min to 1h produced higher background and did not improve the sensitivity.

The hybridization of parallel blots with digoxigenin-labeled M13 showed that with the colour substrate developement the bands were sharper and therefore the separation of distinct fragments was improved. The disadvantage of the colour precipitation is the difficult reprobing of the membranes, but for certain applications where no rehybridization is required the colorimetric detection can still be the preferable method.

REFERENCES

Allefs JJHM, Salentijn EMJ, Krens FA, Rouwendaal GJA (1990) Optimization of non-radioactive Southern blot hybridization: single copy detection and reuse of blots. Nucl Acids Res 18:3099-3100

Carlson DP, Superko C, Mackey J, Gaskill ME, Hanssen P (1990) Chemiluminescent detection of nucleic acid hybridization. Focus 12:9-12

Giles AF, Booth KJ, Parker JR, Garman AJ, Carrick DT, Akhavan H, Schaap AP (1990) Rapid, simple, non-isotopic probing of Southern blots for DNA-fingerprinting. In: Polesky HF, Brinkmann B (eds) Advances in Forensic Haemogenetics 3, Springer, Berlin, p 40-42

Lewin B (1987) Genes, 3rd edn. Wiley, New York

Westneat DF, Noon WA, Reeve HK, Aquadro CF (1988) Improved hybridization conditions for DNA-fingerprints probed with M13. Nucl Acids Res 16:4161

Precision and Accuracy in the Analysis of VNTR Polymorphisms for Paternity Testing

S.C. Reavis, T. Schlaphoff, R. Martell and E.D. du Toit

Provincial Laboratory for Tissue Immunology, Cape Town, South Africa

INTRODUCTION

Single locus VNTR DNA profiling has become an important technique in the identification of parentage. Due to the complex multi-step nature of the VNTR assay, a degree of variability exists in the determination of band sizes. Unacceptable levels of measurement error may adversely effect conclusions regarding inclusion and exclusion of alleged fathers, as well as the establishment of accurate population allele frequency data bases. Possible sources of error are poor separation of large bands, poor visualization of small bands, variation in electrophoretic mobility between gels (inter-assay error) or across a single gel (intra-assay error), and observer error in measurement of band migration distance. The recommended method for determining the level of error for a chosen VNTR assay system is repetitive analysis of human genomic DNA samples (Budowle 1991). Inter and intra-assay precision was determined by repetitive analysis of volunteer DNA using eight commercially available VNTR probes. In order to gauge the accuracy of band sizing techniques we performed repetitive analysis of DNA from the HeLa human cell line.

MATERIALS AND METHODS

DNA was extracted from peripheral blood leucocytes of eight volunteers, and digested with a range of enzymes. The digests were electrophoresed, Southern transferred and hybridized using standard methods, (Maniatis 1982) with the eight probes listed in Table 1. Of the enzymes tested, only Pvu II gave band sizes within a 2.0 to 15.0 kb. size range with all probes, and this enzyme was used throughout the remainder of the trial. For inter-assay precision, the eight volunteer DNA samples were electrophoresed on ten gels, and the membranes hybridized sequentially with the eight probes. For intra-assay precision, DNA from a single individual was electrophoresed in twenty wells of a single gel. This was repeated three times for three different individuals for a total of nine gel runs. These membranes were hybridized with the Mucin-HVR probe. In all gels, an analytical sizing marker (Promega) which displays 30 bands over a 30 kb. size range was included in every fifth well

Advances in Forensic Haemogenetics 4
Edited by Ch. Rittner and P. M. Schneider
© Springer-Verlag Berlin Heidelberg 1992

of each gel. In lane one of each of the gels used for inter-
assay precision, 5ug of Puv II digested HeLa cell DNA
(Amersham) was included. Band migration distance was
determined by measurement with a ruler to the nearest 0.5 mm by
two independent readers. Sizes of unknown DNA fragments were
calculated according to the hyperbolic method as suggested by
Southern (1979), using a spreadsheet program. Each band was
reported as an average of the repeated measurements.

INTER- AND INTRA-ASSAY PRECISION

TABLE 1. Inter-assay Precision

PROBE[1]	MEAN RANGE[2]	CV(%) RANGE	PAIRED MEASUREMENTS[3]
D16S85	2.06-5.06	0.38-1.02%	0.60%
Mucin	3.47-5.92	0.36-0.92%	0.60%
Ha-Ras	2.73-4.18	0.36-0.93%	0.53%
DXYS14	3.65-15.7	0.57-2.42%	0.72%
D2S44	2.85-5.31	0.33-1.07%	0.61%
D14S13	3.93-5.97	0.45-1.02%	0.57%
D10S24	3.18-5.76	0.39-1.01%	0.66%
D17S26	6.40-12.7	0.77-3.72%	0.79%

[1]Probes D16S85, Mucin, Ha-Ras, and DXYS14 were supplied by
Amersham; probes DS244, D14S13, D10S24, and D17S26 were
supplied by Promega.
[2]The range is given for 16 means (2 bands reported per
individual) from 10 repeated gel runs for each probe.
[3]The standard deviation was calculated from 160 repeated
measurements per probe and expressed as a percentage of the
mean band size.

TABLE 2. Intra-assay Precision

SUBJECT[1]	MEAN RANGE[2]	CV(%) RANGE	PAIRED MEASUREMENTS[3]
1a	5.10-5.12	0.61-0.68%	0.29%
1b	3.75-3.80	0.66-0.72%	0.31%
2a	4.16-4.30	0.68-0.84%	0.42%
2b	4.08-4.25	0.51-0.92%	0.55%
3a	5.64-5.85	0.88-0.92%	0.38%
3b	3.33-3.49	0.64-0.80%	0.56%

[1]All subjects were heterozygous, hybridization was with the
mucin probe.
[2]The mean range is given for the 3 means for each band from
each individual. For each mean n=20.
[3]The standard deviation was calculated from 60 repeated
measurements per allele and expressed as a percentage of the
mean band size.

Values for inter-assay precision are reported in Table 1. Two
bands were sized for each of the eight individuals (single

homozygous band patterns were recorded as two bands of
identical size), and means and standard deviations were
calculated for each of the sixteen bands from the results of
the ten gel runs. This was repeated for each of the eight
probes tested using the same ten membranes for each probe (i.e.
each of the ten membranes were stripped and re-hybridized eight
times). Inter-assay precision is reported as a coefficient of
variation (CV), and this was calculated from the means and
standard deviations for each of the sixteen bands. It was
arbitrarily decided that if a probe demonstrated a CV range
greater than 2.0% then it would be rejected for use with this
gel/enzyme system. The probes DXYS14 and D17S26 detected
several bands greater than 12 kilobase pairs with corresponding
CVs which exceeded the acceptable upper limit. This appeared
to be due to inadequate separation of marker DNA in that size
range, making it difficult to achieve consistent observer
agreement on mobility measurements. For the other six probes,
the CVs ranged from 0.33% to 1.07%. The percent error for the
160 repeated measurements is the standard deviation calculated
from the difference in the two measurements, expressed as a
percentage of the mean band size. Values ranged from 0.53% to
0.79% indicating a close agreement between the two readers.
There was minimal deviation of band migration across a single
gel as evidenced by the intra-assay precision values in Table
2.   The CVs ranged from 0.51% to 0.92% for 20 measurements per
allele, and the CVs for 60 repeated measurements per allele
were all less than 0.6%.

INTER-ASSAY ACCURACY

TABLE 3. Inter-assay Accuracy [1]

PROBE[2]	MEAN[3]	S.D.	REPORTED[4]	DIFFERENCE[5]
D16S85	8.90	0.08	9.00	1.1%
D16S85	3.41	0.03	3.20	6.3%
Mucin	5.81	0.03	6.00	3.2%
Mucin	3.79	0.02	3.50	7.9%
Ha-Ras	2.94	0.02	2.80	4.9%
DXYS14	9.63	0.08	10.0	3.8%

[1]Band sizes detected for a Pvu II digest of the HeLa cell line
were compared to band sizes reported for four probes.
[2]Probes listed twice detected heterozygous loci.
[3]The means are calculated from the average value for 10
repeated measurements.
[4]Band sizes reported by probe supplier (Amersham) to 100 base
pairs.
[5]Size difference reported as a percentage of the average band
size.

Bands detected for a Pvu II digest of the HeLa cell line for
each of the probes tested are reported in Table 3. The percent
differences between the mean values and reported values ranged
from 1.1% to 7.9% of the average band size.

CONCLUSIONS

In estimating band sizing precision, it was found that the greatest source of error was in measuring identical bands in different gels (inter-assay error). Here the probes DXYS14 and D17S26 demonstrated CVs in excess of 2.0%, and they were excluded for further use with Pvu II. The remaining 6 probes produced inter-assay CVs less than 1.1%. Measurement error in sizing identical bands within a single gel (intra-assay precision), and the variation between repeated readings, were found to be comparatively low. Laboratories have reported precision values ranging from 0.6% to 2.0% of the measured band size (Baird, et al., 1986; Gjertson, et al., 1990). The methods described in this report have demonstrated a comparable level of precision. Furthermore, based on these results, an overall band sizing error of 2.0% would seem to be adequately conservative for use in determining the exclusion or non-exclusion of accused putative fathers, and in constructing band frequency binning charts. The determination of band sizing accuracy using the HeLa cell line revealed differences of 1.1% to 7.9% between the mean band sizes measured in this laboratory, and values reported by the supplier of four of the probes tested. This rather large discrepancy was most likely due to differences in analytical techniques. The results did however reveal that size estimates were similar (differences of 100 to 400 base pairs). Also the mean values determined by us will serve as an internal assay reference source in an ongoing quality control program.

REFERENCES

Baird M, Balazs I, Giusti A, Miyazaki L, Nicholas L, Wexler K, Kanter E, Glassberg J, Allen F, Rubinstein P, Sussman L. (1986) Allele frequency distribution of two highly polymorphic DNA sequences in three ethnic groups and its application to the determination of paternity. Am J Hum Genet 39:489-501

Budowle B, Giusti AM, Wayne JS, Baechtel FS, Fourney RM, Adams DE, Presley A, Deadman HA, Monson KL (1991) Fixed-bin analysis for statistical evaluation of continuous distributions of allelic data from VNTR loci, for use in forensic comparisons Am J Hum Genet 48:841-855

Gjertson DW, Hopfield J, Lachenbruch PA, Mickey MR, Sublett T., Yuge C., Terasaki PI (1990) Measurement error in determination of band size for highly polymorphic single-locus DNA markers. In: Polesky HF, Mayr WR (eds) Advances in Forensic Hemogenetics, Vol 3. Springer, Berlin-Heidelberg, p3

Maniatis T, Fritsch EF, Sambrook J (1982) Molecular cloning. A Laboratory Manual. Cold Spring Harbor Laboratory Press, Cold Spring Harbor

Southern EM (1979) Measurement of DNA length by gel electrophoresis Anal Biochem 100:319-323

A SIMPLE METHOD TO PREVENT INHIBITION OF TAQ POLYMERASE AND HINFI RESTRICTION ENZYME IN DNA ANALYSIS OF STAIN MATERIAL

W. Pflug*, G. Mai, G. Wahl, S. Aab, B. Eberspächer, U. Keller
Landeskriminalamt Baden-Württemberg, Stuttgart, Germany

Introduction

In forensic science case work DNA analysis of restriction fragment length polymorphisms (RFLP's) and amplified fragment length polymorphisms (AmpFLP's) have become the most powerful methods. But when working with different stain material (i.e. bloodstains, semenstains or vaginal secretions) which may be found on a variety of clothing and other objects, these carriers may interfere with the extraction and subsequent purification of DNA. In some of these cases this prevents restriction and/or amplification. Especially when analyzing cigarette tips restriction with HinfI and amplification with Taq polymerase may be inhibited. The addition of bovine serum albumin (BSA - Serva, Heidelberg) to the reaction mixture can decrease or overcome these inhibition problems.

Methods

DNA extraction and purification was carried out by standard protocols using Phenol/Chloroform reagents. Restriction of DNA was done with restriction enzyme HinfI (Boehringer, Mannheim). Amplification of Apo B 3'-Polymorphism (Boerwinkle et al., Schnee and Pflug) was carried out using 40 pmol of primers, 0.2 mM dNTP's in reaction buffer (10 mM Tris/HCl, pH 8.4), 2.5 mM MgCl$_2$, 50 mM KCl and a final volume of 50 μl, Taq Polymerase (2 U/reaction) came from Cetus Perkin Elmer. After an initial denaturation step of 2 min 27 cycles were carried out: 90 sec denaturation at 94° C, 90 sec annealing of the primers at 61° C, 2 min chain extension at 72° C. Amplified fragments were separated in 2 % agarose at 4 V/cm for about 7 hours.

Results

In our preliminary tests we added an equal amount (about 500 ng) of the same control DNA to each proteinase-K-digest for standardisation. Thus we got equal and good visible amounts of DNA after electrophoresis and staining with Ethidium bromide. **Prior** to the restriction an aliquot (1/10 volume) was taken from each DNA extract for the amplification of the Apo B 3'-region. Each aliquot was first split into two samples comprising one part and 9 parts respectively for parallel amplification. The total amount of DNA for ampflification was therefore about 45 ng and 5 ng respectively. The results show, that BSA can completely avoid inhibition of HinfI restriction enzyme. Dialysis of the DNA prior to restriction had no positive effect but led to a loss of DNA (Fig. 1A). Comparable results can be demonstrated for Taq Polymerase (Fig. 1B).

Advances in Forensic Haemogenetics 4
Edited by Ch. Rittner and P. M. Schneider
© Springer-Verlag Berlin Heidelberg 1992

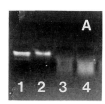
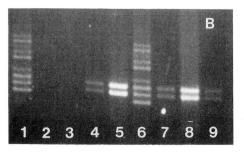

Fig. 1: Control DNA (500 ng aliquots) mixed with proteinase-K digest of
cigarette tips and subsequent:

A restriction with HinfI: -DNA (1); standard restriction
assay (2); standard assay + dialysis +0,1 % BSA (3); standard
assay + 0,1 % BSA (4)

B Amplification of Apo B fragments: marker (1,6); standard
amplification assay containing 5 ng and 45 ng of control-DNA
respectively (2,3); standard assay + dialysis + 0,1 % BSA
(4,5); standard assay + 0,1 % BSA (7,8); pure control-DNA (9)

The addition of BSA to the DNA extract prevents inhibition and gives a
clearly visible band pattern of Apo B-fragments. Without BSA no amplification occurs. The effect of BSA takes place within a concentration of
0,5 % - 0,005 %.

In addition, Fig. 2, shows the amplified Apo B fragments of DNA extracted
from cigarette tips used by different individuals. The DNA extract was
divided into two parts and 0,1 % BSA was added to one part.
As shown in Fig. 2 only the reaction mixture supplemented with BSA gives
a clearly visible band pattern.

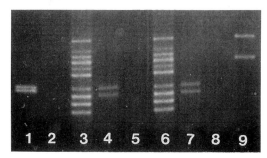

Fig. 2: Amplification of DNA extracted from cigarette tips smoked by
different individuals: with 0,1 % BSA (1, 4, 7) and without BSA
(2, 5, 8); marker consisting of a mixture of different Apo B
fragments (3, 6); pos. control (9)

We often got comparable results regarding inhibition effects of Taq Polymerase with DNA extracts coming from vaginal secretions (supernatants of
semen/vaginal secretion mixtures) and sometimes with bloodstains from
dirty clothing or other objects. By adding BSA we were able to overcome

these inhibition effects. Fig. 3 shows the PCR results of some blood-stains. The amplification mixtures without BSA do not show any signals even on x-ray films after blotting and subsequent hybridisation with non-radioactive chemiluminescence labeled probe.

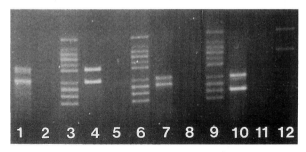

Fig. 3: Amplification of DNA extracted from bloodstains: aliquots
        supplemented with 0,1 % BSA (1, 4, 7, 10) and without BSA (2, 5,
        8, 11) were analyzed; marker (3, 6, 9); pos. control (12)

References

Boerwinkle, F, Xiong, W, Fourest, E and Chan, L (1989) Rapid typing of
    tandemly repeated hypervariable loci by the polymerase chain reaction:
    Application to the apolipoprotein B 3'hypervariable region
    Proc. Natl. Acad. Sci., 86, 212 - 216

Schnee, J and Pflug, W (1990) Apolipoprotein B 3'Length Polymorphismus:
    Frequency distribution of the Alleles in the German population
    First Int. Conference of DNA Fingerprinting, University of Bern

Optimal Size Calling Methods for Electrophoretic Analysis Utilizing Internal Size Standards

K. Corcoran*, E. Mayrand*, J. Robertson*, T. Shaefer** and M. Kronick*

*Applied Biosystems, Inc., Foster City, CA, USA
**Applied Biosystems, GmbH, Weiterstadt, Germany

A technically demanding problem in analytical genetics is quantitative matching of electrophoretic bands. The number usually associated with a match in forensic science is the size of the nucleic acid molecule in base pairs. Unfortunately, there are many inherent difficulties in the accurate quantitative determination of the size of DNA fragments.

A significant problem associated with size determination is lane-to-lane variation in DNA mobility due to differences in such parameters as salt concentration, amount of DNA loaded, thermal gradients, band location on the gel, and ethidium bromide band shifting effects. By utilizing the fluorescence emission differences of two different dyes, it is possible to place the size ladder in the same lane as the unknown. The ladder fragments and the sample DNA are labeled with the two different fluorophores, respectively. To eliminate errors due to lane-to-lane differences, we have utilized such an in-lane size ladder, which fluoresces in red, to construct a standard curve with which we calculate the sizes of products from PCR reactions utilizing either blue, green, or yellow fluorescing 5'-end labeled primers.

Another problem of major concern is that DNA fragments may interact with the gel matrix in ways that are governed by their DNA sequence, so that mobility is no longer just a function of size. Thus, when such a scenario is operative, two fragments of the same size in base pairs may not co-migrate; whereas, two fragments of dissimilar size may migrate at the same rate. In this communication, we present two size ladders, each of which possesses a band that migrates in an anomalous manner.

Using red labeled fragments from an Alu I digest of pBR322, we constructed calibration curves and calculated the lengths of the Collagen 2A1 VNTR alleles using four different approaches. Calibration curves are obtained from either a cubic splines or second order curve fitting procedure. We also determined the sizes of the alleles using the reciprocal relationship between fragment length and mobility described by E. M. Southern (Edinburgh), using either three points from the size ladder (local form), or all the points (global form). We calculated the sizes of the alleles first with all the restriction fragments included in the size ladder and then calculated using the ladder lacking the 695 bp fragment, which runs as a 708 bp band on agarose gels. We examined DNA samples from 100 unrelated Caucasians for the VNTR locus Collagen 2A1 using the PCR and primers labeled at the 5'-end with fluorophores. The samples were run on 2% agarose gels for 6 h in the Applied Biosystems Model 362 Fluorescent Fragment Analyzer.

The data obtained from 8 samples are depicted in Table 1. It is apparent from the data in the Table that the cubic splines and second order least squares curve fitting procedures yield significantly different results when the size ladder contains the 695 fragment. The results obtained with the reciprocal method are quite different, too, depending on whether a local or global approach is utilized. Note that the sizes obtained with the cubic splines and local Southern methods are similar, as are the data obtained with the second order least squares and global Southern methods.

Advances in Forensic Haemogenetics 4
Edited by Ch. Rittner and P. M. Schneider
© Springer-Verlag Berlin Heidelberg 1992

Table 1. Size Calls of the Collagen 2A1 VNTR Alleles Calculated with the Alu pBR322 Size Ladder either *Containing* the 695 bp Fragment or *Without* the 695 Fragment

| lane | With the 695 Fragment | | | | Without the 695 Fragment | | | |
	cubic splines	2nd order least squares	Southern local	global	cubic splines	2nd order least squares	Southern local	global
1	684	668	679	667	671	670	671	668
2	685,696	670,705	680,696	669,703	673,709	672,707	673,709	670,705
3	685	670	681	668	673	672	673	670
4	685,695	669,702	680,695	668,700	672,706	672,704	672,705	669,701
5	685	669	681	668	673	672	673	669
6	619,685	602,668	641,680	601,667	602,672	605,671	603,672	660,669
7	686,710	671,744	682,705	670,743	675,750	674,747	675,750	671,745
8	686	671	681	669	674	674	674	671

The two repeats reported for Collagen 2A1 from sequencing work are 31 and 34 bp, respectively. When we look for a repeat size pattern in the data set obtained with the complete size ladder, we only see a reasonable correlation with the reported repeat length in the data set obtained with either the second order least squares or the global Southern methods: a repeat of about 30 bp is readily apparent. The data obtained by the other two methods, however, give no indication of what the repeat length might be. In fact, this set indicates there might be partial alleles! Examination of 80 other DNA samples from non-related individuals yielded results similar to those presented here. Also in the Table, we show the results obtained from the four calculations when the anomalously running 695 fragment was deleted from the size ladder by the software. Now, all four methods yield similar results. It is apparent that the repeat pattern is indeed about 30 base pairs.

Figure 1 illustrates two size ladders obtained from restriction digests of either plasmid or phage DNA. Shown are curve fits to the data by either the cubic splines or second order least squares methods. Upon examination of the cubic splines curves, one observes a point, which acts as an origin of irregularity in the flow of the line, caused by the fact that the cubic splines line must pass through each point. Now, if the DNA of unknown length falls within the boundary of the irregularity, it is obvious that the estimation of its size will be weighed by the effect of the anomalously running band of the size ladder on the form of the calibration curve. The second order curves form smoothly flowing lines, and no single point seems to influence the shape of the curve. Rather, one can see that the 695 fragment in the Alu I pBR322 curve and the 508 fragment in the Pst I Lambda curve migrate atypically during electrophoresis, because they lie somewhat off the line describing the best fit. The sequence of these fragments probably contain some subtle feature that causes an unusual interaction with the gel matrix.

Next, we let the software ignore the point corresponding to the fragment that seems to be irregular and see if the cubic splines curve becomes similar to that described by the second order least squares method. In the series of curves depicted in Fig. 2, the fragments 695 and 508 are deleted from the Alu I pBR322 and Pst I Lambda ladders, respectively. The cubic spline curve fits of these methods are shown in the figure and it is observed that theh approach the form of the second order curve fits illustrated in Fig. 1. This result explains why the sizes of the Collagen 2A1 alleles presented in Table 1 are dissimilar with the cubic splines and the second order least squares methods: the alleles fell in the region of irregularity on the calibration curve.

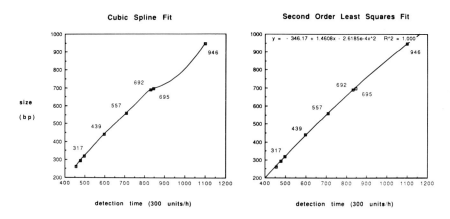

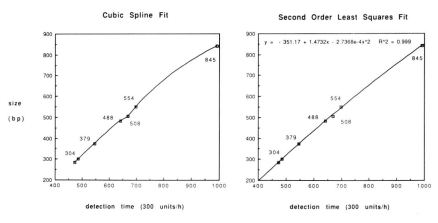

Fig. 1. Two examples showing different curve fitting procedures do not always yield similar results (shown above). Details are given in the text

Fig. 2. Removal of bands with irregular mobility from the size ladder can cause different curve fitting methods to yield similar results (shown on the right). See the text for details

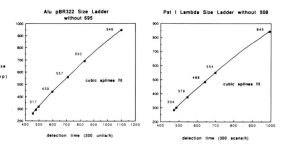

EXTRACTION OF DNA FROM COAGULATED BLOOD SAMPLES

Richard Scheithauer, Hans-Joachim Weisser

Institute for Forensic Medicine
University of Freiburg, Albertstr. 9, 7800 Freiburg, FRG

INTRODUCTION

In forensic medicine, blood samples available for case work are
coagulated predominantly. Following routine manuals, yield of
DNA is irregular and sometimes low.

MATERIALS

■ 9 blood samples of ca. 10 ml were taken from one donor at one
time. No anticoagulating agent was present. Tubes were stored
vertically for one night at room temperature. Following
procedures are shown in the figure.

*Subdivision of
blood samples*

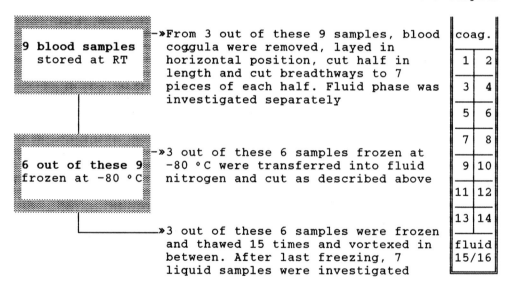

■ Other samples were dried as a whole and grinded.

METHODS

■ All samples were incubated overnight in an extraction buffer
(Bär et al. 1988) containing 400 µg/ml Proteinase K at 56 °C.

■ Just one series was pretreated prior to DNA extraction with
Protease Type VIII from *bacillus licheniformis* for 5 h at 37 °C
with a concentration of 400 µg/ml (7 pieces of the coagula each
of the first three blood samples stored at RT and cut half in

Advances in Forensic Haemogenetics 4
Edited by Ch. Rittner and P. M. Schneider
© Springer-Verlag Berlin Heidelberg 1992

length; pieces No. 2,4,6,8,10,12, and 14 and the fluid phase 16; see figure).

▌ Deproteinization by one phenol/chloroform/isoamyl alcohol and one chloroform/isoamyl alcohol extraction. The isolated DNA was resuspended in 40 µl TE pH 7,4, applied on a membrane filter (Type VM, pore size 0,05 µm; Millipore) and dialyzed for 2 h against TEN buffer pH 7.4 (10 mM Tris-HCl, 1 mM EDTA, 10 mM NaCl) at RT (Gill 1987).

▌ DNA concentration was determined by UV spectrophotometry (260 nm)

RESULTS

	Series 1a Stored at RT Not pretreated	Series 1b Stored at RT Pretreated	Series 2 Stored at -80 °C Fluid nitrogen
coag.			
1 2 →»»	2,37	2,98	3,11
3 4 →»»	2,87	3,25	3,64
5 6 →»»	2,59	3,43	3,64
7 8 →»»	3,00	3,28	2,83
9 10 →»»	2,93	3,19	3,75
11 12 →»»	3,26	3,82	4,60
13 14 →»»	2,57	3,61	3,51
fluid 15/16 →»»	1,07	1,03	

	Series 3 15 freeze/ thaw cycles	Series 4 Dried blood coagula	Series 5 Dried blood fluid phase
All samples	6,44	2,17	1,16

Average amount of DNA obtained from pieces of coagula and remaining fluid in µg/100 mg liquid blood

CONCLUSIONS

■ No characteristic distribution of DNA concentration was found in blood coagula, although blood samples were stored in vertically standing tubes immediately after removal

■ Yield of DNA recovered from coagula is irregular

■ Pretreatment of coagula with a protease prior to extraction showed slight effect

■ Liquid phase contains only little DNA

■ Drying and grinding blood is not advantageous

■ Reproducible high yield was obtained after numerous freeze/thaw cycles and vortexing in between

REFERENCES

Andersson M, Böhme J, Andersson G, Möller E, Thorsby E, Rask L, Peterson PA (1984) Genomic hybridization with class II transplantation antigen cDNA probes as a complementary technique in tissue typing. Human Immunol 11:57-67

Baechtel FS (1988) Recovery of DNA from human biological specimens. Crime Lab Digest 15:95-96

Bär W, Kratzer A, Mächler M, Schmid W (1988) Postmortem stability of DNA. Forensic Sci Int 39:59-70

Gill P (1987) A new method for sex determination of the donor of forensic samples using a recombinant DNA probe. Electrophoresis 8:35-38

Jeanpierre M (1987) A rapid method for the purification of DNA from blood. Nucl Acid Res 15:9611

Kanter E, Baird M, Shaler R, Balazs I (1986) Analysis of restricition fragment length polymorphisms in deoxyribonucleic acid (DNA) recovered from dried bloodstains. J Forensic Sci 31:403-408

Kunkel LM, Smith KD, Boyer SH, Borgaonkar DS, Wachtel SS, Miller OJ, Breg WR, Jones HW, Ray JM (1977) Analysis of human Y-chromosome-specific reiterated DNA in chromosome variants. Proc Natl Acad USA 74:1245-1248

Prinz M, Berghaus G (1990) The effect of various stain carriers on the quality and quantity of DNA extracted from dried blood stains. Z Rechtsmed 103:191-197

Investigation of variation in fragment size determinations found when using single locus DNA probes

J.A. Thomson, T. Fedor*, M. Gouldstone*, P.J. Lincoln, C.P. Phillips, D. Syndercombe Court, V. Tate*, and P.H. Watts

Department of Haematology, The London Hospital Medical College, Turner Street, London E1 2AD, UK
University Diagnostics Ltd, Gower Street, London WC1E 6BR, UK*

When using single locus probes the assignment of a fragment's size is relatively straight forward, but it is essential to have knowledge of the variability that can occur in that assessment before the results can be fully interpreted. When 'matching' consideration must be taken of whether the samples were run on the same gel, on different gels within the same laboratory, or on different gels in different laboratories.

We have made assessments of variability of results by comparing bands from mother-child pairs, run in adjacent tracks of the same gel, and by repeated testing of the same DNA sample on different gels within the same laboratory. Also we have used a series of blood samples to prepare DNA autoradiographs in two separate laboratories using four probes. We have used both a ruler and image analysis methods to size the fragments on both sets of autoradiographs.

METHODS

3μg samples of <u>Alu1</u>-digested DNA from whole blood samples were electrophoresed, blotted and hybridised by each laboratory's standard methods. The probes used were 3'α-HVR, MR24/1, Muc-7 (Amersham Int), TBQ7 and YNH24 (Promega Corp). Fragment sizes were estimated, either using a ruler or by image analysis (Biotrac: Foster and Freeman), using the local form of the reciprocal relationship $c=(m-m_o)(L-L_o)$ as described by Elder and Southern (1987). The DNA size markers used were a 14-rung ^{35}S-labelled ladder (Amersham Int).

RESULTS

A series of 394 pairwise comparisons of fragment sizes of corresponding bands in mother-child pairs were made. The differences in the measured fragment sizes of these pairs are expressed as percentages of the child's fragment size (Fig. 1). Based on these results we consider that a named man is a possible father if he has a fragment within +/-2.5% of the paternal fragment in the child. This 2.5% corresponds to a confidence interval of 99.999%.

Advances in Forensic Haemogenetics 4
Edited by Ch. Rittner and P. M. Schneider
© Springer-Verlag Berlin Heidelberg 1992

Table 1. Cases not resolved by conventional testing alone

CONVENTIONAL TESTING   DNA TESTING

Possible exclusion evidence   Result

	PI (Conventional)	No. probes excluding	PI (DNA)
No exclusions - 2 other children in family excluded	15	Excluded 3/4	
No exclusions - incomplete test	2	Excluded 2/5	
Probable Rh exclusion	3	Excluded 3/4	
Fy 2^{O} order exclusion	10	Excluded 3/4	
EAP 2^{O} order exclusion	2	Excluded 5/5	
PLG 2^{O} order exclusion	24	Excluded 3/3	
Gc 2^{O} order exclusion	10	Excluded 4/4	
HLA only exclusion - B and C loci	11	Excluded 5/5	
Glo 1^{O} order exclusion	3	Excluded 3/4	
ESD 1^{O} order exclusion	350	Excluded 3/4	
Fy 2^{O} order exclusion	110	Not excluded 0/4	100
PLG 2^{O} order exclusion	36	Not excluded 0/4	500

The cases were not randomly selected. All cases are initially
investigated using the conventional systems. DNA testing is
performed only when these fail to produce sufficient evidence
to resolve the case, or when specifically requested. The cases
chosen for DNA testing are therefore biased towards those with
low PI values, or those with only one system showing an
exclusion of paternity after investigation of conventional
polymorphisms.

Figure 1. illustrates that, using DNA testing alone (and with a
wide +/-5% window to interrogate the database), paternity
indices of greater than 100 were achieved in virtually all
cases, provided at least four of the probes selected for this
study were used. The combined use of these DNA probes and
conventional polymorphisms gives consistently high PIs and
corresponding RCPs: all cases (often selected for their low PI
values) where no exclusion was found, gave an RCP of >99.9%
when at least four probes had been successfully applied.

An estimation of the power of exclusion has been made for each
probe by constructing false trios whereby mother-child pairs
are compared with an unrelated man's sample on the same gel
using the +/-2.5% band match criteria. Results from 335 false
families (see Table 2) show a combined exclusion rate of
99.99989% (which increases to 99.999997% when combined with the
expected exclusion rate for conventional tests). 63 men
(18.8%) were not excluded by one out of the range of probes
used, but only 3 men (0.89%) had not been excluded when at
least two probes were used. Use of further probes excluded all
false fathers.

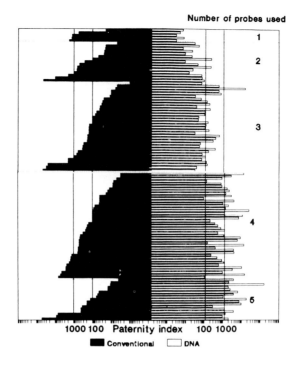

Fig. 1. Comparison of paternity indices provided by
conventional testing and up to five single locus probes (n=114)

Table 2. Exclusion rates for DNA probes

	Muc 7	3'α-HVR	MR24	YNH24	TBQ7
False trios created	269	83	275	257	138
Exclusion rate	88.5%	85.8%	97.1%	94.9%	95.6%

OPTIMIZATION OF THE DIGOXIGENIN/CHEMILUMINESCENCE METHOD FOR THE VNTR DETECTION

Dimo-Simonin N, Brandt-Casadevall C, Gujer H-R

Institut universitaire de médecine légale, Bugnon 21
1005 Lausanne, Switzerland

INTRODUCTION

The non-isotopic digoxigenin method provides a feasible alternative to the radioactive-system for the human VNTR determination. Initially, the digoxigenin probes were used in conjunction with colorimetric detection of DNA fragments [1, 2].Then, it was shown that direct chemiluminescent detection enhanced the sensitivity. Furthermore, reprobing was easier with this technique since no colorimetric precipitate needed to be removed [1, 3, 4, 5]. On the other hand, direct chemiluminescence with AMPPD seemed to be more efficient and more flexible compared to luminol-based enhanced chemiluminescent system [6]. However the remaining problem of limited sensitivity is caused by the background from non specific binding of the anti-digoxigenin-alkaline phosphatase conjugate [7].

The aim of our investigation was to improve the resolution of the VNTR band patterns detection. In this respect, we have optimized parameters such as capillary transfer, fixation, hybridization, stringency washes and detection.

METHOD

3 μg saline-extracted genomic DNA was digested with Hinf I (5U/μg) and size-fractionned on a 0.8 % agarose-gel (Seakem-Gold) for 20h at 35V. It was then transfered by capillary blotting to charged nylon membranes (Sigma) and hybridized with 12 ng/mL digoxigenin-labeled pYNH24 probe (Promega). The DNA-fragments were detected with a chemiluminescent system (AMPPD or CSPD - Tropix).

Parameter optimization :

Capillary transfer to charged nylon membranes (Sigma) with Quick-draw blotting paper (Sigma) for 2h in :
- NaOH 0.4 M
- 10xSSC
- NH$_4$Cl 1M

Fixation :
- UV 245 nm for 15 or 30 sec
- UV 302 nm for 2 min
- baking at 80 °C for 30 min
- UV 302 nm for 2 min and baking at 80 °C for 30 min after a brief alkaline denaturation step followed by neutralization

Hybridization at 68 °C for 20h in 5xSSC / 0.1% N-Lauroylsarcosine / 0.02% SDS with 2.5% I-Light blocking reagent (Tropix) and
- 5% dextran sulfate or,
- 2%, 4%, 6% PEG

Stringency washes in :
- 2xSSC / 0.1% SDS, twice for 5 min at room temperature and 0.1xSSC / 0.1% SDS twice for 15 min at 68 °C
- 2xSSC / 0.1% SDS, twice for 5 min at room temperature and 0.5xSSC / 0.1% SDS twice for 15 min at 68 °C
- 1xSSC / 5% SDS, twice for 20 min at room temperature

Advances in Forensic Haemogenetics 4
Edited by Ch. Rittner and P. M. Schneider
© Springer-Verlag Berlin Heidelberg 1992

Chemiluminescent detection with 0.1 mg/mL AMPPD in :
  - 0.05M Na$_2$CO$_3$/NaHCO$_3$ and 1mM MgCl$_2$ at pH 9.5
  - 0.1M Diethanolamine (DEA) / 1mM MgCl$_2$ and 0.02% NaN$_3$ at pH 10 with and without enhancer substances as albumin and PEG

Chemiluminescent detection with 0.1 mg/mL CSPD (Tropix) in 0.1M DEA buffer at pH 10

RESULTS AND DISCUSSION

Capillary transfer (2h) in 10xSSC with Quick draw blotting paper (Sigma) resulted in the maximal signal/noise ratio. Alkali transfer seemed to be incompatible with digoxigenin-YNH24, and NH$_4$Cl transfer generated a greater background.

Cross-linking at 302 nm enhanced the signal of the bands with respect to baking at 80 °C and decreased the background with respect to UV at 245 nm [8, 9]. It is important to determine the amount of irradiation required in order to prevent the overirradiation of the membrane and to produce the maximum hybridization signal.
Alkali treatment after UV and baking fixation decreased the sensitivity and increased the background (Fig.1).

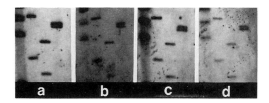

Fig. 1. Cross-linking:

a: at 302 nm
b: at 302 nm after alkali treatment
c: at 80 °C
d: at 80 °C after alkali treatment

Hybridization achieved with the I-light blocking reagent (Tropix) produced optimal results. Hybridization with 5% dextran sulfate reduced background and sensitivity. Hybridization with 2% and 4% PEG decreased the resolution, while using 6% PEG, the sensitivity as well as the background were increased (Fig.2). The greater sensitivity can be attributed to the volumetric exclusion of the probe from the polymer solution and so their effective concentration is increased. On the other hand, a viscous solution can produce a high background [10].

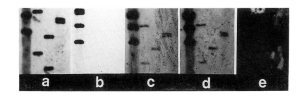

Fig. 2. Hybridization at 68 °C for 20h in 5xSSC and 2.5% I-Light blocking reagent : **a)** with 0.1% N-Lauroyl-sarcosine and 0.02% SDS, **b)** with 2.5% dextran sulfate, **c)** with 2% PEG, **d)** with 4% PEG, **e)** with 6% PEG

Post-hybridization washing with 1xSSC and 5% SDS, twice for 20 min at room temperature gave the best resolution. The background was greatly reduced, and consequently film exposure of 16h and more enhanced the signal of the bands against a relatively clear background. On the other hand washing with 0.5xSSC at 68 °C resulted in almost the same sensitivity but against increased background. In general, the washing conditions should be as stringent as possible [10]. In our assays, we have determined empirically that with low stringency washes (1xSSC instead 0.1xSSC at room temperature) and a higher SDS concentration (5% instead 0.1%), maximal sensitivity without additional bands, and lower background were obtained (Fig.3).

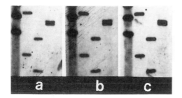

Fig. 3. Stringency washes in :
a) 2xSSC / 0.1%SDS, twice for 5 min at RT and 0.1xSSC / 0.1% SDS twice for 5 min at 68 °C
b) 2xSSC / 0.1% SDS, twice for 5 min at R.T. and 0.5xSSC / 0.1% SDS, twice for 15 min at 68 °C
c) 1xSSC / 5% SDS, twice for 20 min at RT

Membrane blocking : increasing the blocking reagent concentration to 2% (instead 1%), eliminating the washing step between the blocking and antibody binding step and diluting the anti-digoxigenin antibody into the blocking solution improved the sensitivity, decreased the noise and thus allowed a longer exposure time.

Chemiluminescent detection with AMPPD (Tropix) in 0.1M DEA buffer at pH 10 significantly increased the sensitivity compared to carbonate buffer at pH 9.5 [11] and we could detect quantities as small as 60 ng of genomic DNA (Fig.4). Furthermore, the addition of 1% albumine seemed to slightly reduce the background with both carbonate and DEA buffers.

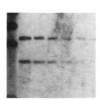

Fig. 4. Genomic DNA titration
detected with digoxigenin-labeled pYNH24 and AMPPD (16h film exposure)
From left to right : 2 μg, 1 μg, 500 ng 250 ng, 125 ng, 60 ng

Chemiluminescent detection with CSPD (Tropix) in 0.1M DEA buffer at pH 10 showed a greater resolution of DNA VNTR-bands in comparison to AMPPD at the beginning of the light-emission (1-3 h after substrate addition) while the genomic patterns were stronger with AMPPD after 16-20h of substrate addition and the lambda-DNA bands were more diffuse (Fig.5). These findings corresponded to results already reported [12].

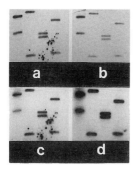

Fig. 5. Chemiluminescent detection
a) with CSPD after 2h.
b) with AMPPD after 2h
c) with CSPD after 16h
d) with AMPPD after 16h

CONCLUSION

The digoxigenin-chemiluminescence is a simple and convenient method for VNTR determination with a sensitivity limit up to 60 ng genomic DNA insofar as the critical parameters previously described are optimized. In this respect, we actually use the following parameters for the detection of the D2S44 locus with digoxigenin-labeled pYNH24:
- capillary transfer to charged nylon membrane Sigma in 10xSSC
- cross-linking at 302 nm for 2 min
- hybridization at 68 °C for 20h. in 5xSSC with 0.1% N-Lauroyl-sarcosine /
  0.02%SDS and 2.5% I-light blocking reagent
- two low stringency washes in 1xSSC and 5% SDS for 20 min each at RT
- membrane blocking in 2 % I-light blocking reagent
- dilution of anti-digoxigenin antibody in blocking reagent
- no washing step between the blocking and antibody binding step
- chemiluminescent detection with 0.1 mg/mL AMPPD or CSPD in 0.1M DEA
  buffer at pH 10

REFERENCES

1. Martin R, Hoover C, Grimme S, Grogan C, Höltke J, Kessler C (1990) A highly sensitive nonradioactive DNA labeling and detection system. Biotechniques 9 : 762-768

2. Dimo-Simonin N, Brandt-Casadevall C, Gujer H-R (1991) Digoxigenin-DNA probes for detecting human VNTR polymorphism. DNA-Technology and its forensic application ed. by Berghaus G, Brinkmann B, Rittner C, Staak M , Springer-Verlag (in press)

3. Brandt-Casadevall C, Dimo-Simonin N, Gujer HR (1991) Recherche en paternité et ADN. J Med Legale Droit Medical (in press)

4. Lanzillo JJ (1991) Chemiluminescent nucleic acid detection with digoxigenin-labeled probes : A model system with probes for angiotensin converting enzyme which detect less than one attomole of target DNA. Anal. Biochem. 194 : 45-53

5. Tizard R, Cate RL, Ramachandran KL, Wysk M, Voyta JC, Murphy OJ, Bronstein I (1990) Imaging of DNA with chemiluminescence. Proc. Natl. Acad. Sci. USA 87 : 4514-4518

6. Beck S, Köster H (1990) Applications of dioxetane chemiluminescent probes to molecular biology. Anal. Chem. 62 : 2258-2270

7. Bronstein I, Voyta JC, Lazzari KG, Murphy O, Brooks E, Kricka LJ (1990) Rapid and sensitive detection of DNA in Southern blots with chemiluminescence. Biotechniques 8 : 310-314

8. Khandjian EW (1987) Optimized hybridization of DNA blotted and fixed to nitrocellulose and nylon membranes. Biotechnology 5 : 165-167

9 Tara AT, Krawetz SA (1990) Parameters affecting hybridization of nucleic acids blotted onto nylon or nitrocellulose membranes. Biotechniques 8 : 478-481

10. Maniatis T, Fritsch EF, Sambrook J (1989) Molecular cloning. A laboratory manual. Cold Spring Harbor Laboratory Publication, New-York, p 9.50

11. Bronstein I, Voyta JC, Lazzari KG, Murphy O, Edwards B, Kricka LJ (1990) Improved chemiluminescent detection of alkaline phosphatase. Biotechniques 9:160-161

12. Martin C, Bresnick L, Juo R-R, Voyta JC, Bronstein I (1991) Improved chemiluminescent DNA sequencing. Biotechniques 11 : 110-113

2.3   Practical Application

PATERNITY ANALYSIS USING THE MULTILOCUS DNA PROBE MZ 1.3

Peter M. Schneider[1], Rolf Fimmers[2], Ulrike Schacker[1] and Christian Rittner[1]

[1]Institut für Rechtsmedizin der Johannes Gutenberg-Universität Mainz, Am Pulverturm 3, 6500 Mainz; [2]Institut für Medizinische Statistik der Universitätsklinik Bonn, FRG

The multilocus minisatellite DNA probe MZ 1.3 detects hypervariable restriction fragment patterns in genomic DNA of man and animals. It can be used for segregation analysis in cases of disputed paternity (Schacker et al., 1991; Rittner et al., 1991a), for identification purposes in forensic medicine and stain analysis (Ogata et al., 1990; Rittner et al., 1991b), as well as in animal breeding for pedigree analysis and verification of inbred strains (Hins & Gruber, 1991). Hypervariable fragment patterns can be generated by using frequently cutting restriction enzymes, e.g. Hinf I, Hae III, Msp I, Mbo I, and Rsa I. A non-radioactive system using the digoxigenin anti-digoxigenin system may be used for the detection of polymorphic fragments (B.E.S.T. Probe MZ 1.3, Biotest AG, Dreieich, FRG). Using this method, less than 1 µg of human genomic DNA can be detected (see Fig. 1). If sufficient genomic DNA is available for study, two parallel restriction enzyme digestions, e.g. using Hinf I and Hae III, should be carried out simultaneously as a control for the possible appearance of unassignable bands due to partially digested DNA (Schacker et al., 1991).

For the application of multilocus DNA probes in paternity testing, two parameters are important and have to be studied separately: 1. the number of non-maternal bands in the child and the presence of all these bands in the putative father, and 2. the band sharing rate to investigate the proportion of identical bands between putative father and child. The number of informative bands can be obtained by directly comparing the DNA profiles of mother and child. In a recent collaborative family study using MZ 1.3 (Schneider et al., submitted), a mean number of 9.8 ± 3.8 informative fragments was observed. A single unassignable band due to a mutation during meiosis was only found in one out of 50 offspring on the basis of 786 meioses. The mean band sharing rate was approximately 20% among unrelated individuals and 57% in parent/child comparisons. A band sharing rate in the range of 40 - 45% may indicate a possible second degree relationship, e.g. when the putative father is the brother of the true father. The band sharing information may also be useful in deficiency cases by including parents, siblings, and legitimate children of a deceased putative father into the analysis (Rittner et al., submitted). In these cases, however, it is advisable to use all available information including blood group analysis.

Advances in Forensic Haemogenetics 4
Edited by Ch. Rittner and P. M. Schneider
© Springer-Verlag Berlin Heidelberg 1992

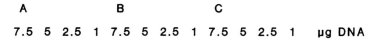

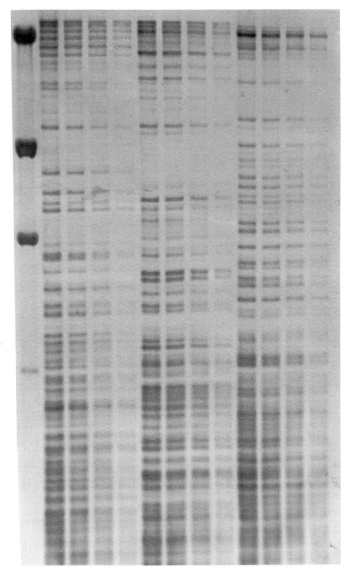

Fig. 1. Hybridisation of the digoxigenin-labelled probe MZ 1.3 to Hinf I-digested genomic DNA samples of three unrelated individuals (A-C). For each individual, total DNA amounts of 7.5 - 1 µg have been loaded. *Left lane:* size marker (*top to bottom:* 23.1/9.4/6.6/4.3 kb)

The data of the collaborative study have been used to determine the frequency distribution of polymorphic fragments detected by MZ 1.3 in a population sample of 694 unrelated individuals. Using a linear scale for the x axis in ln(kb) units which is proportional to the migration distance of DNA fragments in the gel, two frequency ranges were observed for fragments > 10 kb and < 10 kb. Thus it was possible to determine two size ranges with mean fragment frequencies of 0.15 (fragments > 10 kb) and 0.3 (fragments < 10 kb). These frequencies can easily be used to calculate probabilities for identity in cases of stain identification or exclusion probabilities in paternity cases based on the number of informative bands in the child (Fimmers et al., this volume). Using an example with seven non-maternal bands in the child (2 bands > 10 kb and 5 bands < 10 kb), the probability that a second unrelated man has the identical set of seven paternal fragments, is 5.47×10^{-5}, i.e. only one in 18,920 individuals. The application of multilocus probe analysis has also been described in a recent study of more than 1700 routine paternity cases using the probes 33.6 and 33.15 (Jeffreys et al., 1991). The authors could demonstrate the reliability of multilocus probes in paternity testing, although their probes exhibit a significantly higher mutation rate than MZ 1.3, They also suggest to use only the non-maternal bands as a basis for decision on paternity.

References

Fimmers R, Schneider PM, Baur MP. Comparison of different methods for the calculation of indices of paternity (this volume)

Hins J, Gruber FP. (1991) Genetisches Fingerprinting von Inzuchtlinien, Auszuchten, transgenen Individuen und 3T3-Zellen von *Mus musculus* mit der Sonde B.E.S.T. MZ 1.3. *J Vet Med* 38: 61-72

Jeffreys AJ, M Turner, P Debenham. (1991) The efficiency of multilocus DNA fingerprint probes for individualization and establishment of family relationships, determined from extensive casework. *Am J Hum Genet* 48: 824-840

Ogata M, Mattern R, Schneider PM, Schacker U, Kaufmann T, Rittner C. (1990) Quantitative and qualitative analysis of DNA extracted from postmortem muscle tissues. *Z Rechtsmed* 103: 397-406

Rittner C, U Schacker, PM Schneider. (1991) DNA fingerprinting as a tool of paternity testing in Germany. In: Berghaus G, B Brinkmann, C Rittner, M Staak (Hrg) *"DNA technology and its forensic application"*. Springer Heidelberg, 20-32

Rittner C, L Penzes, M Prager-Eberle, U Schacker, PM Schneider, U Jordan, V Schmidt, D Busse, HE Hildebrand, E Koops. (1991) DNA-Spurenanalyse. *Kriminalistik* 7: 439-442

Rittner C, MP Baur, G Rittner, PM Schneider. (1991) Zum Beitrag des DNA-Gutachtens in Fällen mit verstorbenen Putativvätern (sog. Defizienz-Fälle). (submitted for publication)

Schacker U, PM Schneider, B Holtkamp, E Bohnke, R Fimmers, HH Sonneborn, Rittner C. (1990) Isolation of DNA minisatellite probe MZ 1.3 and its application to DNA 'fingerprinting' analysis. *For Sci Int* 44: 209-244

Schacker U, T Kaufmann, PM Schneider, C Rittner. (1991) Reliability of restriction enzyme digestions of genomic DNA for the generation of DNA fingerprints. In: Berghaus G, B Brinkmann, C Rittner, M Staak (Hrg) *"DNA technology and its forensic application"*. Springer Verlag Heidelberg, 103-108

Schneider PM, Fimmers R, Bertrams J, Birkner P, Braunbeck K, Bulnheim U, Feuerbach M, Henke L, Iten E, Prinz M, Simeoni E, Rittner C. Biostatistical basis of individualization and segeration analysis using the multilocus DNA probe MZ 1.3: results of a collaborative study. (submitted for publication)

ANALYSIS OF AUSTRALIAN, BLACK, CAUCASIAN, CHINESE AND AMERINDIAN POPULATIONS WITH HYPERVARIABLE DNA LOCI

I. Balazs, J. Neuweiler, R.C. Williams[1], C. Lantz[2]

Lifecodes Corporation, Valhalla, NY

SUMMARY

Population genetic studies in australian aborigine, american black, chinese, caucasian and amerindian populations were performed with several highly polymorphic DNA loci. PstI-digested samples from random individuals were hybridized to probes recognizing 5 hypervariable loci (i.e. D2S44, D4S163, D14S13, D17S79, D18S27). Results showed that the american black population had the highest level of heterozygosity (92%) followed by caucasian (89%) and chinese (84%). In australians it was 78% while in the various amerindian populations it varied from 74 to 84%. In general, the distributions of DNA fragments show that the most common polymorphic DNA fragments of a locus were within the same size range in all populations. The distinguishing feature of each population was the relative frequency of particular group of alleles. Some of these allele groups showed statistically significant differences between some of the populations. For example, alleles >9.0 Kb in size, in D14S13, or from 4.5 to 4.7 Kb, in D18S27, were two or more times more rare in caucasians than in the other populations.

INTRODUCTION

The high level of heterogeneity found in several DNA loci containing variable number of tandem repeats has made them an extremely useful tool for the identification of individuals. Although the most of the initial evaluation of this type of loci was performed in the American caucasian or black population (Baird et al. 1986, Balazs et al. 1989, Chimera et al. 1989) other smaller populations have been examined (Flint et al. 1989, Kidd et al. 1991). The purpose of this report is to extend these studies to Chinese, Australian aborigine and several Amerindian populations of North America.

MATERIALS AND METHODS

Blood samples. DNA from North American caucasian and black individuals were obtained from samples submitted for paternity testing. Chinese samples represent Han individuals from different regions of China. Australian aborigines were collected from individuals in the Northern Territories. Samples of Amerindians from USA were

---

[1] Arizona State Univ., Dept. Antropology, Tempe, AZ
[2] Laim Dear Reservation, MT

Advances in Forensic Haemogenetics 4
Edited by Ch. Rittner and P. M. Schneider
© Springer-Verlag Berlin Heidelberg 1992

collected at three different indian reservations representing, Cheyenne, Navajo and Pima tribes. Samples from "Maya" individuals were collected in Mexico, in the Yucatan peninsula (Kidd et al.1991). DNA isolation, digestion with PstI, fractionation and hybridization was performed as described by Balazs et al.(1989).

RESULTS AND DISCUSSION

Analysis for several VNTR loci, in different populations shows similar size range distributions of DNA fragment sizes. The largest world populations (i.e. caucasian, black, chinese oriental) have the broadest distribution and highest heterogeneity in fragment sizes. This is partly reflected in the average heterozygosity of the 5 markers examined. The three major ethnic groups show the highest level of heterozygosity (i.e. black: 0.92; caucasian: 0.89; chinese: 0.83). However, native north american populations show a range of values from 0.72 to 0.84. This indicates that the variety of alleles in these four amerindian populations remains high. The heterozygosity of australian aborigines is similar to those of amerindians (i.e: 0.78).

The distinguishing feature of each population is the relative frequency of certain group or size ranges of DNA fragments. For example: in D2S44 DNA fragments in the 10 to 11 Kb size range are 2 to 3 times more common in amerindian, australians and chinese than in caucasians. D17S79 alleles, in the size range of 3.9 to 4.1 Kb and for D18S27 alleles, from 4.5 to 4.7 Kb, are 2 to 3 times more rare in caucasians than in all the other populations. D14S13 has a broad distribution of DNA fragment sizes in all populations, but alleles from 9 to 16 Kb in size are more common in australian, chinese and amerindian populations than in american black and caucasians. The most common D4S163 alleles were found between 6 and 9 Kb. Other rare alleles were found from about 3.4 to <6 Kb and from >9 to 16 Kb in size.

In summary, the analysis of several VNTR loci indicate that these genetic markers are very heterogeneous and highly informative in a large variety of populations. In addition, the application of more rigorous quantitative analysis of this type of data may be a useful tool for population genetic studies.

REFERENCES

Baird M, Balazs I, Giusti A, Miyasaki L, Nicholas L, an others (1986) Allele frequency distribution of two highly polymorphic DNA sequences in three ethnic groups and its application to the determination of paternity. Am J Human Genet 39:489-501

Balazs I, Baird M, Clyne M, Meade E (1989) Human population genetic studies of five hypervariable DNA loci. Am J Human Genet 44:182-190

Kidd JR, Black FL, Weiss KM, Balazs I, Kidd KK (1992) Studies of three amerindian populations using nuclear DNA polymorphisms. Human Biology, in press

Flint J, Boyce AJ, Martinson JJ, Cleg JB (1989) Population bottlenecks in polynesia revealed by minisatellites. Hum Genet 83:257-263

The Application of DNA-Polymorphisms in Paternity Testing

M. Basler, W. Sprecher, M. Rink, and K.-S. Saternus

Insititute of Legal Medicine, Georg-August-University, Windausweg 2, D-3400 Göttingen

INTRODUCTION

Most cases of disputed paternity can be adequately resolved by testing the conventional blood group, serum and enzyme systems, perhaps completed by testing the HLA system. The analysis of DNA polymorphisms is a very useful additional system for distinguishing falsly accused non-fathers from "true" fathers and for providing convincing evidence in favour of paternity in cases of non-exclusions. The purpose of this presentation is to report the results from some extraordinary paternity cases in which the analysis of DNA polymorphisms greatly helped clear up the paternity.

MATERIALS AND METHODS

Routine paternity testing consisted of the conventional serological analysis of the red cell antigen systems ABO, MNSs, Rhesus, Kell, P, Duffy, Kidd, Lutheran and Colton, the serum proteins Gm, Km, Hp, Gc, C3, Bf, Tf, PLG and Pi, the red cell enzymes acP, PGM_1, AK, ADA, 6-PGD, GPT, EsD and GLO, and leucocyte antigens HLA A, B, C by means of standard techniques.

DNA was extracted from EDTA-blood using a non-organic solvent procedure or, in some special cases, by phenol-chloroform extraction. After quantification and control for high molecular weight, 6 µg DNA were digested with the restriction enzymes Hae III or Hinf I at a concentration of 5 U/µg DNA following the manufacturer's specifications. Fractionation of DNA was performed by electrophoresis in 1% agarose, followed by Southern blotting and hybridisation with ^{32}P-labelled DNA probes, YNH24 (Promega), MS31 and g3 (ICI, Cellmark diagnostics). The radioactive fragments were visualized by autoradiography.

RESULTS

Case I: The parentage of a putative father as well as of a putative mother of two children was disputed. Investigations of the conventional systems resulted in a single second-order exclusion for both of the parents to child I. The parentage of child II was excluded for both in the HLA system. DNA polymorphisms resulted in two exclusions of the putative mother to child I and three exclusions to child II. For the putative father, only one exclusion was found to child I. Paternity was excluded, but consanguinity has to be assumed.

	Rhesus	Kidd	Gm	Km	HLA
Child I	CcD.Ee	Jk(a-b+)	(1,2,-3,-11,21)	(1,3)	A2,A28; B51,B60; Cw3
Child II	ccD.EE	Jk(a+b+)	(1,2,-3,-11,21)	(-1,3)	A3,A31; B7,Bw75/w76; Cw1,Cw3
P. Mother	CcD.Ee	Jk(a-b+)	(-1,-2,3,11,-21)	(1,3)	A2,A29; B14,B51; Cw8
P. Father	CCD.ee	Jk(a+b-)	(1,-2,3,11,21)	(1,-3)	A1,A28; B35,B51; Cw4

Advances in Forensic Haemogenetics 4
Edited by Ch. Rittner and P. M. Schneider
© Springer-Verlag Berlin Heidelberg 1992

Locus Probe	D2S44 Hae III/YNH24	D7S21 Hinf I/MS31	D7S22 Hinf I/g3
Child I	2.0 - 1.7 kb	5.7 - 4.2 kb	5.4 - 3.4 kb
Child II	3.7 - 3.3 kb	5.6 - 4.1 kb	6.3 - 5.4 kb
Putative Mother	2.1 kb	7.1 - 6.9 kb	7.1 - 4.5 kb
Putative Father	3.7 - 0.8 kb	5.6 kb	10.8 - 5.4 kb

Case 2: An apparent "silent" allele transmittance was observed at the acP locus. No exclusion occured in the HLA system. Investigating Hae III/YNH24 polymorphism, a fragment of different size was found for the putative father and the child, whereas no exclusion occurred in Hinf I/MS31 and Hinf I/g3 (Fig. 1). The reason for the similarity but exclusion was that the putative father had sent his brother to the blood test.

	acP	HLA
Child	acP B	A2,A29; B35;B51; Cw4
Mother	acP B	A2,A3; B8,B51; Cw7
Putative Father	acP A	A24,A29; B35,B44; Cw2,Cw4

Locus Probe	D2S44 Hae III/YNH24	D7S21 Hinf I/MS31	D7S22 Hinf I/g3
Child	3.2 - 1.1 kb	6.8 - 5.7 kb	6.7 - 5.2 kb
Mother	1.7 - 1.1 kb	6.7 - 5.7 kb	6.1 - 5.2 kb
Putative Father	2.9 - 1.9 kb	6.8 - 6.2 kb	6.7 - 6.1 kb

Case 3: The putative father died before the birth of the child. Blood investigation of the deceased was unsuitable as he received blood transfusions before he died. Therefore, muscle and tendon specimen were investigated by DNA polymorphisms (Fig. 2). Combining the results of these DNA polymorphisms and those of the conventional blood group systems of his mother, a plausibility of paternity W > 99.999% was obtained.

	Kell	acP	HLA
Child	Kk	BC	HLA A11,Aw33; B17,B60; Cw3
Mother	kk	AB	HLA A3,A11; B35,B60; Cw3,Cw4
Mother of the dead Putative Father	Kk	BC	HLA A2,Aw33; B17,B35; Cw3,Cw4

Locus Probe	D2S44 Hae III/YNH24	D7S21 Hinf I/MS31	D7S22 Hinf I/g3
Child	3.0 - 1.8 kb	6.5 - 4.6 kb	3.1 - 1.7 kb
Mother	1.8 kb	7.5 - 4.6 kb	6.8 - 3.1 kb
Putative Father	3.0 - 1.8 kb	6.5 - 4.6 kb	3.0 - 1.7 kb
Mother of the P.F.	3.0 - 1.6 kb	6.3 - 4.6 kb	3.0 - 1.7 kb

Fig. 1

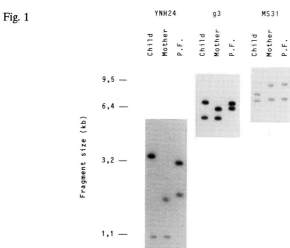

Fig. 2

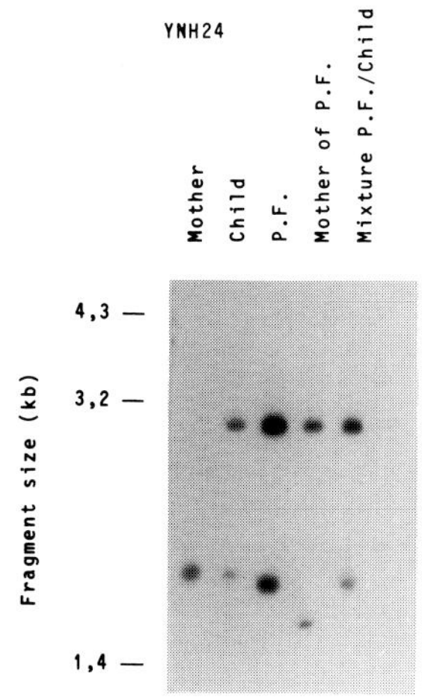

Allele Frequency in the Population of Spain Using Several
Single Locus Probes

E. Valverde, C. Cabrero[1], A. Diez[1], A. Carracedo and
T. Borrás[1]

Institute of Legal Medicine
University of Santiago de Compostela
Galicia, Spain

INTRODUCTION

Studies to determine allele frequency of single locus probes
have been carried out for some of the world's populations. We
have delayed the construction of our database of spanish
populations until solid electrophoretic and statistical
criteria were accepted. Once the EDNAP group approved a
laboratory protocol which has been widely accepted by European
laboratories, we have carried out this study, and therefore we
present the results for the probes YNH24 (HinfI, HaeIII),
MS43a (HinfI), MS31 (HinfI) and TBQ7 (HaeIII).

METHODS

DNA was extracted from whole blood by a high salt method
(Cabrero et al) and digested with HinfI or HaeIII. The
resultant fragments were electrophoresed on agarose gels
(0.7%) at 55V, according to the EDNAP group protocol. After
electrophoresis, DNA was transferred via capillary to nylon
membranes, hybridized with ^{32}P labeled probes, and exposed in
autor adiography cassettes for 2-3 days.
Bands were measured independently by two operators using a
densitometer (Elscript400, Hirschmann), and the data generated
were translated to bp values using a computer program based on
the Elder and Southern method (1987).

RESULTS

    Figures 1, 2 and 3 show frequency data for YNH24, MS43a
and MS31, respectively, using HinfI as restriction enzyme, and
Figures 4 and 5 show frequency data for YNH24 and TBQ7, using
HaeIII as restriction enzyme.
    Accumulated frequency data was analyzed using the
"sliding window fit method" proposed by Gill et al.(1990). For
all probes the sliding window was 2x the match guideline of
2.8 Kb%, i.e. 5.6 Kb%. Frequencies are calculated by summing
the positions of the raw data in 5.6 Kb% block with the mean
value moving 5 bp per interval.

    Frequency tables have been generated based on these
criteria (details of these tables can be seen in Table 1 and
2). The statistical analysis of single locus probes and band
matching in our practical caseworks is carried out with the
'conservative' approach of Gill et al.(1991) using these
frequency tables.

1 Dept. of Molecular Biology of Pharmagen Corp
Calera 3, 28760 Madrid, Spain

Advances in Forensic Haemogenetics 4
Edited by Ch. Rittner and P. M. Schneider
© Springer-Verlag Berlin Heidelberg 1992

Table 1. Detail of a frequency table corresponding to probe MS43a (HinfI as restriction enzyme)

WINDOW CENTRE (bp)	FREQUENCY	WINDOW CENTRE (bp)	FREQUENCY
8247.5	0.14184	9922.5	0.17021
8252.5	0.14184	9927.5	0.17021
8257.5	0.14539	9932.5	0.17376
8262.5	0.14539	9937.5	0.17376
8267.5	0.14539	9942.5	0.17021
8272.5	0.14184	9947.5	0.18085
8277.5	0.14184	9952.5	0.17730
8282.5	0.13830	9957.5	0.17730
8287.5	0.13475	9962.5	0.18085
8292.5	0.13475	9967.5	0.18085
8297.5	0.13475	9972.5	0.18440
8302.5	0.13121	9977.5	0.17730

Table 2. Detail of a frequency table corresponding to probe YNH24 (HinfI as restriction enzyme)

WINDOW CENTRE (bp)	FREQUENCY	WINDOW CENTRE (bp)	FREQUENCY
2542.5	0.04950	2882.5	0.09406
2547.5	0.04950	2887.5	0.09901
2552.5	0.04950	2892.5	0.11386
2557.5	0.04950	2897.5	0.11386
2562.5	0.04950	2902.5	0.11386
2567.5	0.05941	2907.5	0.10891
2572.5	0.06931	2912.5	0.11881
2577.5	0.07426	2917.5	0.12376
2582.5	0.07426	2922.5	0.12376
2587.5	0.08416	2927.5	0.11881
2592.5	0.07921	2932.5	0.11881
2597.5	0.08416	2937.5	0.12871

Population data from different spanish populations seem to have similar profiles and so, these frequency tables can be used for practical casework. Nevertheless, since the sample for some populations is too small, a data file was created in our program for further examination of accumulated data.

REFERENCES

Cabrero C, Diez A, Borras T (to be published) Short and inexpensive non enzimatic procedure to isolate genomic DNA from human blood
Elder JK, Southern E (1987) In: Bishop MJ, Rawlings CJ (eds) Nucleic acid and protein sequence analysis. IRL Press, Oxford, pp 165-1   Oxford, pp 165-172
Gill P, Evett IW, Woodroffe S, Lygo JE, Millican E, Webster M (1991) Databases, quality control and interpretation of DNA profiling in the Home Office Forensic Science Service. Electrophoresis 12: 204-209

Gill P, Werrett DJ (1990) Interpretation of DNA profiles using a computerised database. Electrophoresis 11: 444-448

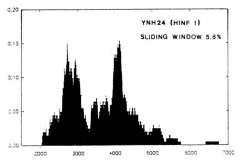

Fig. 1

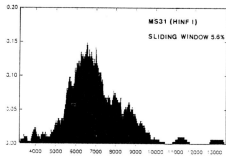

Fig. 2

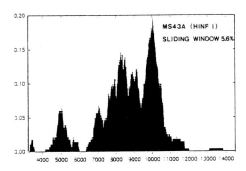

Fig. 3

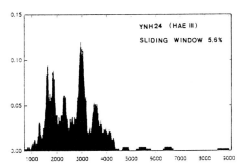

Fig. 4

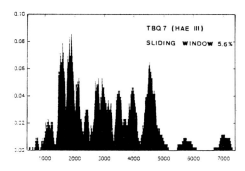

Fig. 5

Figs. 1-5. Frequency distribution of probes YNH24, MS43a and MS31

DNA FINGERPRINTS OF FAMILIES FROM BEJSCE/SOUTH-EAST POLAND

T. Dobosz*, P. Koziol, K. Sawicki, M. Szczepaniak, J. Jagielski, C. Vogt, S. Szymaniec

* Institute of Forensic Medicine, Wroclaw, Poland

Introduction

The paper is a preliminary report on DNA studies in population of Bejsce/Kazimierza Wielka district, Kielce province, South-East Poland. This population is very good known, because family data from church registers are preserved from 1550, completly from 1679. The data have been used for reconstruction of family pedigrees and relationships. The additional informations about Bejsce and its population are presented by Sawicki et al. (4). DNA samples from 17 families numbering 95 persons were prepared using the salt precipitation method and tested after digestion with Hinf I and Hae III using BIOTEST B.E.S.T. Probe MZ 1.3. Additionaly, the blots were reprobed with the oligonucleotide probe $(CAC)_5$. The study showns that almost all families from Bejsce are related, contemporary or in the past.

Material and methods

The preliminary studies were started with 17 families (95 persons), but the ultimate results were obtained only for 6 families (31 persons). The blood samples were collected in 1989 by cubical vein puncture. The samples of about 5 to 20 ml were immediately mixed with sodium citrate and stored at -18° C for almost 2 years. DNA was prepared by phenol method (Kunkel et al., 3) and after digestion by restriction enzymes tested electrophoretically on agarose gels. For $(CAC)_5$, gels were dried. The hybridisation were performed using the Epplen and Zischler method (2) with P^{32} labelled probe. The hybridisation with MZ 1.3 were performed according to Biotest method (1), with nylon membrane Southern capillary blots.

Results and discussion

The figure shows the results of investigation of 6 families. The study has shown that almost all tested families are related, contemporary or in the past. We intend to test the whole population of Bejsce (about 200 families with 1000 members) for obtaining the final results.

Advances in Forensic Haemogenetics 4
Edited by Ch. Rittner and P. M. Schneider
© Springer-Verlag Berlin Heidelberg 1992

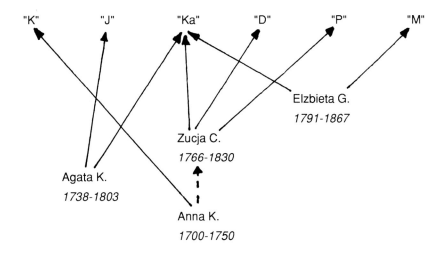

Fig. Genealogy of tested families (female ancestors)

References

1. BEST-Probe MZ 1.3 Digoxigenin. 1990. Manual of Biotest AG

2. Epplen J., Zischler H. 1990. In "DNA fingerprinting with oligonucleotide probe", Fresenius Diagnostic Booklet

3. Kunkel L., Smith K., Boyer S., Borgaonkar D., Watchel S., Miller O., Brew W., Jones H., Rory J. 1977. Proc. Natl. Acad. Sci. USA, 74: 1245

4. Sawicki K. Parish of Bejsce as a source of unique material for population genetic study. 1991. Adv. in Forensic Haemogen. Vol. 4 (in press)

PATERNITY TESTING WITH FIVE VNTR SYSTEMS IN DANES

Hanna E. Hansen & Niels Morling

Institute of Forensic Genetics, University of Copenhagen,
11 Frederik Den Femtes Vej, DK-2100 Copenhagen Ø, Denmark

INTRODUCTION

This study presents the results of examinations with five VNTR systems in Danish paternity cases. The efficiency of the five systems, the reliability of exclusions, and the mutation rates of the systems have been examined. The linkage relationship between the systems D7S21 and D7S22 has been investigated through family studies.

MATERIAL AND METHODS

The material comprised 174 cases of disputed paternity in which all parties were unrelated Danes, 84 mother-child pairs, and 32 families with 70 children. The techniques used for DNA preparation, electrophoresis, autoradiography, and calculation of kilobase values have been described previously (Morling & Hansen, 1992). The restriction enzyme was *Hinf*1. The systems used were: D7S22 (g3), D5S43 (MS8), D7S21 (MS31), D12S11 (MS43) (Wong et al 1987), and D2S44 (YNH24) (Wyman & White 1980).

RESULTS AND DISCUSSION

No paternity case was evaluated before DNA from all the parties could be run side by side on the same gel. Since migration distances never exceeded 1.25 mm between bands identical by descent in mothers and children (Morling & Hansen 1992), exclusion of paternity was established when the distance between the paternally derived band of the

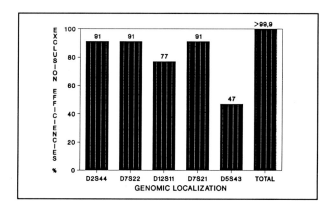

Fig. 1. Exclusion efficiencies of five VNTR systems in 53 Danish paternity cases

Advances in Forensic Haemogenetics 4
Edited by Ch. Rittner and P. M. Schneider
© Springer-Verlag Berlin Heidelberg 1992

child and the nearest band of the alleged man exceeded 1.25 mm. Examinations with VNTR systems were carried out at the second step of the routine paternity investigations, and consequently a comparatively large number of non-excluded men was found in the present material.

The combined efficiency of the five VNTR systems used exceeded 99.9 % (fig. 1). All 53 alleged men, excluded as the fathers by one or more of 12-15 conventional marker systems, were also excluded by at least two of the VNTR systems used. In another eight cases, the alleged men were excluded only by the VNTR systems. In six other cases, two alleged men were full sibs, and two VNTR systems provided the only exclusions of a brother in four of these cases, while two VNTR systems and the HLA-A,B-system excluded one brother in one case, and only the HLA-system gave guidance in the last case.

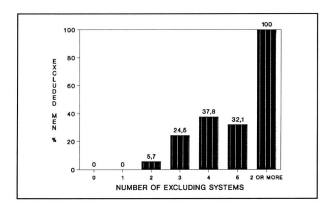

Fig. 2. Exclusion efficiencies of VNTR combinations in 53 Danish paternity cases

The systems D2S44, D7S22, and D7S21 could exclude paternity for 48 (91%) of the 53 men who were excluded by the conventional marker systems. D12S11 and D5S43 were found to be less efficient, excluding 41 (77%) and 25 (47%) men, respectively.

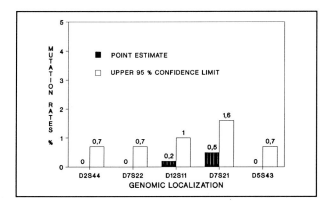

Fig. 3. Mutation rates of five VNTR systems (557 informative meioses)

The presence of parent-child exclusions due to possible mutations was examined in 258 mother-child-pairs and 32 families with 70 children. Presuming that 159 alleged men were the biological fathers since their paternity could not be excluded by any of the 12-15 conventional marker systems or by 2-5 VNTR systems, 557 meioses were obtained. Four cases of exclusions of a parent by only one VNTR system were observed: A mother and a family father, respectively, were excluded by D7S21, and in two paternity cases, the alleged men were excluded by D7S21 (PI = 4740) and by D12S11 (PI = 227), respectively. This leads to observed mutation frequencies of 0.2% for D12S11 and 0.5% for D7S21. No mutations were observed in the D2S44, D7S22, and D5S43 systems (fig. 3).

Table 1. Linkage analysis of D7S21 (MS31)-D7S22 (g3) in 22 families with 2-5 children

	Observed number of:		
Informative haplotypes:		**Recombinants:**	
Maternal	57	21	(36.8%)
Paternal	51	13	(25.5%)
Total	108	34	(31.5%)*

*) $chi^2 = 7.4$, $p < 0.01$

The linkage relationship between D7S21 (MS31) and D7S22 (g3) was examined in 22 families with 57 children (Table 1). The deviation from the 0.5 ratio was significant (p < 0.01). The estimate of the recombination distance between the two loci was about 32 cM.

CONCLUSION

With the five VNTR systems used, a combined exclusion efficiency exceeding 99.9% was found. Because of the chance of mutations exclusion of paternity should not be based on mismatch in only one system.

REFERENCES

Morling N, Hansen HE (1992) Matching criteria for paternity testing with VNTR systems. Advances in Forensic Hemogenetics 4, Springer-Verlag, Berlin Heidelberg, (this issue)

Wong Z, Wilson V, Patel I, Povey S, Jeffreys AJ (1987) Characterization of a Panel of highly variable minisattelites cloned from human DNA. Ann Hum Genet 51:269-88

Wyman AR, White R (1980) A highly polymorphic locus in human DNA. Proc Natl Acad Sci USA 77:6754-6758

Comparison of Population Genetics of the Single Locus Probes pS194 and pL427-4

W. Martin*, H.H. Hoppe, M. Muche, Institut für Blutgruppenserologie und Genetik, Hamburg und L. Henke, Labor für forensische Blutgruppenkunde, Düsseldorf

Summary

Comparing population genetics of different laboratories for the single locus probes pS194 (D7S107) and pL427-4 (D21S112) it became evident that considerable differences of the distributions for the calculated KB values of the fragments were present. The forms of the distribution curves were identical for the same population, but deviations of the determined KB-values for the fragments were found according to the technique used. On the example of the two probes, these deviations can be shown to be linear corresponding to the electrophoresis technique: particularly according to the agarose concentration and -less- to the amount of DNA applied. By that, we have the possibility to combine population genetic data of different laboratories using different techniques after linear correction of the distribution tables or curves. Since this interdependence is valid for all probes, it is quickly possible to compile relatively extensive population genetic tables as a reliable basis for the statistical evaluation in cases of disputed paternity.

Introduction

Fragment size distributions of digested human DNA hybridized with different probes showed deviations in the calculated KB values owing to the techniques used. Dykes et al. could show that dependence especially exists upon the concentration of the agarose gel used for the run and the amount of DNA incorporated into the gel (Fig. 1). This interdependence seemed to be linear in the ranges of agarose concentration and amount of DNA usually used. The goal of our investigation was to find out how different population genetic studies with deviations in the KB values can be corrected and combined in order to get large fragment size distributions for different probes as a basis for a safe statistical evaluation in paternity testing.

DNA-Determinations
Change of kB Values Depending on Agarose Conc. and Amount of DNA Applied

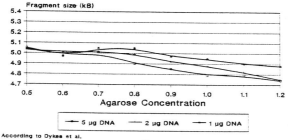

According to Dykes et al.

Fig. 1

Advances in Forensic Haemogenetics 4
Edited by Ch. Rittner and P. M. Schneider
© Springer-Verlag Berlin Heidelberg 1992

Material

Fragment size distributions of the probes pS194 (D7S107) and pL427-4 (D21S112) from Dykes (Denver, USA, Lab 1) and our own laboratory (Hamburg, Germany, Ham) are compared. The sample sizes were: pS194 n=1903 (Lab 1) and n=225 (Ham); pL427-4 n=330 (Lab 1) and n=100 (Ham).

Results and discussion

The deviations in the distributions are evident as shown in Fig. 2 (pS194) and Fig. 3 (pL427-4). Since the peaks of the distribution curves are obviously in the same distance from eachother, the reason for this shift must be a technical one. Experiments showed that changes in the agarose concentration not only led to differences in the running distance but also in the fragment sizes determined. Simple linear correction of the deviations in fragment size determinations gives identical distribution curves as shown in Fig. 4 and Fig. 5.

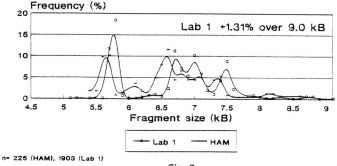

pS194/PST I Polymorphism
Comparison HAM - Lab 1
(kB values +0.1)

n= 225 (HAM), 1903 (Lab 1)

Fig. 2

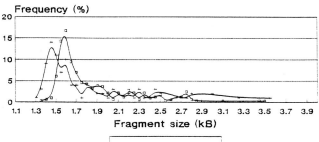

pL427-4/PST I - Polymorphism
Comparison Ham - Lab 1
(kB values +0,05)

n - 330 (Lab 1), 100 (HAM)

Fig. 3

The KB value for the correction can easily be ascertained by determining the KB value of the distance of the main peak of a distribution curve. Persisting small differences in distributions will not influence the correctness of the statistical evaluations , since these calculations have to be done with a certain range (e.g. ± 2% KB) of the actual KB value determined for a fragment. If, in addition, the calculations are performed with a minimum frequency of 0.01, possible errors are eliminated, while the information remains high enough as to the proof of paternity.

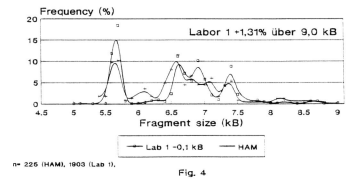

pS194/PST I Polymorphism
Comparison HAM – Lab 1 -0.1 kB
(kB values +0.1)

n= 225 (HAM), 1903 (Lab 1),

Fig. 4

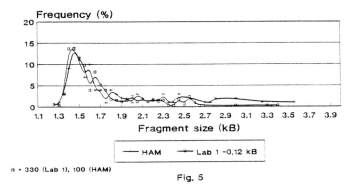

pL427-4/PST I - Polymorphism
Comparison HAM – Lab 1 -0,12 kB
(kB values +0,05)

n = 330 (Lab 1), 100 (HAM)

Fig. 5

As the examples of the probes pS194 and pL427-4 show, it is possible to combine population genetic data of different laboratories using different techniques after linear correction of the distribution tables or curves. Since this interdependance is valid for all probes, it is quickly possible to compile relatively extensive population genetic tables as a reliable basis for the statistical evaluation in cases of disputed paternity.

Comparison of Minisatellite DNA Probes and Blood Group, Protein, and Enzyme Markers in Paternity Cases

G. Mauff, G. Pulverer, Ellen Mühlenbrock, L. Kochhan, Annemarie Klein, Käthe Volz, Annette Bräutigam, K. Hummel, R. Fimmers, and M. P. Baur

Institut für Medizinische Mikrobiologie und Hygiene, Universität zu Köln, Goldenfelsstr. 21, 5000 Köln 41, Germany; Institut für Blutgruppenserologie, Freiburg; Institut für Medizinische Statistik, Dokumentation und Datenverarbeitung, Universität Bonn

INTRODUCTION

Multilocus and single locus minitsatellite probes have been applied to the paternity expertise for some time (Jeffreys et al., 1985; Dykes et al., 1988; Henke et al., 1990; Jeffreys et al., 1991). They are now considered as very useful tools in complex cases of disputed paternity. There are, however, still controversal opinions concerning their application in the standard trio case. In the present study we have been interested in a comparision between the use of single locus minisatellite DNA probes (SLP) and conventional blood group, enzyme, and serological markers under routine conditions.

MATERIALS AND METHODS

In 50 paternity cases with three individuals and four cases with four individuals (two children or two men involved) the paternity expertise was carried out according to German federal regulations. In addition, the genetic markers C3, BF, PLG, ORM1, the subtypes of HP, GC 1, PGM1, TF C, BF F, and in some cases A2HS, PGP and C6 were investigated. Genomic DNA was digested with HinfI, submitted to eletrophoresis and Southern blotting, and hybridized with the DNA probes MS1, MS31, MS43, g3, and MS8 (ICI Diagnostics) as described elsewhere (Wong et al., 1987). For the detection of probe-specific fragments a non-radioactive digoxigenin-dUTP labeled flourescence AMPPD Kit (Boehringer Mannheim) was used, and initially compared with a radioactive ^{32}P assay.

The probability of paternity in the standard expertise as well as in the SLP expertise was calculated according to Essen-Möller (Essen-Möller, 1938). For the DNA expertises the likelihood values were calculated using upper 95 % confidence limits as conservative estimates for the allele frequencies derived from the non-related German adults of the total number of cases.

RESULTS AND DISCUSSION

In the technical evaluation the fluorescent assay was seen to be superior in time, sensitivity and reprobing as compared to the ^{32}P assay, but comparable in experimental effort to the conventional expertise without HLA.

The distribution of SLP fragments among the nonrelated individuals followed published frequencies for Caucasoids (Fig. 1). Remarkable, however, was the wider spectrum of fragments besides the major 6.6 kb fragement of MS8 and the lower frequency for the major 6.4 kb fragment of MS31, and also a lower frequency for the 1.7 kb fragment of g3. This may be related to the limited number of individuals tested here, and to the method of attributing fragment sizes. The rate of heterozygous individuals was in agreement with published frequencies: MS1 0.99, MS31 0.96, MS42 0.95, g3 0.97, and MS8 0.89.

Advances in Forensic Haemogenetics 4
Edited by Ch. Rittner and P. M. Schneider
© Springer-Verlag Berlin Heidelberg 1992

Concordance in exclusion of paternity between the SLP's and standard markers was seen in 17 cases (Fig. 2). In two cases with a single exclusion in the standard expertise all five SLP's were informative. In no case less than three SLP's showed exclusion of paternity. No exclusion was observed with minisatellites or with standard markers alone.

Thirty-six men not excluded by the two procedures had probabilities of paternity between 96.0 % and 99.99 % with conventional markers, between 98.77 and 99,99 % with SLP's (Table1).

Table 1. Comparison of the probability of paternity based on conventional markers and SLP's (no. of cases)

P	conventional markers	SLP's
> 0.9999	24	33
0.9973-0.9999	5	2
0.9900-0.9973	4	0
0.9600-0.9900	3	1

We conclude from our data that with the non-radioactive detection system minisattellites are reliabel for the paternity expertise. Although higher probability values were obtained with results from minisatellites there was no major improvement in the verbal statement of paternity for the non-excluded men. In view of the limited experience with DNA probes as compared conventional to markers and a similar technological effort, we consider that for the presence their application should be confined to complex cases such as involvement of related men, deficiency cases single exclusion in the standard expertise or unsatisfactory probability values.

For biostatistical evaluations more extensive data on SLP frequencies in different populations are needed. They were recently published for a larger West German population sample (Henke et al., 1991). But due to the absence of standardized procedures laboratory specific frequencies for single locus minisatellites may still some time be necessary.

REFERENCES

Dykes D, Watkins P, Bowden D, Polesky H (1988) Identifying DNA RFLP's in routine paternity cases: Non-isotypic methods of detection. In: Mayr WR (ed) Advances in Forensic Haemogenetics 2. Springer, Berlin Heidelberg New York London Paris Tokyo

Essen-Möller E (1938) Die Beweiskraft der Ähnlichkeit im Vaterschaftsnachweis. Theoretische Grundlagen. Mitt Anthrop Ges (Wien) 68: 9-53

Henke L, Paas H, Hoffmann K, Henke J (1990) Zum Einsatz von DNA-Polymorphismen in der Abstammungsbegutachtung. Z Rechtsmed 103: 235-248

Henke L, Cleef S, Zakrzewska, Henke J (1991) Population genetic data determined for five different single locus minisatellite probes. In: Burke T et al. DNA Fingerprinting: Approaches and Applications. Birkhäuser, Basel

Jeffreys AJ, Brookfield JFY, Semeonoff R (1985) Positive identification of an immigrant test case using human DNA fingerprints. Nature 317: 818-819

Jeffreys AJ, Turner M, Debenham P (1991) The efficiency of multilocus DNA fingerprint probes for individualization and establishment of family relationships, determined from extensive casework. Am J Hum Genet 48: 824-840

Wong Z, Wilson V, Patel I, Povey S, Jeffreys AJ (1987) Characterization of a panel of highly variable minisatellites cloned from human DNA. Ann Hum Genet 51:269-288

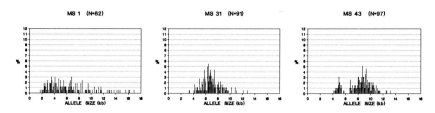

Figure 1: Allele Frequencies of SLP's in Caucasoids (Cologne area)

Figure 2: Exclusion of Paternity: 5 LSP evaluated (N=17cases)

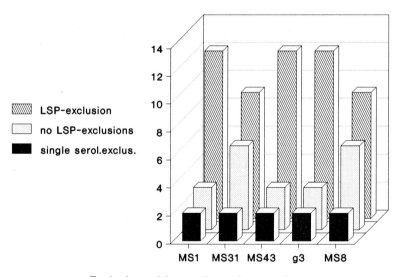

Exclusion with 1 to 7 serolog. markers

Allele frequency distribution of two VNTR polymorphisms
(YNH24/ D2S44; Alpha globin 3'HVR/D16) in Italy

V.L. Pascali, M.Dobosz, M.Pescarmona,E. d'Aloja, and A. Fiori

Immunohematology laboratory, Institute of Forensic Medicine,
Catholic University, Rome, Italy

INTRODUCTION

Variable number of tandem repeats (VNTRs) are a class of
polymorphisms whose degree of variability is still unrivaled
among human genetic markers. Forensic applications of VNTRs
require detailed studies on the population genetics of these
systems. Since most hypervariable profiles exhibit arrays of
continuous Kb measures, a standardized protocol and a
computerized repository of laboratory data are higly desirable
in order to achieve reliable gene frequencies.
The creation of an Italian repository of VNTR frequencies is
presently under way, under the auspices of the Italian working
section (GEFI) of the Society of Forensic Hemogenetics. A
computer algorithm for storage and management of continuous
data has been developed (Pascali et al, 1991) and will be
used for storage, retrieval and analysis of VNTRs data. Data
are presently being collected by a a network of 12 Italian
laboratories, which are expected to investigate individuals
from several regions of Italy. Participating laboratories will
follow a standard experimental procedure and share the same
archive.
This project is presently being developed. Here we present a
first collection of data generated in our laboratory following
the model proposed to the collaborative group. These data are
liable to represent the distribution of two common VNTRs
(D2S44; alpha globin 3'HVR) in Central-Southern Italy and will
be enlarged as long as results from other laboratories will be
available.

MATERIALS AND METHODS

Genomic DNA was extracted, enzymatically restricted (HinfI)
and analysed according to a standard protocol of Southern blot
hybridization (Schneider et al, 1991).
Submarine gels for YNH24 were electrophoresed to meet the best
resolution available in a range from 1 Kb to 5 Kb. Separate
sets of experiments with shorter electrophoretic runs were
required for 3'HVR, because of the high frequency of small
fragments (down to 0.38 Kb) generated in this system.
Hybridization of the resulting filter blots was carried out

Advances in Forensic Haemogenetics 4
Edited by Ch. Rittner and P. M. Schneider
© Springer-Verlag Berlin Heidelberg 1992

with YNH24 (D2S44) (Wong et al, 1987) and alpha globin 3'HVR (D16) (Jarman et al, 1986) specific probes, under high stringency conditions. Length measures were assumed from the autoradiograms by a digitizing tablet. Predictions of Kb values were based on the reciprocal method by Elder and Southern (1987). Lengths and migrational distances of a commercial size marker (1kbladder, Boehringer) were used for measuring unknown sizes of bands.

RESULTS AND DISCUSSION

The distribution of the allelomorphic fragments in the two VNTR systems is shown in Fig.1 and Fig.2. The following features are worthwhile mentioning for each system.

YNH24/D2S44

Data on this system were drawn from 518 chromosomes, screened from 259 unrelated individuals and 83 families. Fragments spanning from 0.5 Kb to 7.84 Kb were identified, with frequencies arranged in a multimodal shape, and a major peak at 2.8 Kb. In this system, only 5 homozygous were detected. This leads to calculate a mean heterozygosity level of 98.5%. Segregation in families did not show any apparent mutation at this locus.

Alpha globin 3'HVR

We screened 360 chromosomes from unrelated individuals. A group of 64 families was also studied. Fragments had a major peak at 0.59 Kb and a plurimodal profile encompassing .38 Kb to 5.46 Kb. The average heterozygosity amounted to 93.3% (12 homozygous out of 180 individuals). No mutational events were seen in the family groups.

REFERENCES

Elder JK, Southern EM (1987) Computer-aided analysis of one-dimensional restriction fragment gels. In Bishop MJ, Rawlings CG (eds.), Nucleic acids and protein sequence analysis, IRL Press, Oxford, pp. 165-172

Jarman AP, Nicholls RD, Weatherall DJ, Clegg JB, Higgs DR (1986) Molecular characterization of a hypervariable region downstream of the human alpha-globin gene cluster. EMBO J 5(8):1857-1863

Pascali VL, d'Aloja E, Dobosz M, Pescarmona M (1991) Estimating allele frequencies of VNTR systems. Forensic Sci Int (in press)

Schneider PM, Fimmers R, Woodroffe S, Werrett, DJ, Bar W et al.(1991) Report of a European collaborative exercise

comparing DNA typing results using a single locun VNTR probe.
Forensic Sci Int 49:1-15
   Wong Z, Wilson W, Patel I, Povey S, Jeffreys, AJ (1987)
Characterization of highly variable minisatellites cloned from
human DNA. Ann Hum Biol 51:269-288

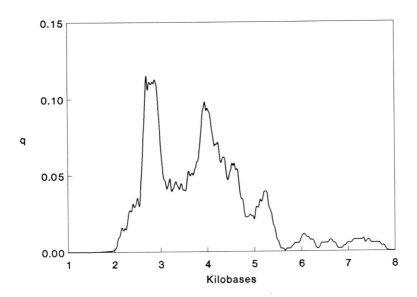

Fig 1. Allele frequency distribution of YNH24

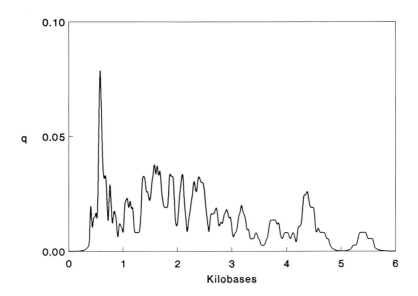

Fig 2. Allele frequency distribution of alpha globin 3'HVR

DNA-Profiling with pHINS310, pMUC7, pMR24/1, pYNH24 and pMS43a for Paternity Testing

T. Rothämel, H.-J. Krüger, W. Keil and H.D. Tröger

Institute for Legal Medicine, Medical University
Institut für Rechtsmedizin der Medizinischen Hochschule
Konstanty-Gutschow-Strasse 8

W-3000 HANNOVER 61, FRG

INTRODUCTION

A huge variety of well established conventional blood group systems is available for paternity testing and still can be extended by acquiring new phenotypic polymorphisms.
Nevertheless DNA-polymorphisms widely come into increasing use as a powerful tool for paternity casework, not at least for their uniform and practicable methodical procedure.
This paper presents a comparison of the results from 12 current routine paternity cases tested with up to 30 red cell antigen & enzyme as well as serum protein polymorphisms with the results achieved by the use of up to 5 SLPs detecting high polymorphic VNTRs: pHINS310, pMUC7, pMR24/1, pYNH24 and pMS43a (Elbein et al 1985; Gendler et al 1987; Yokoi et al 1990; Odelberg et al 1989; Wong et al 1987).
The order, in which the conventional markers actually were tested, was as follows: AB0, MNS, RH, KEL, FY, HP, GC, GM, KM, ACP1, PGM1, ADA, AK1, PGD, ESD, P1, GLO1, JK, LU, TF, B, C3, PI, F13A, F13B, GPT1, C6, C8 1, HSGA, PLGN, ORM1.

METHODS

DNA of 12 triplets (child, mother, putative father) was prepared by proteolytic digestion of pelleted white blood cell nuclei, organic extraction and ethanol precipitation. The HinfI-fragments were separated in 1% agarose gels (20*20cm) at 30V/110mA for 24h and alkali blotted to charged nylon membranes. Probes were labeled with P32 dCTP by multi-primed extension, blots were exposed to Amersham MP-films with two intensifying screens at -28 degrees Celsius or to Amersham beta-max-films at ambient temperature for 5 days. Fragment lengths were calculated according to the method of Elder & Southern (1987), the plausibility of paternity ("W"-value) was calculated using the formulae of Mayr (1972) with a sliding window of +/- 3 sigma. "Allele"-frequencies for pHINS310, pMUC7 and pMR24/1 were taken from our own population data (n=207), frequencies for pYNH24 (Odelberg et al 1989) and pMS43a were provided by PROMEGA and CELLMARK.

RESULTS

The 12 cases from paternity testing revealed 10 constellations including the putative father. The corresponding values for the probability of paternity achieved by either the VNTR-markers or the conventional polymorphisms as well as both in combination are scaled up in table 1 and shown in figure 1. Profiling with only 3 probes resulted in "W"-values which only in 2 cases exceeded 99.73% whereas in 6 cases the values were ranging from 98.01% to 99.67%. "W"-values clearly beyond

Advances in Forensic Haemogenetics 4
Edited by Ch. Rittner and P. M. Schneider
© Springer-Verlag Berlin Heidelberg 1992

99.73% could be calculated by probing trios with 5 VNTR-markers. There also were 2 cases in which the alleged father could be excluded both with the conventional and the DNA-markers (I. all 5 probes / II. 4 probes lacking pHINS310). Figure 2 gives an example for trios tested with pMR24/1.

	pHINS310 pMUC7 pMR24/1	pHINS310 pMUC7 pMR24/1 pYNH24 pMS43a	conv. markers/ number of systems	conv. markers + 3 SLPs	conv. markers + 5 SLPs
1	96.2656		99.9200/26	99.9970	
2	99.7695		›99.9990/26	›99.9999	
3	98.0111		99.8500/29	99.9970	
4	99.9826		99.9800/26	›99.9999	
5	98.6873		99.7500/30	99.9967	
6	98.4363		99.9600/26	99.9994	
7	98.8605	99.9700	99.9920/26	99.9999	›99.9999
8	99.6064	99.9816	99.9930/26	›99.9999	›99.9999
9	95.4593	99.7967	99.9650/26	99.9983	›99.9999
10	99.6751	99.9857	›99.9990/26	›99.9999	›99.9999

Table 1   Pobability of paternity ("W"-values): Conventional polymorphisms vs DNA-profiling with 3 or 5 SLPs

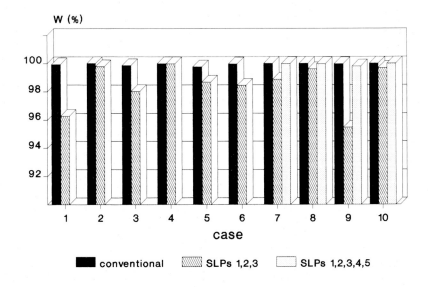

Fig. 1 Probability of paternity ("W"-values): Conventional vs DNA-markers

DISCUSSION

DNA-profiling with 5 SLPs in paternity testing seems to be sufficient to achieve "W"-values exceeding 99.73 % - results which are comparable to the values calculated from a large range of conventional markers. If classical blood grouping and DNA-analysis are combined VNTRs can assist a reduced set of chosen conventional markers to lift the probability of paternity to values beyond 99.73 % and, regarding their enormous exclusion potential, can help to detect falsely alleged fathers.

Fig. 2 Probing trios (child, mother, alleged father) with pMR24/1: (from left to right) trio 1; 2; 4; 6 reveal inclusions whereas 3 and 5 show exclusions (standard ladder = PROMEGA "wide range"; the anode is at the top)

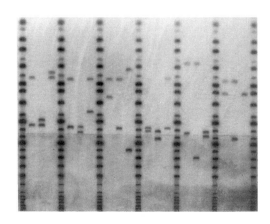

REFERENCES

Elbein S, Rotwein P, Permutt MA, Bell GI, Sanz N, Karam JH (1985) Lack of association of the polymorphic locus in the 5'-flanking region of the human insulin gene and diabetes in American blacks. Diabetes 34:433-439

Elder JK, Southern EM (1987) Computer-aided analysis of one-dimensional restriction fragment gels. In: Bishop MJ, Rawlings CJ (eds) Nucleic acid and protein sequence analysis. IRL Press, Oxford, pp 165-172

Gendler SJ, Burchell JM, Duhig T, Lamport D, White R, Parker M, Taylor-Papadimitriou J (1987) Cloning of partial cDNA encoding differentiation and tumor-associated mucin glycoproteins expressed by human mammary epithelium. Proc Acad Natl Sci USA 84:6060-6064

Mayr WR (1972) Grundlagen zur Berechnung der Vaterschaftswahrscheinlichkeit im HL-A-System. Z Immun Forsch 144:18-27

Odelberg SJ, Plaetke R, Eldridge JR, Ballard L, O'Connell P, Nakamura Y, Leppert M, Lalouel JM, White R (1989) Characterization of eight VNTR loci by agarose gel electrophoresis. Genomics 5:915-924

Wong Z, Wilson V, Patel I, Povey S, Jeffreys AJ (1987) Characterization of a panel of highly variable minisatellites cloned from human DNA. Ann Hum Genet 51:269-288

FREQUENCY DATABASES FOR THE DNA PROBES MS1, MS31, MS43A, AND YNH24, DERIVED FROM CAUCASIANS, AND AFRO-CARIBBEANS IN THE LONDON AREA

C. Buffery, F. Burridge, M. Greenhalgh, S. Jones, and G. Willott

Metropolitan Police Forensic Science Laboratory, 109 Lambeth Road, London, United Kingdom, SE1 7LP

INTRODUCTION

DNA from blood samples submitted to Metropolitan Police Forensic Science Laboratory have been analysed with the probes MS1, MS31, MS43A and YNH24 using the restriction enzyme Hinf I. Frequency databases have been prepared from more than 1000 Caucasian and more than 500 Afro Caribbeans in order to assess the evidential significance of matching DNA profiles.

METHOD

The protocol used was developed in this laboratory and is based on the method of Smith (1990) and Gill (1987, 1990) with certain modifications.

DNA was extracted from 150μl aliquots of liquid blood. Phenol and phenol/chloroform extractions were performed to purify the DNA. Following a partial restriction stage the DNA was then quantified using a Hoefer TKO100 DNA fluorometer. Complete restriction of 500ng DNA (typically 1-3μl) was carried out with Hinf I at 37°C overnight. Pre- and post-restriction samples were analysed on a 1% agarose minigel to test the quality of the extracted DNA and the efficiency of restriction. Samples showing incomplete restriction were further purified and re-restricted.

Size separation of restricted DNA was achieved by electrophoresis in a 0.7% agarose gel running in TBE buffer at 70 volts. Electrophoresis continued until a 2.3 kb λ/HindIII fragment had migrated 15cm from the origin (approximately 18 hours).

Following denaturation the DNA was transferred onto a nylon membrane using a vacuum transfer apparatus. DNA was fixed by baking the membrane at 80°C for 2 hours or ultra-violet irradiation.

DNA probes MS1, MS31, MS43A (Cellmark Diagnostics) and YNH24 (Promega Corporation were radiolabelled by ^{32}P dCTP by the random priming technique using Amersham's oligo-labelling kit. Unincorporated nucleotides were removed by gel filtration through a 1ml Sephadex G50 column. Using a modified Church and Gilbert protocol (1984), prehybridisation for 5 minutes was followed by hybridisation with radiolabelled probe at 65°C overnight. The membranes were rinsed with 2xSSC, 0.1% SDS followed by longer washes with 0.1xSSC, 0.1% SDS. Autoradiography was carried out at -70°C for 1 to 10 days. Membranes were stripped of probe before re-hybridisation with another.

Advances in Forensic Haemogenetics 4
Edited by Ch. Rittner and P. M. Schneider
© Springer-Verlag Berlin Heidelberg 1992

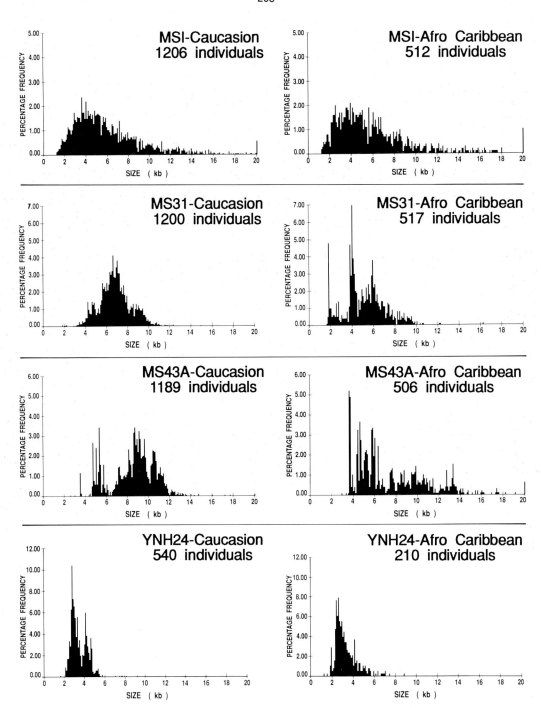

Distribution of MSI, MS31, MS43A and YNH24 alleles
For Caucasians and Afro Caribbeans in the London area
(Histograms reproduced here by kind permission of Forensic Science International)

All autoradiographs were analysed using a video-based scanning system developed in this laboratory (Catterick et al. 1991; Buffery et al. 1991) which utilises the Elder and Southern (reciprocal method, local form [1987]) for band size calculation with reference to molecular weight markers at three differing positions on the autoradiograph. Data points were recorded at 0.01 kb intervals and binned to 0.1 kb for generation of the histograms.

RESULTS AND DISCUSSION

Careful quantity estimation of purified DNA resulted in uniform band intensities which ensures greatest accuracy and reproducibility of sizing using the video scanning system.

The histograms generated by our data show good correlation with previously published, smaller data collections where loci and restriction enzyme are in common (Smith et al.1990; Gill et al. 1991; Brinkman et al. 1991; Odelberg et al. 1989).
The major ethnic groups do demonstrate differences in their allele distributions but alleles of exceptionally high frequency have not become apparent.

Interestingly, MS1 which has the highest observed mutation rate (0.052 per gamete [Jeffries et al. 1988]) displays the least variability between ethnic groups. Hence MS1 is considered to be an extremely powerful forensic probe and is likely to be less sensitive than other loci to the effects of population substructure.

References

Brinkmann B, Rand S and Wiegand P (1991) Population and family data of RFLP's using selected single and multilocus systems. Int. J. Leg. Med., 104: 81-86

Buffery C, Catterick T, Greenhalgh M, Jones S and Russell JR. (1991) Assessment of a video system for scanning DNA autoradiographs. Forensic Sci. Int., 49: 17-20

Catterick T and Russell JR (1991 in press) The Development of a video scanner for forensic DNA autoradiographs. Lab. Microcomputer

Church GM and Gilbert W. (1984) Genomic Sequencing. Proc. Natl. Acad. Sci. USA, 81: 1991-1995

Elder JK and Southern EM (1987) Computer aided analysis of one dimensional restriction fragment gels. In: Bishop MJ and Rawlings CJ (eds) Nucleic acid and protein sequence analysis. IRL Press, Oxford, pp 165-172

Gill P, Lygo JE, Fowler SJ and Werrett DJ. (1987) An evaluation of DNA fingerprinting for forensic purposes. Electrophoresis, 8: 38-44

Gill P, Woodroffe S, Lygo JE and Millican ES. (1991) Population Genetics of Four Hypervariable Loci. Int. J. Leg. Med., (in press)

Gill P, Sullivan K and Werrett DJ. (1990) The analysis of hypervariable DNA profiles: problems associated with the objective determination of the probability of a match. Hum. Genet., 85:75-79

Jeffreys AJ, Royle NJ, Wilson V and Wong Z. (1988) Spontaneous mutation rates to new length alleles at tandem repetitive hypervariable loci in human DNA. Nature, 332: 278-281

Odelberg SJ, Plaetke R, Eldridge JR, Ballard L, O'Connell P, Nakamura Y, Leppert M, Lalouel JM and White R. (1989) Characterization of eight VNTR Loci by Agarose Gel Electrophoresis. Genomics 5: 915-924

Smith JC, Newton CR, Alves A, Anwar R, Jenner D and Markham AF. (1990) Highly polymorphic minisatellite DNA probes. Further evaluation for individual identification and paternity testing. J. Forensic Sci. Soc., 30: 3-18

AN EVALUATION OF SINGLE LOCUS PROBES IN CASEWORK

F.J.Burridge, M.J.Greenhalgh and G.M.Willott

Metropolitan Police Forensic Science Laboratory,
109 Lambeth Rd. London SE1 7LP
United Kingdom

INTRODUCTION

 DNA profiling using Single Locus Probes has been in use in casework at the Metropolitan Police Laboratory since November 1988. The probes used are D1S7 (MS1), D7S21 (MS31), D12S11 (MS43A) AND D2S44 (YNH24). These together with the restriction enzyme Hinf1 enable us to produce results that are compatible with other members of the European DNA Profiling group (EDNAP).
 Since 1988 approximately 2800 blood samples and 1000 case stains have been examined. Results from these tests have now been analysed and it has been possible to draw some useful conclusions regarding the suitability of various types of staining for DNA profiling.

TYPES OF CASES EXAMINED

 DNA profiling provides extremely powerful evidence in body fluid cases but it is expensive and relatively time consuming. Hence it has been necessary to restrict its use to the more serious cases. (table 1.) There are many examples where the body fluids present are suitable for profiling but they have not been examined because of these restrictions.

Table 1.   Case types examined in 1990 at the Metropolitan Police Laboratory

CASE TYPE	NUMBER OF CASES	%
MURDER	79	16
RAPE	272	55
INDECENT ASSAULT	76	15
BUGGERY	33	6
ASSAULT	18	4
MISCELLANEOUS	19	4

A wide range of body fluids are acceptable for DNA profiling assuming that intact nucleated cells are present. A high priority is placed on serious sexual assaults and semen is the most commonly encountered type of stain followed by blood. Details of the success rates with different items are given in Table 2.

SEMEN STAINING

 The most numerous semen stained exhibits are vaginal swabs. The success rate with this type of item is very high.(a positive result is defined as obtaining a profile which is different from that of the donor of the swabs). The high success rate is probably due to the good quality of the DNA and the absence of contaminants that can inhibit restriction. Many swabs where there were only very low numbers of spermatozoa visible under microscopic

Advances in Forensic Haemogenetics 4
Edited by Ch. Rittner and P. M. Schneider
© Springer-Verlag Berlin Heidelberg 1992

Table 2. Exhibit types and success rates in 1990

EXHIBIT TYPE	SUCCESS RATE %
semen staining:	
INTERNAL VAGINAL SWABS	92
ANAL SWABS	56
KNICKERS	90
FABRIC/CLOTHING	72
SALIVA/MOUTH SWABS	43
CONDOMS	50
blood staining:	
DENIM	27
KNIVES	83
SHIRT MATERIAL	75
OTHER CLOTHING	53
LEATHER	43
saliva:	
CONTROL SALIVA SAMPLES	59
CIGARETTE ENDS	4
hairs:	
PLUCKED HAIR CONTROL SAMPLES	95
SHED HAIRS FROM CASE ITEMS	16

examination and which yielded less than 100 ng of DNA still gave good quality profiles. For this reason it is difficult to set a lower limit of semen concentration for profiling acceptability. In virtually all cases involving semen the preferential extraction method for separating spermatozoa from epithelial cells is used. Staining in the crutch of knickers also gives a high success rate and this is an option when there is no semen on vaginal swabs.

The lower rates of success with semen on anal swabs and in saliva samples probably reflects the fact that the levels of semen are often much lower. However semen profiles have been obtained from saliva samples taken up to 4 hours after an act of oral sex. Condoms are sometimes encountered in casework and they give an unusually low success rate considering the amount of semen present. This may be due to the fact that semen inside a condom will remain liquid and degrade more quickly than a stain on a dry substrate or that spermicides present in some condoms could inhibit restriction.

BLOOD STAINING

The percentage success obtained from blood staining is less than that from semen. DNA concentration in blood is much lower so a larger stain will be required and the more fragile nature of white blood cells compared with spermatozoa is likely to lead to faster degradation of DNA in bloodstains. The most suitable substrates for bloodstaining such as knife blades can be easily swabbed and the blood concentrated. Diffuse bloodstains on clothing are difficult to extract and concentrate. The normal protocol uses direct extraction of stain material with SDS and proteinase K . This is very efficient with small concentrated stains but with diffuse stains it yields a large volume of dilute DNA which is more awkward to process.

Denim has been included as a separate category because of the difficulties encountered with restricting the DNA that has been extracted. The dye present in the denim is extracted along with the DNA and it can be difficult to remove. It appears to strongly inhibit restriction enzymes as do the dyes present in some other dark coloured fabrics. Attempts have been made to remove these contaminants with further solvent extractions, dialysis and preparative electrophoresis. These methods have not always been entirely successful. If DNA is excessively coloured after purification it is re-dissolved in 0.2 m sodium acetate and then re-precipitated with ethanol. This often makes sufficient difference to allow the sample to be restricted successfully.

The same reasons probably account for the lower number of positives in the "other clothing" and "leather" categories whereas success with blood on shirt material which is colour fast and has probably been washed many times previously is relatively good.

SALIVA STAINING

Saliva contains cells that are constantly being shed from the lining of the mouth. In cases where blood or hair samples are not available, saliva may be used as a control sample.

Attempts to prepare profiles from saliva stains on cigarette ends etc have met with low success. The small volume of saliva present in stains makes them unlikely to work and no attempts to carry out DNA profiling are made unless a reasonable number of cells can be seen using the microscope.

There have been many requests to attempt profiling of saliva present on vaginal swabs following sexual assaults. The situation here is complicated by the presence of a second body fluid (vaginal) in large excess. As it is not possible to separate the cell types by a preferential extraction a mixed profile will result. The profile of the vaginal material is likely to be very much stronger than that of any saliva and secondary bands may well appear during the long autoradiograph exposures necessary for the weak saliva profile. Therefore at present, profiling on this type of exhibit is not performed.

HAIRS

Plucked head hairs are frequently used as control samples. A sufficient quantity of good quality DNA is usually obtained from approximately 10 hairs. However the success rate with shed hairs recovered from items such as hats and masks is much lower.

CONCLUSIONS

DNA profiling has been remarkably successful at providing very strong evidence from seminal stains especially those from vaginal swabs and knickers. Blood stains have given profiles in the majority of cases although dark coloured fabrics can cause difficulties. Success with saliva stains has been considerably lower. In the absence of a blood sample control, the use of plucked hairs is more likely to give a DNA profile than a saliva sample.

On DNA typing of hard tissues

Hammer, U., U. Bulnheim, R. Wegener
Institute of Legal Medicine, University of Rostock, Germany
O-2500 Rostock 1, Friedrich-Engels-Str. 108

INTRODUCTION

DNA preparation from tissues is necessary for forensic and pathological case work. Various methods for handling tissues and
samples have been described. Mostly it's possible to receive
muscles, lymph nodes or other organs from autopsy material in
sufficient quantities and good quality. The amount of degraded
DNA correlates directly with the duration of the postmortem
period (Bär 1988). Tissues with a high content of fibers and
minerals such as skin, tendon, also prostata and uterus, cartilage, bone and tooth (root) are more resistant to environmental
factors and can protect cells and their DNA longer than other
parenchymatous tissues as brain, muscle or liver.
In this paper are shown first experiences in DNA preparation of
hard an solid tissues, the yield and quality of DNA in dependence
of storage time and give some methodological advices.

MATERIAL

Specimens of all tissues from the same 40 years old male accident
victim who died immediatly. Cadaver was kept at 4^{0} C.
Prepared tissues samples:
- skin with complete lamination (without subcutis)
- tendon (Achilles tendon)
- cartilage (hyalin from joints, elastic from epiglottis, fibro-
  cartilage from intervertebral disk)
- bone from the skull
- teeth from the dentist

METHODS

Storage conditions:
Fresh cutted tissue pieces from autopsy material, frozen at
-80^{0} C immediatly, after one, after two and after three weeks
storage time in tubes at room temperature.
- The pieces were rasped in frozen conditions to aliquots of
  appr. 500 mg and stored again in the freezer till steps of
  cell lysis. We used a rasp with a very deep and rough profile
  for getting chips of bone or teeth or a pappy mass of skin,
  tendons and cartilages. All kinds of tissues had to rasp
  quickly because the material thaws within one minute and you
  will get only smear.
  For rasping the small pieces of hyalin cartilage they should
  be embedded in frozen water because of their very smooth
  surface.

Advances in Forensic Haemogenetics 4
Edited by Ch. Rittner and P. M. Schneider
© Springer-Verlag Berlin Heidelberg 1992

- Before lysis with Proteinase it is useful to decalcify the
  rasped bones and teeth:
  For one aliquot of 500 mg take 40 ml of high molar EDTA.
  Gently shaking overnight at 50° C (look at established methods
  in histological labs).
  After decalcification wash two times with isotonic sodiumchloride.
- Lysis with various concentrations and combinations of Pro-
  teinase K, Collagenase A (Boehringer) and Hyaluronidase
  (Dessau).
  For one aliquote mix gently with 10 ml of 0,01 M Tris-HCl
  (pH 7,6), 0,01 M EDTA, 0,1 M NaCl (pH 8,0) and 2 % SDS.
  Before addition of SDS it is useful to shake vigorously the
  mixture for getting a homogenious distribution of all tissue
  particles.
- Deproteinization two times with phenol-chloroform (1:1) and
  once with chloroform-isoamylalcohol (24:1).
- At least remove the upper phase because of impurities at the
  wall of the tubes such as insoluble minerals, filling substances
  of teeth, rests of tissue after incomplete lysis.
- DNA precipitation, digestions with restriction enzyme (Hinf I)
  and electrophoresis with known and established procedures.
- Hybridisation and visualization with the Digoxigenin labelled
  B.E.S.T.-Probe MZ 1.3.

RESULTS

1. Total yield of DNA from fresh prepared tissues (Table 1, Fig. 1).
2. We found clear less postmortal degradation of DNA prepared from
   hard and solid tissues compared with parenchymatous tissues
   (Fig. 2).
3. DNA from bone can be obtained with and without decalcification.
   After decalcification we got a higher yield of DNA (appr. 100 %).
   DNA in a tooth can only be recovered from the pulp and the
   directly surrounded parts of the dentin.
4. For all kinds of tissues the amount of Proteinase could be
   limited to 2 mg/500 mg rasped material. Less than 1 mg gave no
   sufficient desintegration and lysis. After testing Collagenase
   and Hylase alone with different concentrations we did not find
   lysis of the samples.
5. Only in combination of Proteinase and 300 units of Hyaluronidase
   it was possible to reduce the amount of Proteinase to less than
   1 mg/500 mg rasped material. Other combinations of Proteinase,
   Collagenase and Hyaluronidase gave no additional effect.
6. There were no fundamental differences in reaction of the
   various kinds of tissue to the enzymes.
7. All kinds of tissues of the same body showed identical band
   patterns.

Table 1.

Total yield of DNA from fresh tissues.
Yield in ug/g tissue

skin	325	bone	300
tendon	187	tooth	5
cartilage	612	prostata	580

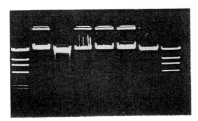

Fig. 1.

High molecular weight control of DNA from
fresh autopsy material: lambda, skin, tendon,
cartilage, bone, tooth, prostata
(from left to right)

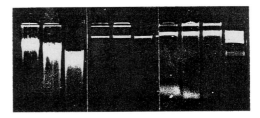

Fig. 2.

High molecular weight control of DNA prepared from
muscle, tendon and bone after storage time of one,
two and three weeks at room temperature
(from left to right)

DISCUSSION

The described mechanic destruction of tissues by rasping is simple
but good for efficiency of digestion with Proteinase. Furthermore there is no danger of contagiousness by microdrops during
homogenization with a conventionel apparatus.
Commonly digestion with Proteinase will be sufficient. Using
of Hyaluronidase and Proteinase together could be important only
for analysis of tissues which are very rich in cells and fibers.
The influence of the enzymes used for cell lysis to activity of
restriction enzymes should be investigated in a further study.
The comparison of enzyme activity between Proteinase, Collagenase
and Hyaluronidase is difficult (definition of units). Thatswhy the
enzyme dosis choosed in our lab should go in control. Using of
Collagenase type "A" was decided after recommendations of
Boehringer. Main contents of the phiols are lyophilized Collagenase and some proteolytic activities.
For DNA analysis after longer postmortem period we recommend preparation of bone or prostata and uterus as showed in this paper.
It is not necessary to take bone marrow; also compact structures
of pelvis or skull are suitable.

REFERENCES

Baird M, Giusti A, Meade E, Clyne M, Shaler R, Benn P,
Glassberg J, Balazs I (1988) The Application of DNA-Print for
    Identification from Forensic Biological Materials. Adv Forens
    Haem 2
Bär W, Kratzer A, Mächler M, Schmid W (1988) Postmortem stability
    of DNA. Forens Sci Int 39: 59 - 70
Gill P, Jeffreys AJ, Werret DJ (1985) Forensic application of
    DNA fingerprints. Nature 318
Mangin PD, Ludes BP (1991) A Forensic Application of DNA Typing:
    Paternity Determination in a Putrefied Fetus. Am J Forens Med
    Pathol 12: 161 - 163
Ogata M, Mattern R, Schneider PM, Schacker U, Kaufmann T,
Rittner C (1990) Quantitative and qualitative analysis of DNA
    extracted from postmortem muscle tissue. Z Rechtsmed 103:
    397 - 406

Use of the Minisatellite Probe MZ 1.3 for Identification and Relation of Dismembered Corpses

W. Huckenbeck, H. Müller

Institute of Legal Medicine, Heinrich–Heine–University, Düsseldorf, FRG

INTRODUCTION

The inquest of dismembered corpses confronts the investigator with several problems. One of them is the identification of parts of corpses and their relation to one or more persons. Putrefaction severely alters the integrity of macromolecules and receptors. We tested the usefulness of the hypervariable minisatellite probe MZ 1.3 for such sorts of examinations. The probe proved to be successful in demonstrating individual bands. The results of in–vitro experiments – including freeze–dried specimens – are discussed.

MATERIAL & METHODS

1. Extraction of DNA : about 1 g specimens of postmortem heartblood, brain cortex, muscle tissue and spleen are homogenized mechanically (Ultra–Turrax, IKA) in 10 ml nuclei lysis buffer containing 10 mM Tris-Cl ph 8, 400 mM NaCl, 2 mM EDTA pH 8. Freeze–dried samples were treated in the same way. Heart blood was incubated with 50mM KCl at 37°C followed by centrifugation (1000xg).This procedure was repeated up to the pellet got white colour. Digest with Proteinase K (500µg/ml) and SDS (final concentration 0.5%., incubation overnight at 37°C, DNA extraction twice in phenol/chloroform/isoamyl alcohol (25:24:1), praecipitation by solding 2 vol. of abs. ethanol, resumption of the DNA pellet in 100 µl TE and incubation at 56°C for one hour; once more praecipitation by adding 20 µl 3M Na–acetate and 500 µl abs. ethanol, one time wash of the DNA pellet in 70% ethanol, resumption of the dried pellet in TE followed by dialysis for 3–4 hours. 2. Digestion of DNA : 50 U of the enzymes Hinf I and Hae III overnight at 37° (at least for 18 hours).

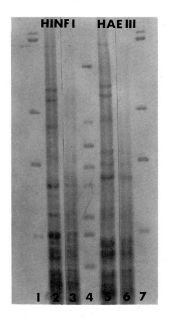

FIG.1a   Burnt Corpse

Lane 1,7 – bacteriophage lamda Hind III marker;
Lane 2,5 – heart blood;
Lane 3,6 – myocard;
Lane 4 – bacteriophage DNA Bst EII marker

Advances in Forensic Haemogenetics 4
Edited by Ch. Rittner and P. M. Schneider
© Springer-Verlag Berlin Heidelberg 1992

3. Electrophoresis: separation of the restriction fragments in a 0.6 % agarose gel (20 X 20 cm) in 1 X TBE at constant voltage (40V) for 27 hours.
4. Southern blot: depurination in 0.3 M HCL for 20 minutes, denaturation in 0.5 M NaOH, 1.5 M NaCl twice for 30 minutes; transfer of the DNA on a lab bench covered with plastic wrap on a nylon membrane (BIODYNE A; Fa. PALL and ONCOR) soaked in denaturation solution for 15 minutes, transfer blot proceeding overnight followed by neutralization of the membrane in 0.5 M Tris-Cl pH 8.0, 1.5 M NaCl for 15 minutes, washing the membrane in 2 X SSC for 10 minutes. Finally the DNA is baked at 80°C for 1 hour.
5. Non-radioactive detection: prehybridization and hybridization with the multi-locus minisatellite probe B.E.S.T. MZ 1.3 digoxigenin according to the method described in the BIOTEST-Manual (Fa. BIOTEST, Dreieich, Germany).
6. Colour development : Incubation with antibody alkaline phosphatase complex solution (Fa. BIOTEST or Fa. BOEHRINGER), 1:5000, for 30-60 minutes, development with BCIP/NBT (BCIP: 50mg/ml DMF; NBT: 75mg/ml 70% DMF).

CONCLUSIONS

DNA-Fingerprinting is a useful method for identification of postmortem tissues (1,2,3,4). According to its original definition the genetic fingerprint requires use of a multi locus probe or quite a number of several single locus probes. Multi locus fingerprinting gives more information per examination and methodical artefacts can be recognized by interpreting the DNA pattern. We tested the multi locus probe B.E.S.T. MZ 1.3 DIGOXIGENIN (BIOTEST) for use in relation of tissues to one or more persons. Some of our results are shown in fig.1 and fig.2. The probe was detected as a useful aid in such cases of identification. Best results can be expected in heart blood, brain cortex and muscle tissue. DNA typing on freeze-dried tissues demonstrates that the method of freeze-drying is a very mild technique for both toxicology and serology.

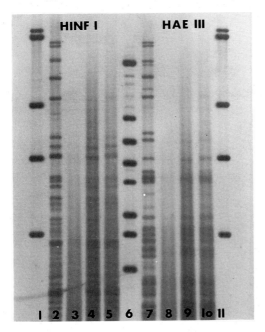

FIG. 1b   Child, 8 weeks old

Lane 1,11 - bacteriophage lamda
Hind III marker
Lane 2,7 - heart blood
Lane 3,8 - spleen
Lane 4,9 - brain cortex
Lane 5,10 - muscle tissue
Lane 6 - bacteriophage DNA Bst
EII marker

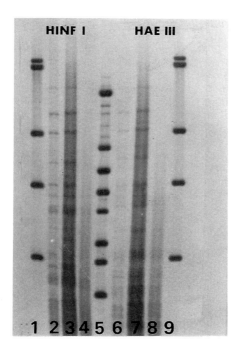

FIG. 2   Freeze-Dried Tissues

Lane 1,9 – bacteriophage
lamda Hind III marker;
Lane 2,6 – heart blood;
Lane 3,7 – brain cortex
Lane 4,8 – muscle
Lane 5 – bacteriophage DNA
Bst EII marker

REFERENCES

1) Nowak, R., Fink, T. (1986) Geschlechtsbestimmung an Leichenmaterial durch Nachweis spezifischer Nukleotid-Sequenzen des Y-Chromosoms nach DNA-Spaltung.
Z. Rechtsmed. 97: 21–28

2) Ogata, M., Mattern, R., Schneider, P.M., Schacker, U., Kaufmann, T., Rittner, C. (1990) Quantitative and qualitative analysis of DNA extracted from postmortem muscle tissues. Z. Rechtsmed. 103: 397–406

3) Pöche, H., Wrobel, G., Schneider, V., Epplen, J.T. (1990) Oligonucleotid-Fingerprinting mit (GTG)5 und (GACA)4 für die Zuordnung von Leichenteilen. Arch. f. Krim. 186/1+2: 37–42

4) Pöche, H., Wrobel, G., Schneider, V., Epplen, J.T. (1990) DNA-Fingerprinting in Katastrophenfällen – Identifizierung einer Brandleiche (Hotelbrand mit 7 Opfern).
(Abstract) Zbl. Rechtsmed. 34,6: 415

RFLP IN CONJUNCTION WITH ANATOMICAL TRAITS IN INDIVIDUALISATION OF BONE

G V RAO & V K KASHYAP*

Central Forensic Science Laboratory
Ramanthapur : Hyderabad   500 013
A. P.   INDIA

ABSTRACT

RFLP of D4S139 and D14S1, loci is used to individualize a tibia bone seized in a homicide case. Bone was sexed with a Y specific probe. Anatomical traits were eleborately studied to conclude identification.

INTRODUCTION

RFLP analysis is an unequivocal approach for individualisation of biological materials. The conclusiveness of evidence depends upon recovery of DNA from sample, number and nature of loci analysed and DNA prints used for comparison. DNA profiles of body fluids their stains and soft tissue are frequently prepared using multilocus or a battery of highly polymorphic locus specific probes and compared with suspects or of his/her parents to fix the identity of sample (Gill P. 1985). Without adequate amount of high mol. wt. DNA and proper controls the DNA profiling is insignificant. The identity of deceased from a bone in similar situation is established with only pAW101 and pH 30 two loci specific probes and using 102(d)2 (Singh L et al 1980) a Y specific probe. Anatomical traits, i.e. age, height and nature of callus present on an old healed fracture of tibia were examined for conclusive identification.

MATERIALS & METHODS

Examination of Bone

A left tibia and a small piece of maxilla containing 5 teeth (3 PM + 2M) seized in a homicide case were X-rayed and examined to ascertain height and age. A callus present on lower extremity of tibia was X-rayed and examined to know nature and time of fracture (Krogman & Iscan 1986).

DNA Extraction and Profiling

The bone marrow (BM) of tibia was scrapped out mechanically into TES buffer. The extracted marrow alongwith blood samples

---

* Author for correspondence to

Advances in Forensic Haemogenetics 4
Edited by Ch. Rittner and P. M. Schneider
© Springer-Verlag Berlin Heidelberg 1992

of mother (M), brother (B), sister (S) was subjected for DNA analysis by standard method (Gautreau et al 1983). 1.0ug DNA from each sample was digested with EcoRI and Hind III separately. DNA samples (BM, M, BM+M, S, B) alongwith human control of known allele composition, lambda size marker were electrophoresed in lane 1 to 7 respectively. After transfer and baking on nylon membrane blots of EcoRI and Hind III digested DNA were hybridized with pAW101 (Nakamura et al 1988) and pH30 (Milner et al 1989) probes respectively. The hybridized blots were washed stringently with 0.1 x SSC, 0.1% SOS and exposed for autoradiography.

Sexing

100ng of bone DNA was dotted on nylon membrane alongwith DNA of M, B & S and known control of both sexes and hybridized with P32 labelled 102(d) 2 Y-specific probe to ascertain sex of source.

Band Matching and Statistical Interpretation

The size of bands in DNA print of bone M, B and S were computed with relative mobilities of DNA size marker. The bands of bone were compared with bands in profiles of M, S and B. The probability of relationship was calculated using (Lynch 1988), a database of allele frequency for South Indian population prepared for both the probes (data unpublished). The probability value of involvement of two persons of a particular age, sex and height and with similar abnormality – like limping as reported in this case of suspected deceased in a homicide case was also calculated. The final conclusion of the identity of source of bone was drawn by considering (i) Probability of relatednes between bone and M, S & B DNA Profiles; and (ii) probability of any other individual of same anatomical traits involved in homicide.

RESULT AND DISCUSSION

On visual comparison of DNA profiles developed by pAW101 with EcoRI restricted DNA and pH30 with Hind III digested DNA, it is clear that one band (12kb) for pAW101 is comparable with a band of mother's profile, other band of bone matches with the non-maternal (paternal) band in one of the two siblings. Similarly, one band (8kb) of bone is comperable with one band of mother's profile, other band matching with the siblings band. Bone marrow DNA did not hybridize with 102(d) 2 probe indicating that bone belongs to a human female. On examination of tibia maxilla and tooth sections and their radiographs, it was found that tibia and maxilla may belong to a human female of 25±5 years age group and 5'.1"±1" height may be having a healed fracture on lower extremity of tibia which may cause limping as in the case of suspected deceased. Since the mean probability of presence of any allele of D4S139 in two unrelated individuals is 3.6×10^{-2} and allele of D14S1 is 2.7×10^{-3}, this suggests that tibia belongs female child of M and true sibling of B&S (probability 1.23×10^{-8}).

A.

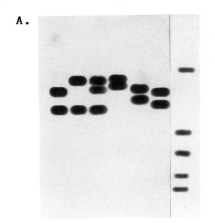

B.

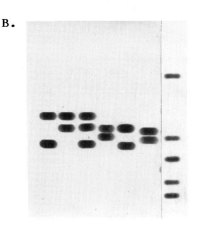

Figure 1(A)&(B): DNA Profile of a bone individualization case. DNA profile of bone marrow : Lane 1; Mother, Sister and Brother : Lane 2,4,5; Bone marrow + Mother : Lane 3; Known control : Lane 6; Size marker : Lane 7; (A) DNA profile with pAW101, (B) DNA profile with pH30

The chance of any other lady of 25±5 age group and 5'.1"±1" of height in India having a 6-8 year old healed fracture in lower end of tibia leading in limping worked out to be 1.8×10^{-7}. From DNA profiling and anatomical traits study, tibia is found to belong to suspected deceased (probability 1.7×10^{15}). It is evident from this study that a bone can be successfully individualized, with RFLP analysis at two loci, provided it bears specific characteristics which are discernable on examination.

REFERENCES

Gautreau C, Rahuel C, Cartron JP and Leucotte G (1983) Comparison of two methods of high molecular weight DNA isolation from human leukocytes. Anal Biochem 134:320-324
Gill P, Jeffreys AJ and Werrett DJ (1985) Forensic Application of DNA 'fingerprints'. Nature 318:577-579
Krogman WM and Iscan MY (1986) The human skeleton in Forensic Medicine. 2nd edn. Charles Thomas, USA
Lynch M (1988) Estimation of relatedness by DNA Fingerprinting. Mol Biol Evol 5:584-599
Milner ECB, Lotshaw CJ, Willems van Dijk, Charmley P, Cancannon P and Schroeder HW (1989) Isolation and mapping of a polymorphic DNA sequence pH30 on chromosome 4(HGM provisional No.D4S139). Nucleic Acids Res 17:4002
Nakamura Y, Carlson M, Krapcho K, Kanamori M and White R (1988) New approach for isolation of VNTR markers. Am J Hum Genet 43:854-859
Singh L, Purdom IF and Jones KW (1980) Sex chromosome associated satellite DNA. Evolution and Conservation Chromosoma 79:137-157

Application of DNA Fingerprinting to Problematical Paternity Cases

T. Kishida, M. Fukuda, Y. Tamaki

Department of Forensic Medicine
Medical College of Oita, Hasama-cho
Oita 879-55, Japan

INTRODUCTION

DNA fingerprinting has found wide application in forensic science practice. This communication describes briefly the results of DNA fingerprinting with minisatellite probes applied to problematical paternity cases with a relatively low probability of paternity or involving silent alleles.

MATERIALS AND METHODS

Typing for Conventional Genetic Systems

Blood samples from paternity trios were tested for 27 conventional genetic systems by routine techniques. The genetic systems used were as follows: 7 red cell antigen systems (ABO, MNS, RH, DI, P, JK, and FY); 14 serum protein systems (GM, KM, HP, TF, GC, PI, A2HS, C6, C7, C81, BF, HF, HI, and F13B); and 6 red cell enzyme systems (ACP, ESD, GPT, GLO1, PGD, and PGM1).

Case Summary

In Case 1, blood samples were tested for 25 genetic systems, exclusive of GM and KM since the child was four months old. The overall probability of paternity exclusion by the 25 systems was 0.9563, yet none of the systems indicated nonpaternity. On the other hand, the overall probability of paternity was 0.4175, which was too low to establish paternity.

In Case 2, typing for 27 genetic systems revealed isolated nonmaternity in the GM system and nonpaternity in the C7 system. Contrary homozygosity was observed in both systems (GM AG/GM AB3ST and C7 1/C7 2). Based on the 25 systems, exclusive of GM and C7, the overall probability of paternity exclusion was calculated at 0.9990 and the overall probability of paternity at 0.9986, which was interpreted as establishing paternity. The results strongly suggested the presence of silent alleles in the GM and C7 systems. In addition, a GC variant with two pairs of double band was found in the mother; therefore, the blood samples of the mother's family were examined

Advances in Forensic Haemogenetics 4
Edited by Ch. Rittner and P. M. Schneider
© Springer-Verlag Berlin Heidelberg 1992

likewise. Unfortunately, we could not examine the alleged father's kindred.

DNA Fingerprinting

DNA samples were isolated from peripheral blood by a phenol-alcohol method and digested with *Hae* Ⅲ (Case 1) or *Hin* f Ⅰ (Case 2). After agarose gel electrophoresis, the digests were Southern-blotted onto nylon membranes. The blots were hybridized with a digoxigenin-labeled MZ 1.3 probe (B.E.S.T.-Probe, Biotest, Frankfurt, FRG) in Case 1, and with an alkaline phosphatase-labeled synthetic Myo probe (SNAP Probe, Molecular Biosystems, San Diego, Ca) in Case 2. The band sharing frequencies were calculated according to the formula of Schacker *et al.* (1990).

RESULTS AND DISCUSSION

Figure 1 shows the DNA fingerprints. In Case 1 (left part), the numbers of shared child/mother and child/alleged father bands were 5 and 4, respectively. The band sharing frequency for the alleged father was calculated at 0.571, and this value was interpreted as establishing paternity.

In Case 2, the results of the family study supported the presence of a GM silent allele and a GC variant suggestive of a gene duplication of two *GC∗1* alleles (Fig. 2). In DNA fingerprinting, the child shared 4 bands each with the mother and the alleged father (Fig. 1, right part). The band sharing frequencies were 0.500 and 0.615, which establishied parent-child relation.

This study demonstrates that conventional genetic systems cannot compete with highly polymorphic DNA loci.

REFERENCES

Schacker U, Schneider PM, Holtkamp B, Bohnke E, Fimmers R, Sonneborn HH, Rittner C (1990) Isolation of the DNA minisatellite probe MZ 1.3 and its application to DNA 'fingerprinting' analysis. Forens Sci Int 44:209-224

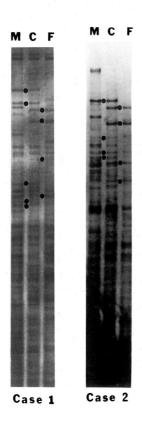

Case 1   **Case 2**

Fig. 1. DNA fingerprints of two families. M = mother, C = child, F = alleged father. Informative bands are indicated by dots

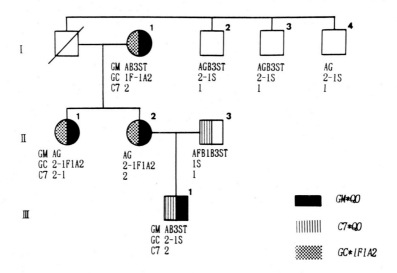

Fig. 2. Pedigree of the family with *GM*QO*, *C7*QO*, and *GC*IFIA2* (Case 2)

Application of conventional polymorphisms and single locus DNA probes in cases of disputed paternity

P.J. Lincoln, C.P. Phillips, D.Syndercombe Court,
J.A. Thomson, P.H. Watts

Department of Haematology, The London Hospital Medical College,
Turner Street, London E1 2AD, UK

A series of 151 cases of disputed paternity have been
investigated using up to 5 single-locus DNA probes and also a
battery of 15-20 systems of red cell antigen, red cell enzyme,
serum protein polymorphisms and also, but rarely, HLA. The DNA
probes used were Muc 7, MR24/1, 3'α-HVR (Amersham Int), TBQ7
and YNH24 (Promega Corp).

We have assessed the combined use of both conventional and DNA
testing in this context. Also the cases have been used to
determine the power of exclusion of wrongly named men by the
construction of false trios.

METHODS

3μg samples of <u>Alu1</u>-digested DNA from whole blood samples were
electrophoresed, blotted and hybridised using the probes named
above. Fragment sizes were estimated by manual measurement of
migration distances using the local form of the reciprocal
relationship $c=(m-m_o)(L-L_o)$ as described by Elder and Southern
(1987). The DNA size markers used were a 14-rung ^{35}S-labelled
ladder. (Amersham Int). A named man is considered a possible
father if he has a band within +/-2.5% of the paternal band in
the child, when the samples have been run on the same gel. The
frequency of occurrence of the paternal band in the child was
estimated from databases compiled in this laboratory using a
window of +/-5% of the paternally contributed band size,
summing the number of bands in this range. Databases are of
150-250 European caucasians.

RESULTS

114 of the 151 cases gave no exclusions on conventional or DNA
testing, using up to 5 probes. Clear exclusions were found
using conventional testing in 25 cases, and all of these were
detected with two or more DNA probes.

In 12 cases the conventional testing did not allow a clear
conclusion to be made but DNA testing was useful (see Table 1).

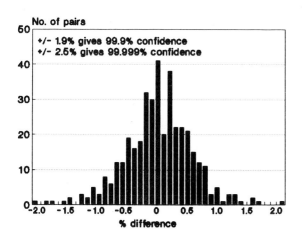

Fig. 1. Frequency
distribution of %
size difference
between 394
mother-child pairs
showing the
within-gel variation
experienced

To assess the variation seen when samples are run on different
gels, two control samples were electrophoresed on 30 gels
carrying case samples. Figure 2 shows the variation for each
of the five probes used. The larger variation seen with
3'⍺-HVR and TBQ7 is due mainly to the very small fragments seen
here. We currently use a window of +/-5% when using databases
or matching samples from different gels, but it is likely that
this window will be altered to reflect the variation seen over
a particular fragment size range.

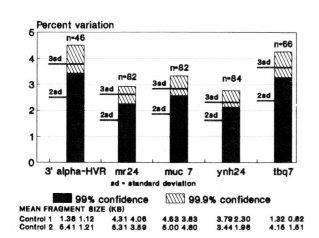

Fig. 2. Bar chart
showing the amount
of between-gel
variation for each
probe

It is important on some occasions to be able to compare samples
that have been processed and measured in different laboratories
using different techniques. The data was examined initially
for outliers by plotting mean fragment size against difference
in fragment size. Five outliers were identified, all relating
to measurement made by image analysis. The discrepancies were
due to wrongly identified bands, poorly resolved bands and
problems associated with sizing when there are not sufficient
ladder rungs. Obviously assiduous checking of results,
whatever method of measurement is used, is essential to avoid
errors. Also, a large between-laboratory difference, in the
sizes of the two very large bands detected, was related to the
different resolution in the large fragment region of the gels
run in the separate laboratories. Therefore it would also seem
that rigorous standardisation is important if there is going to
be a meaningful exchange of results or sharing of databases.

Figure 3 shows that, when results from the two laboratories
were compared, there was minimal variation (around +/-1.5%) in
measurements produced by manual (ruler) and automatic (image
analysis) methods of measurement and both performed similarly.
Figure 4 shows that, using this set of probes, up to a +/-5%
variation can occur in fragment sizes obtained from tests
conducted in two different laboratories.

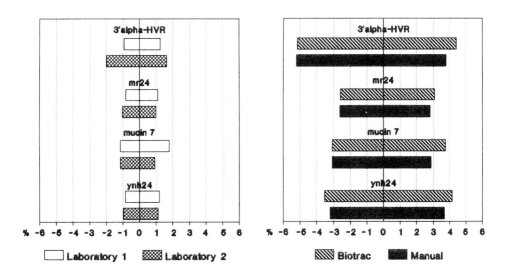

Fig. 3. 99% confidence
intervals for the between
measurement method %
differences

Fig. 4. 99% confidence
intervals for the between
laboratory autoradiograph %
differences

MS1, MS31 AND MS43A SINGLE LOCUS PROBES: A PRELIMINARY STUDY IN THE BASQUE POPULATION AND ITS APPLICATION IN PATERNITY TESTING

S. Alonso*, A. Castro, A. García-Orad, P. Arizti, G. Tamayo**, M. Martínez de Pancorbo

Servicio de Diagnóstico de la Paternidad Biológica del País Vasco: Dpto. de Biología Celular y Ciencias Morfológicas*, Dpto. de Medicina Legal**. Facultad de Medicina y Odontología. Campus de Leioa, Vizcaya, SPAIN

INTRODUCTION

Traditionally, phenotype markers have been used to establish identity and biological paternity. At the present time polymorphisms in minisatellite regions, such as those revealed by single locus probes, may solve all filliation matters with a much higher fiability (Jeffreys et al. 1985a, 1985b; Rose et al. 1988; Valentin 1980).

In this work the results obtained from the study of loci D1S7, D7S21 and D12S11 in a small sample of Basque population are shown in order to set a data base with the frequency of the alleles detected on these loci with the probes MS1, MS31 and MS43A going, which will enable us to establish biological paternity using these DNA polymorphisms in our population. Using these probes we also studied five mother-child-alleged fathers selected among those we have been requested to solve till now.

MATERIAL AND METHODS

Four micrograms from each individual were digested with Hinf I and the fragments obtained, fractionated by electrophoresis in 0.7% agarose gels. Single locus probes were provided already labeled with the NICE system (Cellmark Diagnostics). Allele sizes for fragments detected with SLPs, were performed taking as a reference the NICE DNA analysis ladder (from BRL) in combination with probe MW100, and using Elder and Southern´s reciprocal method. K562 cell line was used as a control. The probability of paternity for each case was calculated using Jeffreys´ method.

RESULTS AND DISCUSSION

The frequency distributions for the alleles detected with single locus probes MS1, MS31, and MS43A are shown in Fig. 1. The size ranges of the fragments (Table 1) are very similar to those found by Smith et al. (1990). The allele number obtained in this sample is lower than that reported in the literature. It might be argued, as Balazs et al. suggest (1989), that these polymorphic loci in our population contain alleles that are smaller than those retained by gels used here. The occurrence of such alleles would result in the detection of an excess number of homozygous individuals relative to those predicted by the frequency of alleles. However, the calculated heterozygosity does not differ statistically from that observed; therefore it seems more probable that this might reflect some differential features of the Basque population. This population has been shown to have gene frequency distributions different from the European ones in several number of studied polymorphic systems (García-Orad et al., 1990; Aguirre et al., 1991). A more extensive population sample will allow us to solve this point.

Advances in Forensic Haemogenetics 4
Edited by Ch. Rittner and P. M. Schneider
© Springer-Verlag Berlin Heidelberg 1992

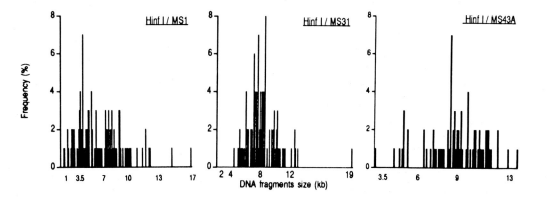

Fig. 1. Distribution of MS1, MS31 and MS43A alleles

Table 1. Observed (Ho) and expected (He) heterocigosities, allele sizes and mean frequencies for three loci

PROBE	Ho	He	Size-range (kb)	Most frequent allele (kb)	q
MS1	0.945	0.965	0.9 - 17	3.8 ± 0.14	0.035
MS31	0.833	0.891	1.9 - 19	8.0 ± 0,28	0.109
MS43A	0.892	0.920	3.4 - 14	8.8 ± 0.31	0.080

Table 2. Discriminatory capabilities of MS1, MS31 and MS43A for identity and paternity pourposes

PROBE	Alleles	$2q-q^2$ [a]	$q^2(2-q)$ [b]	Pex [c]
MS1	4 2	0.0688	0.0024	0.952
MS31	19	0.2061	0.0224	0.893
MS43A	18	0.1536	0.0123	0.887

[a] Band sharing probability
[b] Inclusion probability
[c] Exclusion probability of paternity

The inclusion probability and the exclusion probability of paternity estimated from the above results are showed in Table2. These parameters confirm the discrimination power of single locus probes MS1,MS31 and MS43A in the Basque Country. In order to test this, five mother-child-alleged father trios were analyzed; the results obtained are shown in table 3. In all the cases, the pattern of inclusion or exclusion of the alleged father, matched that observed using the conventional systems.

The results obtained with the application of these probes, points their power of exclusion up, and confirm the possibility of obtaining very high probabilities of paternity. Thus, we continue elaborating a more complete data base which will enable us to use these probes for identity and paternity purposes in our population.

Table 3. Results on five cases tested with MS1, MS31 and MS43A probes and conventional systems

	Exclusion				
Case	MS1	MS31	MS43A	P P	Exclusion with conventional systems
#1	-	-	-	0.995	
#2	+	+	+	-	Gc, ACP, PGM
#3	-	-	-	0.948	
#4	+	+	-	-	Rh, ADA, GLO
#5	-	-	-	0.989	

ACKNOWLEDGEMENTS: This work has been supported by a grant from the Basque Government (PGV 9041-1). MS1, MS31 and MS43A single locus probes have been kindly supplied by Cellmark Diagnostics (Abingdon U.K.).

REFERENCES

Aguirre AI, Vicario A, Mazón LI, Martínez de Pancorbo M, Estomba A, Lostao C (1991) Acid phosphatase, adenosin deaminase and esterase D polymorphisms in the Spanish Basque population. Hum Hered 41:93-102

Balazs I, Baird M, Clyne M, Meade E (1989) Human population genetic studies of five hypervariable DNA loci. Am J Hum Genet, 44:182-190

Elder JK, Southern EM (1983) Measurement of DNA fragments length by gel electrophoresis. Anal Biochem 128:227-231

García-Orad A, Arizti P, Esteban JL, García-Orad C, García-Arenzana C, Constans J, Martínez de Pancorbo M (1990) Gene Geography 4:43-52

Jeffreys AJ, Wilson V, Thein SL (1985a) Individual-specific "fingerprints" of human DNA. Nature 316:76-79

Jeffreys AJ, Brookfield JFY, Semeonoff R(1985b) Positive identification of an immigration test-case using DNA fingerpritns. Nature 317: 818-819

Rose SD, Keith TP (1988) Aplication of DNA probes in parentage testing. American Clinical Laboratory

Smith JC, Anwar R, Riley J, Jenner D, Markham AF (1990) Highly polymorphic minisatellite sequences: allele frequencies and mutation rates for five locus-specific probes in a Caucasian population. J Forensic Sci 30:19-32

Valentin J (1980) Exclusions and attributions of paternity: practical experiences of forensic genetics and statistics. Am J Hum G 32: 420-230

Wong A, Wilson V, Patel I, Povey S, Jeffreys AJ (1987) Characterization of a panel of highly variable minisatellites cloned from human DNA. Ann. Hum. Genet. 51: 269-288

DNA FINGERPRINTING WITH PROBES 33.15 AND 33.6 IN POPULATION FROM THE BASQUE COUNTRY

S. Alonso*, A. Castro, A. García-Orad, P. Arizti, G. Tamayo**, M. Martínez de Pancorbo

Servicio de Diagnóstico de la Paternidad Biológica del País Vasco. *Dpto. de Biología Celular y Ciencias Morfológicas y **Dpto. de Medicina Legal. Facultad de Medicina y Odontología. Universidad del País Vasco. 48940 Leioa, Vizcaya, SPAIN

INTRODUCTION

Some minisatellite areas dispersed through the human genome show a high level of genetic variability which makes them useful for identity and paternity purposes. This great variability in the number of repetitions among loci from different individuals, determines the probability of finding two unrelated people with an identical restriction profile to be minimum (Jeffreys et al. 1985a, Jeffreys et al. 1985 b).

As the application of these probes gives a high power of resolution, we have chosen multilocus probes 33.6 and 33.15 to carry out a study on a sample of resident population from the Basque Country. The obtained results will enable us to use these probes for Legal Medicine purposes in our population.

MATERIAL AND METHODS

The studied sample consisted of 50 unrelated individuals. Eight micrograms from each individual were digested with Hinf I and the obtained fragments fractionated by electrophoresis in 0.7% agarose gels. DNA from K562 cell line was used as control. The multilocus probes were labeled by the repeat unit multipriming system (Cellmark Diagnostics), using $\alpha^{32}P$ dGTP. The mobilities of the restriction fragments were measured using a videodensitometer.

RESULTS AND DISCUSSION

The average number of bands per individual obtained with probes 33.15 and 33.6 is shown in Table 1. Fragments were classified according to different size ranges to analyze them in the size class which gave the best resolution for each probe. Our results show that probe 33.15 resolves more fragments within the region of lowest size (in kb), while probe 33.6 reveals more fragments in the highest size class.

The probability of bandsharing between two unrelated individuals $(2q-q^2)$ is shown in Table1. These results are similar to those obtained by Jeffreys et al. (1985c) and Gill et al. (1987) who previously found the probability of sharing one band to be higher for the smallest minisatellite fragments.

Advances in Forensic Haemogenetics 4
Edited by Ch. Rittner and P. M. Schneider
© Springer-Verlag Berlin Heidelberg 1992

The band-sharing distribution between two individuals fits a binomial distribution for both probes individually ($X^2{}_{5\,d.f} = 2.822$ for 33.15 and $X^2{}_{5\,d.f} = 2.579$ for 33.6). Both probes show very high heterozygosities (Table 2), which points out that they are extremely resolutives for identity and paternity testing purposes, since the combination of both probes reveals that the probability of all bands matching between two unrelated individuals is 1.403×10^{-21}.

Table 1. Similarities of DNA fingerprints between random pairs of individuals, using multilocus probes[*]

DNA fragments size (kb)	Fragments per individual ± s.d.	$2q-q^2$	q
PROBE 33.15			
23.13 - 9.42	1.6 ± 1.1	0.20	0.10
9.42 - 6.56	3.0 ± 1.3	0.29	0.14
6.56 - 4.37	7.2 ± 1.6	0.21	0.10
Mean no. of bands: 11.8 ± 2.6			
PROBE 33.6			
20 -10	4.3 ± 1.5	0.48	0.24
10 - 6	3.4 ± 1.5	0.34	0.17
6 - 4	6.2 ± 2.0	0.18	0.09
Mean no. of bands: 13.9 ± 3.9			

[*] Data were obtained from a sample of 43 unrelated Basque Country individuals

Table 2. Mean allele frequencies (q), heterozygosities (H), and mean probability of two unrelated individuals sharing all fragments ($2q-q^2$), detected by probes 33.15 and 33.6

	PROBE 33.15	PROBE 33.6	33.15+33.6
q	0.087	0.103	0.095
H	0.913	0.897	0.905
$2q-q^2$	7.674 E-10	1.829 E-10	1.403 E-21

The band-sharing distribution between two individuals follows a binomial distribution for both probes individually ($X^2{}_{5d.f.} = 2.822$ for 33.15 and $X^2{}_{5d.f.} = 2.579$ for 33.6). Both probes 33.15 and 33.6, show very high heterozygosities.

In order to test the exclusion power of these probes in paternity testing, 5 trios mother-child-alleged father selected among those we have been requested to resolve until now were studied. The results obtained from the DNA fingerprints in each paternity case are shown in Table 3. In cases 1, 3 and 5, bandsharing between the mother and the child was that expected ($\approx 62,6\%$). However, the children did not show any father-specific band, excluding case 5, in which the child showed only one father-specific band.

In cases 2 and 4, the expected mother-child bandsharing was confirmed. A high number of shared-bands between alleged fathers and children was also found. In case 2, all the child´s bands were assigned, and in case 4 there remains just one unassigned band, which is supposed to be a mutant one. As the data did not exclude the alleged fathers, probe 33.6 was also applied to cases 2 and 4. The use of this probe resulted in the band assignaments shown in Table 3. Also in this table, the calculated probabilities of paternity for each probe and for each mother-child-alleged father trio are summarized. The analysis of these five cases studied agreed to the results previously obtained through the study of the conventional markers (table 4). In all the cases where these markers had excluded paternity, probes 33.15 and 33.6 also did it. This exclusion was particularly evident in case 5 where after the analysis of 19 protein systems and red cell groups, exclusion could only be stated by the HLA system. The probabilities of paternity obtained with multilocus probes 33.15 and 33.6 were much higher than those obtained through conventional markers. This makes the application of these probes to be of great interest also in the Basque Country.

Table 3. Assigned bands and Pp in paternity cases using probes 33.15 and 33.6

| Case | Parents' shared bands | Child's bands | | | | Pp |
		Mother specific	Father specific	Shared bands	Unassigned bands	
Probe 33.15						
#1	3	6	0	3	6	
#2	3	6	5	3	0	0.9998
#3	4	5	0	4	7	
#4	1	6	3	1	1	0.6992
#5	4	5	1	2	8	
Probe 33.6						
#2	10	2	3	8	0	0.7574
#4	4	7	10	4	0	0.9999
Probes 33.15+33.6						
#2	13	8	8	11	0	0.999943
#4	5	13	13	5	1	0.999991

Table 4. Results in five cases tested with conventional systems

CASE	SYSTEMS WITH OBSERVED EXCLUSION	Pp
#1	MNSs, Gc, PGM1, ADA	
#2	Not observed	0.952
#3	MNSs, GLO, AK	
#4	Not observed	0.996
#5	HLA A, B, C	

ACKNOWLEDGEMENTS: This work has been supported by a grant from the Basque Government (PGV 9041-1).

REFERENCES

Gill P, Lygo JE, Fowler SJ, and Werret DJ (1987) An evaluation of DNA Fingerprinting for forensic purposes. Electrophoresis 8:38-44

Jeffreys AJ, Wilson V and Thein SL (1985a) Hypervariable "minisatellite" regions in human DNA. Nature 314: 67-73.

Jeffreys AJ, Brookfield JFY and Semeonoff R(1985b) Positive identification of an immigration test-case using DNA fingerpritns. Nature 317: 818-819.

Jeffreys AJ, Wilson V andThein SL (1985c) Individual-specific "fingerprints" of human DNA. Nature 316:76-79

Casuistic: The Use of DNA–Fingerprinting in Cases of Affiliation
Without Mother

W. Huckenbeck, H.Müller, M. Prinz

Institute of Legal Medicine, Heinrich–Heine–University, Düsseldorf*

INTRODUCTION

We report a case of affiliation which can be assigned to the problem area
of the so called deficiency cases. The mother and the putative father
both were dead. For the examinations the putative father was exhumed
after a period of four weeks. The mother had died years earlier,
exhumation seemed to be pointless. The following samples were taken from
the putative father's corpse: heart blood, muscle, brain and bone marrow.
The conventional serological typing resulted in an isolated exclusion (AcP
system). The use of the hypervariable minisatellite probe MZ 1.3. gave no
satisfying result (bandsharing: about 30 %). Only the use of single locus
probes confirmed the exclusion from paternity.

CASUISTIC

A fortyeight–year–old man wanted to be accepted as illegitimate son of a
ninetyone–year–old man, who had died two weeks ago. The natural mother
was already passed away since five years. The civil division was
interested about the chance that serological examinations would produce
conclusive results in this paternity case. We proposed to exhume the
corpse as soon as possible which was carried out four weeks after death.
In spite of winter time the corpse had attained an advanced status of
putrefaction. Samples could be taken from heart blood, muscle, brain and
bone marrow.

EXAMINATIONS & RESULTS

From the very beginning we pursued a two–line examination: typing of
the conventional markers and DNA fingerprinting. The conventional
markers found are shown in table 1. Only 15 markers could be determined
in the corpse's blood. The remaining 11 markers (in laboratory routine
use) were destroyed by putrefaction. In the HP*system the results were
inconsistent with paternity: child HP*1 and putative father HP*2. Because
of the known inconstancy against putrefaction we did not excluded a
destroyed HP*1 band in the post mortem blood. The second obvious
exclusion was found in the acP*system: child acP*B and putative father
acP*A. To our opinion one can always expect a disappearing *A pattern
before destruction of the *B pattern. Nevertheless this exclusion had to
be appreciated properly, especially because of the possible existence of
a silent allele. In spite of the putrefaction non–degraded DNA could be
isolated from heart blood and muscle tissue. The use of the multi locus
probe Digoxigenin MZ 1.3

TAB. 1	CONVENTIONAL SEROLOGICAL MARKERS
Child: 0, MNss, CcD.e, K–, HP*1, GC*1s, Gm $^{-1,-2,3,10,-21}$, Km $^{-1,3}$, acP*B, PGM₁*a1, AK*1, ADA*1, EsD*1, 6–PGD*A, GLO*2, PGP*2–1 Putative father: A1, MNss, c.Ee, K–, Hp*2, Gm $^{-1,-2,3,10,-21}$, Km $^{-1,3}$, acP*A, PGM₁*a3a1, AK*1, ADA*1, EsD*1, 6–PGD*A, GLO*2–1, PGP*3–1	

TAB.2	DNA-FINGERPRINTING : a)p YNH 24; b)pL336		
Enzyme		Child	Putative Father
a)			
Pst		10.900 +/- 0.33 Kb	12.750 +/- 0.38 Kb
		10.250 +/- 0.31 Kb	11.500 +/- 0.35 Kb
HINF I		2.825 +/- 0.08 Kb	4.650 +/- 0.14 Kb
		2.250 +/- 0.07 Kb	3.100 +/- 0.09 Kb
Hae III		1.700 +/- 0.05 Kb	3.750 +/- 0.11 Kb
		1.225 +/- 0.04 Kb	2.075 +/- 0.06 Kb
b)			
Pst		3.24 Kb	6.76 Kb
		3.09 Kb	4.65 Kb

(BIOTEST, Germany) led to the electrophoretical results shown in figure 1. The evaluation gave no definite conclusion: the band sharing rates were 36%, 43,9% and 35,5%.
Only the use of single locus probes [pYNH 24 (PROMEGA), pL 336, (COLLABORATED RESEARCH INCORPORATED)] led to reproducible and definete results. These results are shown in figure 2 and described in table 2.
The dead putative father could unambiguously excluded from paternity.

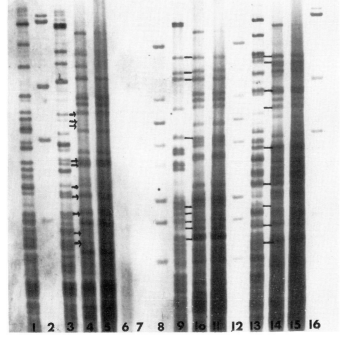

FIG. 1 MZ 1.3 DIGOXIGENIN : Lane 1 – genomic DNA control; Lane 2,16 – bacteriophage DNA HIND III; Lane 3,9,13 – Child; Lane 4,10,14 – P.f. heart blood; Lane 5,11,15 – P.f. muscle tissue; Lane 6 – P.f. bone marrow, degraded; Lane 7 – P.f. brain cortex, degraded; Lane 8,12 – bacteriophage Bst EII

CONCLUSIONS

In this reported case experiences show that DNA examinations principally should be included in so called deficiency cases. To the conventional serological examinations DNA fingerprinting is an important supplement. 10 years ago this paternity case would not have been solved definitly. Additionally the reported case shows that multi locus probes and single locus probes should be used parallel to achieve an expanded spectrum of examinations.

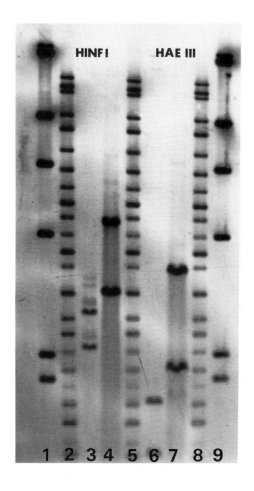

FIG. 2 : Use of pYNH 24

Lane 1,9 – bacteriophage DNA HIND III marker
Lane 2,5,8 – analytical marker DNA Wide Range #DG 1931 (PROMEGA)
Lane 3,6 – Child
Lane 4,7 – Putative Father, muscle tissue

* and Institute of Legal Medicine, University of Cologne

RESULTS OF DNA ANALYSIS FROM SIX FORENSIC SCIENCE LABORATORIES IN GERMANY

W. Pflug, Landeskriminalamt Baden-Württemberg, Stuttgart *
J. Teifel-Greding, Landeskriminalamt Bayern, München
S. Herrmann, Landeskriminalamt Berlin
M. Gerhard, Landeskriminalamt Niedersachsen, Hannover
R. Wenzel, Landeskriminalamt Rheinland-Pfalz, Mainz
H. Schmitter, Bundeskriminalamt, Wiesbaden

Introduction

In 1987 a DNA working group of three german forensic science laboratories was founded in order to establish the DNA analysis in routine case work. The members of this group came from the state labs of Berlin, of Baden-Württemberg, Stuttgart, and the federal lab (BKA) in Wiesbaden. In october 1989 these three laboratories started to use DNA analysis in case work. Scientists of other german state labs (table 1) started DNA profiling in 1990 or at the beginning of 1991 after having been trained by members of the working group. The results of DNA analysis in this paper are based on the work of six forensic science labs in Germany.

Methods

A modified version of Gill's method for DNA preparation and separation by electrophoresis in 0,8 % agarose gels was used (Gill et al.). Hybridization was carried out according to Smith et al. Single locus probes MS 1, MS 31, MS 43 A and G 3 (Wong et al.) from ICI/Cellmark were used sequentially. Allele sizes of DNA fragments were calculated by reference of DNA size markers labelled with ^{35}S (Amersham).

Results

Table 1 shows that a total number of 216 cases was analyzed with the DNA profiling method by the six above mentioned laboratories from october 1989 till march 1991.
The majority have been rape cases. Although even small and very aged stains (up to several years old) were used, DNA profiles have been obtained in approximately 78 % of these cases. A match of suspect samples with crime stains was observed in 55 % and an exclusion of all suspects in about 19 % of the cases.
No results were obtained in about 22 % of the cases due to insufficient or totally degraded DNA isolates. No suspects were known in 4 % of the cases. These data are comparable to those of other European labs.
Table 2 and Table 3 show the data from the forensic science lab in Stuttgart, where a comparison between conventional stain analysis (for example ABO, PGM, Gc etc.) and DNA results was done. The importance of the DNA method is clearly shown by the fact, that in rape cases within the group of suspects which could be excluded by DNA profiling (Table 3) more than 50 % could not be excluded by conventional systems alone. In one extreme case a suspect was incriminated by ABO, PGM and Gc systems (frequency 1 : 1000) but could be excluded by DNA analysis (Fig. 1).

Advances in Forensic Haemogenetics 4
Edited by Ch. Rittner and P. M. Schneider
© Springer-Verlag Berlin Heidelberg 1992

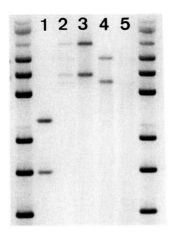

Fig. 1: Exlusion of a suspect by RFLP analysis using probe MS 43 A.

lane 1: suspect (OSe / PGM 1+ / Gc 2)
lane 2: stain of semen/vaginal secretion
lane 3: stain of semen (H, Le b / PGM 1+ / Gc 2)
lane 4: victim (BSe / PGM 1+1- / Gc 2-1S)
lane 5: supernatant of stain in lane 2

At the left and the right side are two ^{35}S-standards (Amersham)

References

Gill, P, Jeffreys, AJ and Werrett, DJ (1985) Forensic application
   of DNA fingerprints.
   Nature, Vol. 318: 577 - 579

Smith, JC, Anwar, R, Riley, J, Jenner, D and Markham, AF (1990)
   Highly polymorphic minisatellite sequences: allele frequencies
   and mutation rates for five locus-specific probes in a Causcasian
   population.
   J. Forens. Sci. Soc. 30 : 19 - 32

Wong, Z, Wilson, V, Patel, I, Povey, S and Jeffreys, AJ (1987)
   Characterization of a panel of highly variable minisatellites
   cloned from human DNA.
   Ann. Hum. Genet. 51: 269 - 288

Table 1   Results of DNA analysis (RFLP-SLP) *

	rape cases	others	Inclusion	Exclusion	DNA neg.	no suspect in case
Landeskriminalamt Baden-Württemberg	61	19	44	18	14	4
Bundeskriminalamt Wiesbaden	38	5	19	10	10	4
Landeskriminalamt Berlin	22	7	15	5	8	1
Landeskriminalamt Niedersachsen	10	30	27	5	8	-
Bayerisches Landeskriminalamt	11	6	8	3	5	1
Landeskriminalamt Rheinland-Pfalz	5	2	5	-	2	-
Sum	147	69	118	41	47	10

* The above case statistics gives only a limited information about the number of analyzed stain material and blood samples. In most cases several stains and blood samples (sometimes up to 20 - 50) were analyzed.

Table 2   Inclusions-suspect sample matches crime stain

weighting of evidence	DNA analysis (RFLP-SLP)	conventional systems (like ABO, PGM, Gc etc.)
must have come >1:1 Million	44	-
could have - very likely to have 1:2 - 1:5000	-	18
not to exclude (suspect phaenotypes allows no differentiation from stain profile)	-	16
no results	-	10

Table 3   Exclusions-suspect sample differs from crime stain

weighting of evidence	DNA analysis (RFLP-SLP)	conventional systems (like ABO, PGM, Gc etc.)
Exclusion	18	6
not to exclude (suspect phaenotypes allows no differentiation from stain profile	-	8
no results	-	4

ALLELE FREQUENCIES FOR FIVE DIFFERENT SINGLE LOCUS PROBES IN A POPULATION OF SOUTH-WEST GERMANY

W. Pflug*, G. Bäßler, G. Mai, U. Keller, S. Aab,
B. Eberspächer, G. Wahl
Landeskriminalamt Baden-Württemberg, Stuttgart, Germany

Introduction

In forensic science case work DNA analysis of restriction fragment length
polymorphisms (RFLP's) has become the most powerful method. Nearly all
labs working in the field of stain analysis prefer single locus probes
(SLP's) because these probes have a better sensitivity than multilocus
probes and offer the possibility of building a database for the alleles
frequency. In routine case work in our lab we use 4 - 5 single locus probes and the results of DNA analysis are reported as frequency data. The
precision of measuring fragment lengths i. e. the differences that may occur for the same individual on different blots was determined and is subsequently taken into consideration. For calculating the frequency we use
the "sliding window" routine, a conservative method of frequency determination (Gill et al.). Up to now the only frequency data for a german population come from the area of Düsseldorf (Henke et al.). To compare the
frequency data from Henke with the distribution in our area of South-West
Germany, we analyzed about 360 unrelated individuals.

Methods

DNA extraction and separation of **HinfI** restricted DNA fragments was carried out by standard methods. Hybridization was done according to Smith et
al. Single locus probes MS 1, MS 31, MS 43 A and G 3 (Wong et al.) from
ICI/Cellmark and YNH 24 (Nakamura et al.) from Promega were used sequentially.
Length of DNA fragments was calculated by reference to a standard curve of
size markers labelled with ^{35}S (Amersham).

Results

Allele sizes and the allele frequency distributions were determined for
the 5 hypervariable loci D1S7, D7S21, D12S11, D7S22 and D2S44 detected by
minisatellite probes MS 1, MS 31, MS 43 A, G 3 and YNH 24. The determination of allele sizes is limited by the resolution of the electrophoresis
system. Fragments differing in mobility by 0,5 mm could be resolved. The
resolution limit and measurement reproducibility ranges from ±100 bp in
the 1,5 - 3,0 kb region of the gel to ±600 bp in the 12 - 15 kb region.
The reproducibility of measurements was confirmed by including an aliquot
of known control-DNA on every gel. For comparison with other statistical
data, actual fragment sizes were approximated to 0,1 kb steps (bins). For
probes MS 1, MS 31, MS 43 A, G 3 and YNH 24 restriction fragments could be
registrated in 151, 78, 87, 116 and 46 bins. In fact this does not give

Advances in Forensic Haemogenetics 4
Edited by Ch. Rittner and P. M. Schneider
© Springer-Verlag Berlin Heidelberg 1992

the allele number, but can serve to estimate the variability of each system. The observed homozygosity was 4,1 % (MS 1), 5,3 % (MS 31), 8,5 % (MS 43), 6,1 % (G 3) and 4,6 % (YNH 24). The frequency profile of all SLP's is in good accordance with the profiles established by Henke et al., Smith et al. and Promega Corp. USA. Differences could only be noticed in the profile of MS 43 (Henke et al.) at about 8 kb and the profile of YNH 24 (Promega Corp. USA) at 3,5 kb.

References

Gill, P, Sullivan, K and Werrett, DJ (1989) The Analysis of Hypervariable DNA Profiles. Problems associated with the Objective Determination of the Probability of a Match. CRSE Report, No. 681

Henke, L, Cleef, S, Zakrzewska, M and Henke, J (1990) Population Genetik Data as Revealed by Means of Five Different Single Locus Probes. First Int. Conf. of DNA Fingerprinting, University of Bern.

Nakamura, Y, Leppert, M, O'Connell, P, Wolff, R, Holm, T, Culver, M, Martin, C, Fujimoto, E Hoff, M, Kulmin, E and White, R (1987) Variable number of tandem repeat (VNTR) markers for human gene mapping. Science, 235, 1616 - 1622

Smith, JC, Anwar, R, Riley, J, Jenner, D and Markham, AF (1990) Highly polymorphic minisatellite sequences: allele frequencies and mutation rates for five locus-specific probes in a Caucasian population. J. Forens. Sci., Soc. 30, 19 - 32

Wong, Z, Wilson, V, Patel, I, Povey, S and Jeffreys, AJ (1987) Characterization of a panel of highly variable minisatellites cloned from human DNA. Ann. Hum. Genet., 51, 269 - 288

Single locus probe profiles obtained from HinfI restricted DNA of a south-west German population

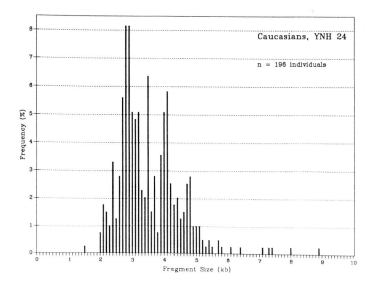

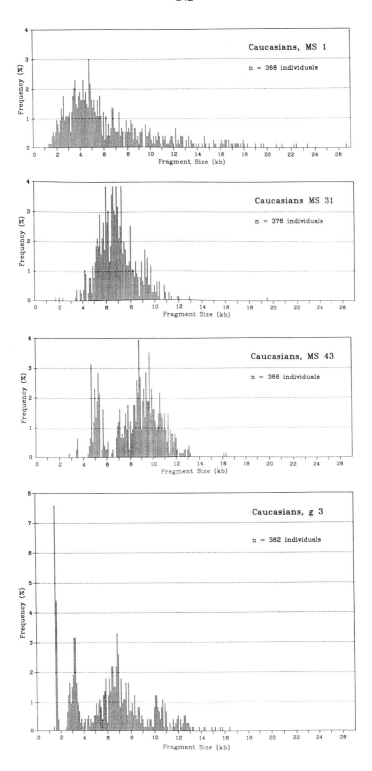

Distribution of variable number of tandem repeat (VNTR) DNA
polymorphism at D2S44 locus in Tuscany (Italy)

R. Domenici[*], I. Spinetti[*], M. Nardone[*], M. Pistello[**] and
L. Ceccherini-Nelli[**]

[*] Section of Legal Medicine, [**] Section of Virology
Department of Biomedicine, University of Pisa, Italy

INTRODUCTION

RFLP (restriction fragment-lenght polymorphism) at the D2S44
locus, detected by the highly polymorphic probe YNH24 (Nakamura
et al. 1987), can be used as an efficient tool in stain and
paternity testing, as long as reliable fragment size frequencies
are available (see van Eede et al. 1991, Gill et al. 1991,
Budowle et al. 1991).

Pascali et al. (1990) and Gasparini et al. (1990) previously
described distribution of allelic frequencies in some Italian
populations (roman with YNH24/PstI, venetian with YNH24/MspI,
respectively).

We report here RFLP frequencies for YNH24/HinfI in a population
sample from Pisa, Tuscany.

MATERIALS AND METHODS

Samples (5 ml) from 100 unrelated healthy blood donors, born in
Pisa province, were collected at the Transfusion Center of S.
Chiara Hospital, Pisa, Italy.

DNA was purified from 500μl buffy coats after haemolysis of
erytrocytes in 1xSSC (twice): pellets were resuspended in NaAc
0.2M containing Proteinase K (0.5 mg/ml) and SDS (0.6%) 56°C
1hr. Extraction was carried out in phenol/chloroform 1:1 and
subsequent precipitation by addition of 2 volumes of ETOH
(twice). Estimation of DNA concentration was carried out by
direct comparison to undigested Lambda DNA loaded in 0.4%
agarose gels at different concentrations. 5 μg DNA restriction
enzyme digestion was carried out at 37°C overnight with HinfI
(3U/μg): fragments were run in 0.8% agarose gel (15x25) in TBE
at constant voltage (30V) for approximately 48 hr until the 4.36
Kb fragment of the Lambda marker had migrated approximately 9
cm. Gel pretreatment, blotting and baking was according to the
conditions recommended from the blotting paper supplier (Schleicher & Schuell). YNH24 probe was random primed labelled with P[32]
d(CTP) and purified on Sephadex G50. Prehybridization, hybridization, washing and autoradiography were carried out as
previously described (Ceccherini-Nelli et al., 1987). The
typing results were recorded manually by the "ruler and pencil"
method. The size of the fragments detected was calculated by
comparison of the known Lamba Hind III digested fragments used
as external marker (Southern 1979).

Advances in Forensic Haemogenetics 4
Edited by Ch. Rittner and P. M. Schneider
© Springer-Verlag Berlin Heidelberg 1992

RESULTS AND DISCUSSION

YNH24/HinfI DNA VNTR polymorphism was examined in 100 unrelated samples; Fig.1 shows some of the results obtained.

Fig.1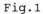

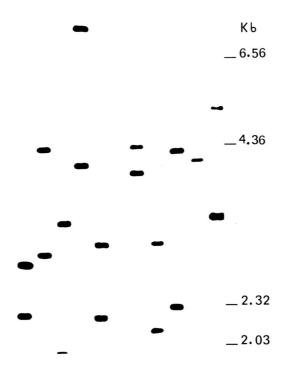

Fig.2

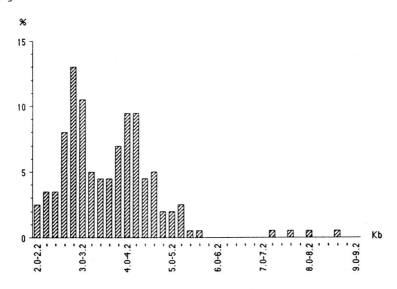

Five individuals showed only one fragment and therefore they were regarded as homozygous (heterozygosity, 95%). Fragment size distribution was continuous in the 2.0-5.5 Kb range. The average measurement error was estimated about 2% . After a conservative approach (see Budowle et al. 1991, van Eede et al. 1991), fragments were grouped at 0.2 Kb intervals. The histogram in Fig.2 illustrates the data and shows a bimodal distribution (in accordance to what reported in the literature) at 2.8-3.0 Kb and 4.0-4.4 Kb. The most common bin frequency estimate for Tuscany population was 13% (this figure was comparable with what shown from Budowle et al. 1991 and van Eede et al. 1991).

ACKNOWLEDGMENTS

Dr. Nakamura is greatly thanked for his kind gift of probe YNH24. The work was supported by the Italian Ministry of the University and Scientific Research.

REFERENCES

Budowle B, Giusti AM, Waye JS, Baechtel FS, Fourney RM, Adams et al. (1991) Fixed-bin analysis for statistical evaluation of continuous distributions of allelic data from VNTR loci, for use in forensic comparisons. Am J Hum Genet 48:841-855

Ceccherini-Nelli L, De Re V, Molaro G, Zilli L, Clemente C, Boiocchi M (1987) Ha-ras-1 Restriction fragment length polymorphism and susceptibility to Colon Adenocarcinoma. Brit J Cancer 56: 1-5

Gasparini P, Trabetti E, Savoia A, Marigo M, Pignatti PF (1990) Frequency distribution of the alleles of several VNTR DNA polymorphism in the Italian population. Hum Hered 40:61-68

Gill P, Evett IW, Woodroffe S, Lygo JE, Millican E, Webster M (1991) Databases, quality control and interpretation of DNA profiling in the Home Office Forensic Science Service. Electrophoresis 12:204-209

Nakamura Y, Leppert M, O'Connell P, Wolff R, Holm T, Culver M et al. (1987) Variable number of tandem repeat (VNTR) markers for human gene mapping. Science 235:1616-1622

Pascali VL, D'Aloja E, Dobosz M, Pescarmona M, Fiori A (1990) Allele frequencies distribution of two VNTR markers (YNH24; YNZ22) in PstI digests from random Italian individuals (population of Rome) Adv Forens Haemogenet 3:68-70

Southern EM (1979) Measurement of DNA length by gel electro-phoresis Anal Biochem 100:319-323

Van Eede PH, Henke L, Fimmers R, Henke J, de Lange GG (1991) Size calculation of restriction enzyme HaeIII generated frag-ments detected by probe YNH24 by comparison of data from two laboratories: the generation of fragment-size frequencies. Forens Sci Int 49:21-31

EXPERIENCES WITH SIX SINGLE LOCUS PROBES IN PATERNITY TESTING

Birgit Brüggemann, Dietlinde Teixidor, Maria Kilp, S. Seidl

Institute of Immunhaematology, University Frankfurt and Red Cross Donor Service Hessen, Sandhofstr. 1, D-6000 Frankfurt 71, Germany

INTRODUCTION

Recent developments in molecular biology allow the rapid detection of specific DNA-polymorphisms and DNA-testing is also used in paternity testing. Two different approaches are in use: Multilocus probes (MLP's) and single locus probes (SLP's). We report our experiences with 6 SLP's in cases of disputed paternity. Apart from DNA-testing most cases were also investigated with the conventional systems (red cell and serum groups, enzyme polymorphisms) and some of them with the HLA-system.

MATERIAL AND METHODS

For DNA-analysis the following biotin labelled SLP's were used: pS 194 (5.0-11.0 Kb), pL 336 (2.0-6.0 Kb), pL 159-1 (4.0-5.5 Kb), pL 355-8 (6.0-8.0 Kb), pL 427-4 (1.4-3.4 Kb) and pR 365-1 (1.3-3.5 Kb).

DNA digest was performed by adding 25 units of Pst I to 10 µg of genomic DNA, followed by gelelectrophoresis (42-66 hours), hybridization for 16 hours, 3x washing, 10 min. incubation with streptavidin, again 3x washings, thereafter alkaline phosphatase followed by 4x washings, finally NBT and BCIP was added. In all cases the bands could be easily identified.

RESULTS AND DISCUSSION

A total of 23 cases of disputed paternity were investigated. In 13 cases in which 6 SLP's were applied no exclusion of the alleged men was observed. In these cases biostatistical calculation was performed using ESSEN MÖLLER probability (W). In 10 of 13 cases (76.92%) the biostatistics revealed $W \geq 99.73\%$. However, when only 3 SLP's were used $W \geq 99.73\%$ was observed in 6 of 13 cases. In 4 cases a remarkable difference exists between 6 and 3 SLP's. For comparison these four cases were investigated with 6,5,4 and 3 SLP's. The data are shown in fig. 1. In two cases (No. 2 and 3) a significant difference exists between the W-values calculated after applying 3 and 6 SLP's, whereas the differences in cases 1 and 4 are rather small. It should also be noted that in cases in which DNA-testing did not result in W-values of $\geq 99.73\%$ the combination with the HLA-system or the conventional systems (red cells, serum groups or enzyme allotypes) gave W-values of $\geq 99.73\%$.

Advances in Forensic Haemogenetics 4
Edited by Ch. Rittner and P. M. Schneider
© Springer-Verlag Berlin Heidelberg 1992

Comparison between 6, 5, 4 and 3 SLP's
in cases of disputed paternity

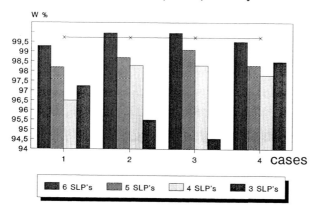

In table 1 10 of 23 cases of disputed paternity are listed with
exclusion. The second collumn shows the number of probes applied
in each case. Except two cases (No. 6 and 38a) exclusion was obtained with two or more SLP's.

Table 1

Exclusion in 10 cases of disputed paternity

Case No.	Probes investigated n	Exclusions n	(%)
4	6	3	(50%)
6	4	1	(25%)
8	5	5	(100%)
10	6	5	(83.3%)
15	5	2	(40%)
20	3	3	(100%)
22	3	3	(100%)
29	5	4	(80%)
33	5	5	(100%)
38a	4	1	(25%)

Table 2 summarizes the exclusion rates obtained with the six SLP's
used in this study. As expected the exclusion rates varied between
the various probes. Probe 427-4 resulted in all cases applied in
exclusion of the alleged men, whereas the lowest exclusion rate
(25%) was observed with probe 365-1. This probe had also the lowest rate (51.70%) as indicated by the manufacturer.

Table 2

Exclusion rates in cases of disputed paternity

Probes	cases investigated	exclusion rate n	exclusion rate %	exclusion rate % (manufacturer)
pL 427-4	10	10	100	83.27
pR 365-1	8	2	25	51.70
pL 355-8	6	3	50	67.82
pL 159-1	11	8	72.7	43.54
pL 336	6	5	83.3	88.88
pS 194	10	7	70	79.08

A case of disputed paternity with consanguinity (uncle-niece) could be clacified by DNA-analysis, excluding the alleged man (uncle) with 4 probes.

SUMMARY

Six SLP's were applied in 23 cases of disputed paternity:

1. Exclusion of the alleged men was observed in 10 cases, including a case with consanguinity between mother and alleged man (uncle/niece).

2. Exclusion rates varied between 25% and 100% of the SLP's applied.

3. In 10 of 13 cases (76.92%) with no exclusion the biostatistical calculation resulted in W-values of $\geq$ 99.73%.

4. When DNA-analysis was combined with the results of HLA-testing or with the data obtained with conventional systems W-values of $\geq$ 99.73% resulted in all cases.

5. DNA-analysis with SLP's is a reliable technique which can be applied in cases of disputed paternity.

Detection of DNA polymorphisms by using α satellite probes:
Application to the forensic identification

M.Yamada, Y.Yamamoto, T.Fukunaga, Y.Tatsuno* and K.Nishi

Department of Legal Medicine
Shiga University of Medical Science
Seta-Tsukinowacho, Ohtsu 520-21, Japan

INTRODUCTION

The α satellite is a complex family of tandemly repeated DNA located at the centromeric regions of human chromosomes. Each chromosome contains some tandem copies of a higher – order repeat unit, comprised of tandem monomer units of 171 bp. It is also reported that the α satellite DNA shows RFLPs based on site variations within and between monomer units (Waye 1987; Willard 1986, 1987).

Here we describe that RFLPs involving α satellite can be a tool of the forensic identification.

MATERIALS AND METHODS

DNAs were prepared from peripheral lymphocytes from healthy Japanese individuals.

The probes, D11Z1, D17Z1 and DXZ1 (α satellite DNAs on 11, 17 and X chromosomes, respectively), were obtained from Oncor and labeled with digoxigenin – dUTP by random primed (DNA Labeling & Detection Kit, Boehringer).

DNAs were digested with BglI, EcoRI, HindIII, MspI, PvuII or XbaI and the fragments were sepatated by agarose gel electrophoresis. After Southern blotting – hybridization procedures, the filters were washed in 0.1 x SSC – 0.1 % SDS at 65 ℃ and the hybrids were detected by enzyme immunoassay.

---

* Present address ; Dept of Legal Medicine, Kobe University
  School of Medicine, Chuo-ku, Kobe 650, Japan.

Advances in Forensic Haemogenetics 4
Edited by Ch. Rittner and P. M. Schneider
© Springer-Verlag Berlin Heidelberg 1992

RESULTS AND DISCUSSION

Fig. 1.
EcoRI – D17Z1
polymorphism

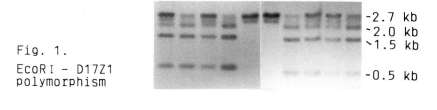

- -2.7 kb
- -2.0 kb
- -1.5 kb
- -0.5 kb

Fig. 2.
PvuII – D17Z1
polymorphism

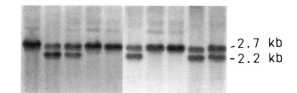

- -2.7 kb
- -2.2 kb

For detecting the RFLPs involving α satellite, genomic DNA from unrelated Japanese individuals was digested with restriction endonuclease and hybridized to the α satellite DNA probe. EcoRI – and PvuII – cleaved genomic DNA gave the

Table 1. Frequencies in a Japanese population

	Fragment	n	Present	Absent
EcoRI – D17Z1	2.0 kb	184	0.45	0.55
	1.5		0.72	0.38
	0.5		0.72	0.38
PvuII – D17Z1	2.2 kb	110	0.47	0.53

n ; number of chromosomes examined.

clear polymorphic variations of chromosome 17 (Fig. 1 and 2). Both the pattern of bands and the relative intensity of each band were reproducible. Table 1 gives the frequencies in a Japanese population of the polymorphic fragment lengths. Mendelian inheritance was also investigated (Fig. 3).

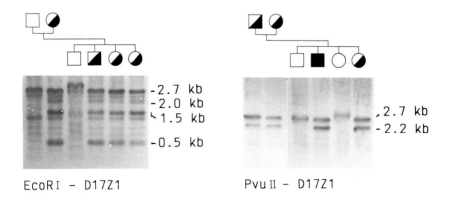

EcoRI - D17Z1   PvuⅡ - D17Z1

Fig. 3. Mendelian inheritance of the polymorphisms

The detection method used was practically enough sensitive and the polymorphisms described here are likely to be available for the individual identification or parentage testing.

REFERENCES

Waye JS, Creeper LA and Willard HF (1987) Organization and evolution of alpha satellite DNA from human chromosome 11. Chromosoma 95:182-188

Willard HF, Waye JS, Skolnick MH, Schwartz CE, Powers VE and England SB (1986) Detection of restriction fragment length polymorphisms at the centromeres of human chromosomes by using chromosome - specific α satellite DNA probes: Implications for development of centromere - based genetic linkage maps. Proc Natl Acad Sci USA 83:5611-5615

Willard HF and Waye JS (1987) Hierarchical order in chromosome - specific human alpha satellite DNA. Trends in Genet 3:192-198

Population genetic studies of six hypervariable DNA-Loci

A. Wilting, U. Hintzen, M.O.Völker, J. Bertrams

Institute of Laboratory Medicine and Microbiology, Elisabeth Hospital Essen, Germany

INTRODUCTION

Until recently, scientific investigations in cases of disputed parentage have relied upon techniques concerning gene products as HLA, red cell antigens, enzyme polymorphism, and proteins. Using recombinant DNA-techniques additional genetic polymorphism can be obtained and further exclude an alleged father from paternity. One group of genetic markers applied in disputed parentage cases refers to as DNA restriction fragment length polymorphism (RFLP). Independent of age, sex, and expression of gene products RFLPs are a helpful tool in typing new borns, children, and semen specimen. At the present time numerous genetic polymorphisms have been identified using various combinations of DNA-probes and restiction endonucleases. One obstacle in applying RFLP-techniques in forensic investigations is the lack of biostatistical evaluation of the detected polymorphism as well as gene frequency data of a given population. Here we report the allele frequency distribution of six hypervariable DNA-loci using probes pS 194, pL 159-1, pR 365-1, pL 355-8, pL 427-4, and pL 336 from ONCOR (distributed in Germany by IMMUCOR). PST I restricted probes were tested with 1200 DNA samples extracted from unrelated individuals from the German Ruhr area.

MATERIALS AND METHODS

DNA from 1200 (200 per probe) EDTA blood samples from unrelated individuals from the German Ruhr area were extracted according to the method of Miller et al. (1988) using non-toxic non-organic treatment. 10 μg of DNA sample were restricted with 140 IU PST I according to standard procedures (Maniatis et al. 1982) and electrophoresed 42 hours at 1.4 V/cm, except for probe pL 336 (66 h). Agarose concentration varied with respect to the applied probes, i.e.: 0.7% pS 194/ 355-8; 0.8% pL 159-1; 0.9% pL 427-4/ pR 365-1/ pL 336. Three biotinylated lambda size markers were loaded on the gel at the most-left, most-right and mid position. DNA samples were depurinated and denatured using 0.25 N HCl and 0.5 N NaOH/1.5 M NaCl, respectively and blotted onto ONCOR Sureblot nylon membranes using a PHARMACIA vacuum blotting device. Each sample was hybridized with six biotinylated single-locus probes in a BACHOFER rotating incubator at 42°C over night. After stringend washing at 52°C (probe pL 336: 70°C) detection was carried out using non-isotopic alkaline phosphatase-streptavidin detection system of ONCOR. Fragment lengths were calculated by biotinylated lambda size markers restricted with Hind III, PSTE II and Sph I ranging from 23.1 to 2.2 kb.

Advances in Forensic Haemogenetics 4
Edited by Ch. Rittner and P. M. Schneider
© Springer-Verlag Berlin Heidelberg 1992

RESULTS AND CONCLUSIONS

As revealed by allele frequency data plots, the 6 hypervariable single-locus probes presented here give satisfying frequency responses over a defined frequency range of 2-6 kb. The following figures show a comparison of the own data and the results obtained by Dykes (unpublished) in a Caucasian population from the United States. There are no striking differences concerning range and pattern of the frequency data produced by five single-locus probes. Some kb-shifts of frequency maxima ranging from 0.0 - 0.3 kb may be due to different evaluation procedures and are within statistical error. As can be depicted from Table 1 there are major differences in the frequency maxima of probes pL 355-8 and pL 159-1: the maximum frequency rate of the German population exceeds the correspondent of the United States by the factor of two.

Further investigations will show if this effect is due to population specificity or depends on the different population sample rate. Therefore biostatistical evaluation of data from disputed parentage cases should be based on the appropriate population allele frequency data.

Table 1. Comparison of frequency data of the tested probes obtained from two different Caucasian populations

Probe	N	Freq. range (kb)	mean freq.	Freq. max. (%)	kb	Heterozy- gocity
pS 194	208	5.2- 9.0	5.8	24.0	6.0	0.85
*	1908	5.0-12.5	1.5	22.0	5.7	0.85**
pR 365-1	208	1.3- 3.3	9.4	38.4	1.8	0.71
*	151	1.5- 3.3	5.35	34.0	1.8	0.66**
pL 355-8	195	5.7- 7.9	9.8	29.2	6.2	0.70
*	218	3.7- 7.4	2.64	15.0	6.2	0.83**
pL 159-1	209	4.0- 5.9	8.9	34.4	4.7	0.62
*	470	3.8- 5.5	5.52	19.0	4.5	0.74**
pL 427-4	224	1.1- 5.7	6.2	30.3	1.5	0.94
*	330	1.2- 3.5	3.9	28.0	1.6	0.94**
pL 336	191	2.1- 8.9	4.1	14.6	2.5	0.97
						0.88**
* Data obtained from Dykes (unpublished)						
** Heterozygocity data published by ONCOR						

254

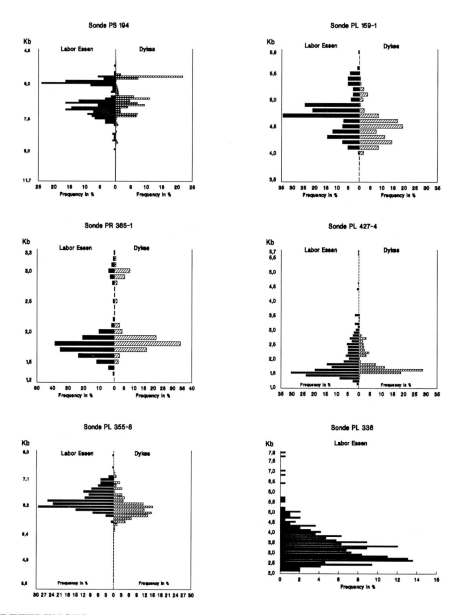

REFERENCES

Maniatis T, Fritsch EF, Sambrook J (1982) Molecular cloning: a laboratory manual. Cold Spring Harbour Laboratory Press, New York

Miller SA, Dykes DD, Polesky HF (1988) A simple salting out procedure for extracting DNA from human nucleated cells. Nucleic Acids Res 16:1215

Minisatellite DNA Probe MZ1.3: Band Sharing Rates Among Siblings and the Part of Informative Bands Among Children

D. Padeberg, U. Hintzen, and J. Bertrams

Institute of Laboratory Medicine and Microbiology, Elisabeth Hospital, Essen, Germany

INTRODUCTION

After Vassart et al. (1987) had demonstrated the possibility to detect hypervariable fragments in human DNA utilizing the wildtype bacteriophage M13, Schacker et al. (1990) managed to isolate a minisatellite probe, called MZ1.3 by screening a human library with a DNA probe, which comprised the complete bacteriophage M13mp18. The 27bp repetitive sequence of MZ1.3 shows variable homology of 53% - 73% to the repetitive sequence of the protein III gene of the M13 genome, whereas it does not indicate a clear homology to the probes 33.6 and 33.15. Yet, it is suitable for producing highly informative fingerprints from human DNA (Schacker et al. 1990). In 1989/90 a collaborative study of eleven European laboratories MZ1.3 (BIOTEST; Art. No. 825020) was initiated in order to test the reproducibilty by different laboratories and to extend the population genetic data (Schneider et al., in preparation). As part of this study we analysed the finger-prints of Caucasian families with three or more children, with respect to the number of informative bands among 186 children and the band sharing rates among siblings.

MATERIAL AND METHODS

Human genomic DNA was isolated from 10 ml EDTA blood with a salting out procedure (saturated NaCl solution) and precipitated with ethanol (Miller et al. 1988). For Southern blot analysis, 10 μg of DNA were digested with 30 units of restriction endonuclease Hinf I (BIOLABS) at 37°C over night. Restriction fragments were separated on a 0.7% agarose gel in TBE buffer at a constant voltage (40 V) for 27 hours. Gel dimensions were 20x25 cm. After electrophoresis and depurination with 0.3M HCl for 30 min, Southern blotting was performed in 0.4M NaOH. The transfer of DNA onto a nylon membrane (Nytran Ny 13, SCHLEICHER & SCHÜLL) was completed after 4 - 6 hours. Alternatively a vacuum blotter with 0.5M NaOH and 1.5M NaCl as transfer buffer was used. Blotting was completed after 2 hours. The membrane was washed in neutralization buffer (1.5M NaCl, 0.5M Tris, pH 8) for 5 min. and followed by a second wash with 6xSSC for 2 min. The dried membrane was baked for 2 hours at 80°C. Nylon filters were prehybridized for 4 hours in 20 ml of hybridization solution (5xSSC, 0,1% N-lauroylsarcosine, Na-salt, 0.02% SDS) and hybridized for 15 hours at 60°C in 20 ml hybridization solution containing the digoxigenin labeled probe MZ1.3. After hybridization the membranes were washed twice in 2xSSC, 0.1% SDS for 5 min, and twice with 0.2xSSC, 0.1% SDS for 15 min. For color development a digoxigenin labeled nucleic acid detection kit (BOEHRINGER MANNHEIM) was used.

Advances in Forensic Haemogenetics 4
Edited by Ch. Rittner and P. M. Schneider
© Springer-Verlag Berlin Heidelberg 1992

RESULTS AND DISCUSSION

For calculation of band sharing rates as 0.5x(n/a + n/b) (n = no. of common bands; a, b = total no. of bands per individual) 222 sibling pairs were compared, which yielded an average band sharing rate for siblings of 63.0% +/- 11.2%. On the other hand 391 parent/ child comparisons yielded a band sharing rate of 59.4% +/- 11.8%, which is in the same order and nearly identical to the rate given by Schacker et al. (1990) (59.9% +/- 7.8%). Accordingly, band sharing rates between parents and children are very similar to the band sharing rates between siblings (Fig. 1 and 2). However it is of interest that the band sharing rates are not proportional to the total number of bands (Fig. 3).

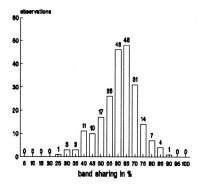

Figure 1: Distribution of all possible band sharing rates (n=222) among 186 children

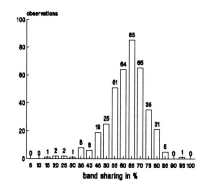

Figure 2: Distribution of band sharing rates (n=391) between parents and children

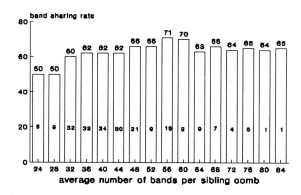

Figure 3: Relations between band sharing rates (n=189) among siblings and total number of bands. The number of observations are given in the columns

All fragments found in 186 children could be associated with parental fragments without finding a new mutation. The average total number of bands was 20.5 ± 6.3, the average number of informative maternal plus paternal bands only 13.4 ± 4.0 (65.4%). Noteworthy bands of all mother-child-father trios within a distance of 0.5 mm consequently were considered to be identical. With regard to the distribution of informative bands (Fig. 4) it is obvious that the number of informative bands is directly proportional to the total number of bands per child. Accordingly it is important to achieve a large number of total bands to reach a maximum of information. Nevertheless, despite of an increased number of informative bands (up to 26 per child) in cases with large numbers of total bands, the relative amount of informative bands decreased from 83.5% to 61.9% (Fig. 5). Further analysis may show whether this observation is significant.

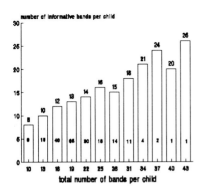

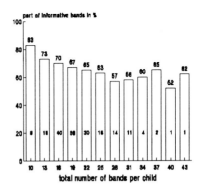

Figure 4: Number of informative bands among 189 siblings dependent on the total number of bands per child. The number of observations are given in the columns

Figure 5: Part of informative bands among 189 siblings dependent on the total number per child. The number of observations are given in the columns

REFERENCES

Miller SA, Dykes DD, Polesky HF (1988) A simple salting out procedure for extracting DNA from human nucleated cells. Nucleic Acid Res 16:1215
Schacker U, Schneider PM, Holtkamp B, Bohnke E, Fimmers R, Sonnenborn HH, Rittner C (1990) Isolation of the DNA minisatellite probe MZ1.3 and its application to DNA "fingerprinting" analysis. Forensic Sci Int 44:209-224
Schneider PM, Fimmers R, Bertrams J, Birkner P, Braunbeck K, Bulnheim U, Feuerbach M, Henke L, Iten E, Osterhaus E, Prinz M, Simeoni E, Rittner C (1991) Biostatistical basis of individualization and segregation analysis using the multilocus DNA probe MZ 1.3: Results of a collaborative study. Hum Genet (submitted)
Vassart G, Georges M, Monsieur R, Brocas H, Lequarre AS (1987) A sequence in M13 phage detects hypervariable minisatellites in human and animal DNA. Science 235:683-684

DNA Fingerprinting in Paternity Testing in Lithuania

V.Naktinis, V. Popendikytė, G. Khvatovitch and G.Garmus

Institute of Applied Enzymology FERMENTAS, Fermentų 8, 232028 Vilnius, Lithuania

The classical methods of personal identification which up till now have been used in forensic and criminologic practice, were mainly based on biochemical and immunobiological practice (i.e. on blood group ABO system, Rh, HNSs, or on serum tests, such as P, Gm, Lewis Hp, or enzymatic system of erythrocytes), as well as dactyloscopic analysis of papillary line comparison.

On the basis of the observations by Vassart, G. et al. (1987) and Dzhincharadze, A. et al. (1987), proving that wild-type M13 bacteriophage DNA could serve as a molecular probe for detection of hypervariable minisatellite regions in human genome, the DNA fingerprinting technique for disputable paternity testing in forensic medicine was applied. The method used included the DNA extraction from the mother, father in dispute and child, digestion with Hinf I (preferentially) or Bsu RI restriction endonuclease, electrophoresisthrough agarose gel, and Southern blot-hydridization to ^{32}P-labeled M13 probe. The latter is prepared from single-stranded M13 DNA by partial synthesizing of the second strand from the forward sequencing primer in the DNA polymerase I Klenow fragment - catalyzed reaction. Since 1990, the DNA fingerprinting method above was approved by Lithuanian authorities for the use in paternity testing. Since the fall of 1990, 28 cases of disputed paternity using M13 probe were studied. The following regularities were observed in the fingerprints obtained: in average, 20 well identifiable DNA fragments were scored for every individual, whereas 6 fragments were shared by all the individuals in the case. For nearly 20% of the cases studied, the number of co-migrating identifiable fragments made up to 10-13. The ambiguity obtained was eliminated by parallel use of restriction endonuclease Bsu RI. Two cases of paternity exclusion were obtained, whereas in one case the exclusion was obtained by DNA fingerprinting only, where no conventional biochemical or blood group marker system was effective

The DNA fingerprint was made using a biotin-labeled M13 DNA fragment. For such a purpose, two primers have been synthesized - TCCTATTGGGCTTGCTATCC and TTTCGGTCATAGCCCCCTTA - surrounding the hybridizing sequence in the protein III gene. The M13 DNA fragment was then labeled with biotin using the amplification reaction by Bellany, R. et al. (1990). For development of the membrane, streptavidin-alkaline phosphatase conjugate and BEIP/NBT (5-bromo-4-chloro-3-indolyl phosphate/Nitro Blue Tetrazolium) was used.

Advances in Forensic Haemogenetics 4
Edited by Ch. Rittner and P. M. Schneider
© Springer-Verlag Berlin Heidelberg 1992

REFERENCES

Vassart G et al. (1987). A sequence in M13 phage detects hypervariable mi-
    nisatellites in human and animal DNA. Science 235:683-684
Dzhincharadze A et al. t. 1987. Genomnaja "daktiloskopija". Dokl. AN SSSR
    295:230-233
Bellamy R et al.(1990) Better fingerprinting with PCR. Trends in genetics
    6:32

DNA typing in forensic casework in Norway:
Strategies and experiences

B. Mevåg, S. Jacobsen, B. Eriksen, and B. Olaisen

Rettsmedisinsk Institutt, Universitetet i Oslo, Rikshospitalet,
027 Oslo 1, Norway

INTRODUCTION

During the last four years, VNTR typing has been offered in forensic
casework as a supplement to traditional diagnostics.

Probes presently used are MS1 (D1S8), YNH24 (D2S44), MS31 (D7S21), and
MS43A (D12S11). Extraction and electrophoresis are performed according
to "EDNAP standards"; e.g. using enzyme HinfI, TBE-buffer and SeaKem
agarose (Schneider et al. 1991). Fragment sizes are determined using
the automated scanning equipment developed at the Metropolitan Police
Forensic Science Laboratory.

At present, the police is charged per sample. When they decide whether
to have carried out a DNA typing, they thus take into consideration
the importance of having the DNA evidence as well as the costs of it.

Here we present some statistical data of our casework illustrating the
development in DNA typing strategy. We also give selected examples illustrating the kinds of cases chosen for DNA analysis by VNTR typing.

CASEWORK STATISTICS

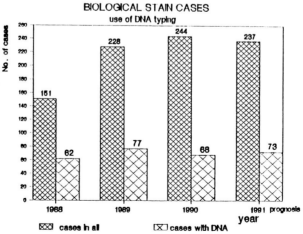

Fig. 1.   The development of the total number of cases with biological
evidence and the number of cases chosen for DNA typing

Advances in Forensic Haemogenetics 4
Edited by Ch. Rittner and P. M. Schneider
© Springer-Verlag Berlin Heidelberg 1992

We have experienced a wide variety of case types. Rapes and other cases involving sexual assaults are the most common ones, but cases under investigation for murder or incest, or body identification cases are also relatively frequently seen.

Choices largely made by the police, have caused that the number of cases chosen for DNA typing has remained constant even if the total number of casework has increased (Fig. 1).

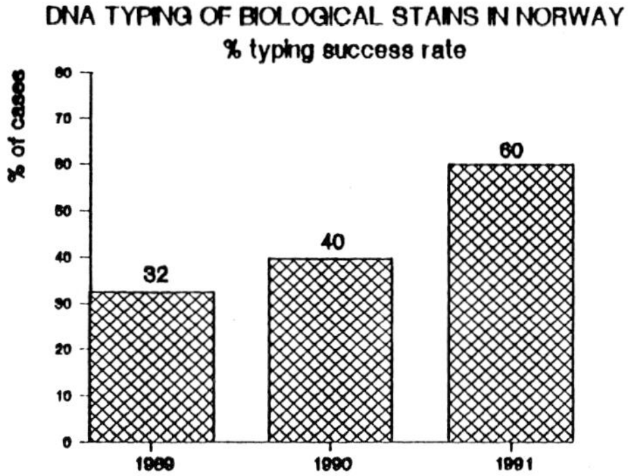

DNA TYPING OF BIOLOGICAL STAINS IN NORWAY
% typing success rate

Fig. 2. DNA typing success rates (per cent of successfully typed cases in cases chosen for DNA typing) in stainwork in Norway

During the last three years, the success rate expressed as the percentage of cases where DNA types was achieved in critical samples, has gradually increased (Fig. 2). High success rates were achieved in stains or material from underwear/clothing, vaginal swabs, organs/biopsies etc. Low success rates were experienced in sigarettes, masks, mouth swabs, rectum swabs, narcotic's syringe, old hairs, and in some fabric.

The overall achievements by DNA typing may be illustrated by the following numbers: In 1989 DNA typing identified 18 offenders and excluded 9 suspects, in 1990 the numbers were 21 and 100, while the prognosis for 1991 is 41 and 22, respectively.

EXAMPLES

1   Hit and run motor car accident

A six year old boy was found killed, obviously hit by a car. The next day a lorry at a slaughterhouse 80 km from the scene of the accident was examined. Samples collected from the tyre and the wheelarch proved to be of human origin. DNA patterns from the stain material matched those from the deceased (Fig. 3).

2   One rapist - several victims

Three rape cases from different parts of the country were linked by technical evidence as well as by similar "modus operandi". DNA analyses of semen stained exhibits in the three cases indicated that one particular man was involved in them all. In addition, in two of the cases, DNA fragments from altogether three more men showed up (Fig. 4).

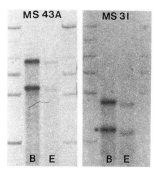

Fig. 3. DNA patterns in a hit and run accident. Probes used are indicated. B: body, E: Exhibit, material from tyre and wheelarch

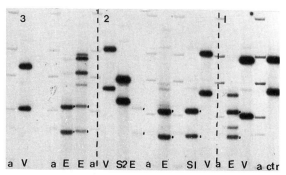

Fig. 4. DNA patterns in three rape cases. A: Amersham ladder, S1, S2, S3: suspects, V: victim, E:exhibit, semen from vag.swabs and underwear

3 Incest - chorion biopsy

A young married woman was sexually abused by her father. After getting pregnant, she did not know whether her husband or her father was the father of her child. A paternity test was requested for guidance as to the continuation of the pregnancy. Chorion villus sampling was performed. DNA typing excluded the grandfather. The woman decided to carry through the pregnancy (Fig. 5).

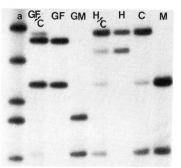

Fig. 5. DNA types in an incest case. GF: grandfather, GM: grandmother, C: chor.vill.biopsy, M:mother, H:husband

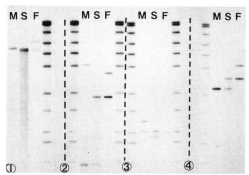

Fig. 6. DNA types in identification. S: burned body, M: mother, F: father

4 Identification of a burned body

DNA type comparisons between DNA from a burned body and blood DNA from parents of the missing person, led to identification (Fig. 6).

REFERENCES

Schneider PM, Fimmers R, Woodroffe S, Werrett DJ, Bär W, Brinkmann B, Eriksen B, Jones S, Kloosterman AD, Mevåg B, Pascali VL, Rittner C, Schmitter H, Thomson JA, Gill P (1991) Report of a European collaborative exercise comparing DNA typing results using a single locus VNTR probe. Forensic Sci. Int. 49:1-15

Determination of Incest in Forensic Casework Using Multi-locus
DNA Profiling

P.L. Ivanov L.V.Verbovaya and M.B.Maljutov[*]

Institute of Molecular Biology USSR Academy of Sciences.
117984 Vavilov str., 32, Moscow, USSR
[*]Moscow State University, 119899, Moscow, USSR

INTRODUCTION

Recently we have described an approach based on computer Monte-
-Carlo simulations of human multi-locus DNA fingerprints, to estimating genetic relatedness between individuals (Ivanov et al.
in press). Briefly, we have developed, through statistical modelling, frequency distributions of similarity between DNA profiles belonging to the known types of relatives. Thus, the probability that the given estimate of similarity is associated
with a particular degree of relatedness could be directly assay-
ed. As we have shown, the model yielded reliable estimates for
detecting consanguinity and distinguishing biological relationships.

In the present study, we used the principle of this treatment to
go on to establish a method for determining incest in forensic
casework.

METHODOLOGY

The large number of "phantom" multi-band DNA profiles were independently computer simulated in the spirit of the model previously described (Ivanov et al.; Maljutov et al. in press) in line
with the basic genetic formalization underlying the DNA fingerprinting technique (Jeffreys et al.1985,1987). These profiles
constitute the parent population for producing offspring phantom profiles. For each randomly chosen pair of profiles which is
considered to be the parent pair, the offspring phantom profile
was simulated, where the inheritance of bands was modelled according to Evett et al.(1989). Then, for this offspring phantom,
the partner profile was randomly chosen to constitute the new
parent pair, and the next degree offspring phantom was generated
as above. Such a cycle can be repeated as many times as needed
for reaching the desired genetic level. On the other hand, instead of random partner one can consider the partner to be relative of prescribed genetic order. Thus, an incest case of any
type could be modelled. The whole procedure was prepared independently L=1000 times to produce statistically acceptable data.

Then, frequency distributions of similarity were computer deve-

Advances in Forensic Haemogenetics 4
Edited by Ch. Rittner and P. M. Schneider
© Springer-Verlag Berlin Heidelberg 1992

loped for pairwise comparisons between DNA profiles of questioned individuals. Statistic relation index, R, was used as an operational measure of similarity (Ivanov and Verbovaya 1990). R is defined as a ratio: the amount of matched bands/total amount of scorable band positions within the pair of profiles A and B: $R = S_{AB}/(n_A + n_B - S_{AB})$, where n_A and n_B are the numbers of component bands in each fingerprint under comparison; S_{AB} is the number of shared bands.

RESULTS AND DISCUSSION

Several types of the extreme parentage cases involving incest were modelled. In Case I, a father and a child is the first--degree relative of the mother (i.g. her father or brother). In Case II, a father of a child is the second-degree relative of the mother (i.g. her uncle or grandfather). The alternative out-bred version of each pedigree in dispute was modelled as well. For each class of cases R frequency distributions were simulated between DNA fingerprints of inbred father and the child and, in parallel, between the corresponding outbred relatives: parent and second- or third-degree offspring (for Case I and Case II, respectively). The results are presented in Fig. 1, where graphic hystograms and approximating normal densities as well as corresponding numerical hystograms are shown.

It is apparent, that R is appreciably higher in parentage cases involving incest when compared with alternative relative pairs from outbred pedigrees. One can consider differences between R value averages as being statistically significant in such kind of comparisons. The mean probability of non-distinguishing between alternative degrees of relatedness in situations as modelled was estimated to be approximately 10%, which corresponds to discriminatory capability of 90%.

It should be noted that incest will also increase the similarity of DNA profiles between the child and the mother (data not shown). However, distinguishing between outbred and inbred maternity cannot be readily made because of intrinsic very short genetic distance. Meanwhile, when the focus is being on paternity, the two hypotheses are fairy distinguishable in the mean. Therefore, the approach is sufficiently informative for establishing incest or, alternatively, for identifying falsely accused relative in the majority of practical cases. On the other hand, inclusionary statistics for particular case can be produced using the tail probabilities for predicted relatedness, as it is illustrated in Case report.

CASE REPORT

By means of this approach, the authors succeeded in determining incest in forensic case when the suspect was charged with violation against his grand-daughter involving impregnation of the victim (Fig. 2).

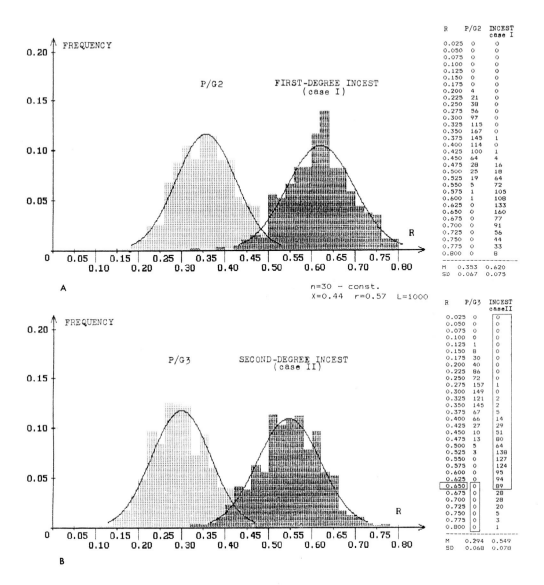

Fig. 1. Monte-Carlo simulations of similarity between human multi-band DNA profiles for alternative degrees of relatedness.
Graphic hystograms, approximating normal densities and numerical
consequences of the treatment are shown.
A: frequency distributions of "MvaI/M13" relation index (R) simulated among parent/second-degree offspring pairs (P/G2), and
corresponding critical relatives as modelled for incest Case I.
B: frequency distributions of "MvaI/M13" relation index (R) simulated among parent/third-degree offspring pairs (P/G3), and among
corresponding critical relatives as modelled for incest Case II.
Parameters of the basic model (Maljutov et al., in press), corresponding means (M) and standard deviations (SD) are indicated.
The data used to detect incest in particular forensic investigation are boxed. For detailes see text

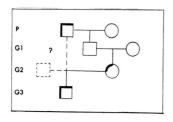

Fig. 2. Scheme for the questioned pedigree

Significantly, that DNA fingerprint test has not revealed any unassigned bands in a disputed trio. In standard paternity dispute, when the parents of the child are nonrelatives, such a result is satisfactory evidence to prove paternity positively. However, family relatedness between the mother and alleged father will obviously increase the possibility that this could have occured by chance. Therefore, as the direct exclusion by parental mismatches cannot be made, the probabilities should be calculated for inclusion estimate.

The critical pair alleged father/son, which should be apriori considered as formal P/G3 (i.e. great-grandfather/great-grandson) yielded R value of 0.65. In the spirit of the approach reported here, this is suggestive of high degree of relatedness and one could argue that the suspect might be rather biological father of the child, than his great-grandfather (Fig.1B). Following the reasoning by Evett and Buckleton (1989), we evaluated the evidence under these two alternative explanations, by calculating the Bayesian likelihood ratio, which in this case exceeded 900.

Such an evidence strongly supports paternity version, and has been accepted by court as satisfactory evidence for establishing incest.

REFERENCES

Evett IW, Werrett DJ, Buckleton JS (1989) Paternity calculations from DNA multi-locus profiles. Journal of the Forensic Science Society 29:249-254

Evett IW, Buckleton JS (1989) Some aspects of the Bayesian approach to evidence evaluation. Journal of the Forensic Science Society 29:317-324

Ivanov PL, Maljutov MB, Verbovaya LV, Savchenko YO (1991) Evaluation of multi-locus DNA profiling using Monte-Carlo simulations. Fingerprint News (in press)

Ivanov PL, Verbovaya LV (1990) Determination of degrees of relatedness for sexual assault case (DNA fingerprinting with M13 probe) Zentralblatt Rechtsmedizin 34:444

Jeffreys AJ, Wilson V, Thein SL (1985) Individual-specific "fingerprints" of human DNA. Nature 316:76-79

Jeffreys AJ, Morton DB (1987) DNA fingerprints of dogs and cats. Animal Genetics 18:1-15

Maljutov MB, Ivanov PL, Savchenko YO, Verbovaya LV (1991) On the approximation of confidence intervals and robustness of relatedness inference based on similarity index of genetic profiles. J.Applied Statistics (in press)

3 Biostatistics and Databases

The Robustness of Models for Evaluating Patterns of DNA Multi-Locus Probes

C.H. Brenner

2300 Grand Canal, Venice, California 90291, USA

INTRODUCTION

DNA multi-locus probe patterns clearly have the potential to be powerful evidence in clarifying issues of identity, paternity, or other questions of kinship. Unfortunately the evidence is difficult to quantify. Any computation rests on assumptions built into a mathematical model. Of the assumptions usually built into models of multi-locus profiles, some are improbable and some -- like independence -- are at best nearly impossible to justify.

Computer simulations and other arguments presented here suggest encouragingly that some of the difficult assumptions may not be essential assumptions.

In particular, in considering independence a distinction has to be made between haplotypes and phenotypes. Of course, there can be 100% independence among the band positions (phenotypic information) only if the underlying haplotypes are also independent. However, redundant information in the haplotypes is by no means reflected in equal measure as redundancy in the phenotypes.

ASSUMPTIONS

The following simplifying assumptions define what will be referred to as the "ideal" multi-locus genetic model:

A. Unambiguity:
    1. There is a <u>discrete</u> collection of possible band positions, rather than a continuum. Therefore one can always make an unequivocal decision as to match / no match, and a correct interpretation of possible double bands.
    2. The patterns are <u>clear</u> in that one can clearly differentiate between a band and a stray mark.
    3. Fragments always <u>manifest</u> bands.
B. Genetic simplicity:
    1. Each position represents a +- system (i.e. + <u>dominates</u> -).

Advances in Forensic Haemogenetics 4
Edited by Ch. Rittner and P. M. Schneider
© Springer-Verlag Berlin Heidelberg 1992

           2.   There is <u>no mutation</u>.
    C.   Independence of bands:
           1.   There is <u>no observable allelism</u> -- bands at two
                different positions won't come from the same
                locus.
           2.   There is <u>no linkage</u> between loci -- neither a
                physical linkage nor statistical correlation.
    D.   Constant band frequency
           1.   There is <u>no overlap</u> between fragment sizes from
                different loci.
           2.   Every fragment size occurs with the <u>same frequen-
                cy</u>.

On the basis of these assumptions formulae can be derived for the
correct likelihood ratio (i.e. significance of the evidence), as
Evett et al (1989) and Hummel et al (1990, "Biostatistical ...")
have done in the case of using the multi-locus pattern of a trio
for evaluation of paternity.   Hummel's analysis includes an
ingenious maximum likelihood method to estimate the parameters
of band frequency, and number of potential band positions (N).
In consequence however, the analysis relies more heavily on the
idealized assumptions.

Formulae for evaluating identity can easily be derived.

Of course no one believes that the ideal model is a correct
description of nature.   However, that does not necessarily
invalidate the calculations.   They may still be approximately
right, or they may be conservative.   Some of the assumptions can
be tested by computer simulations, or by explicit analysis.

<u>Constant Band Frequency</u>

For evaluating identity, this is a conservative assumption as can
be shown by calculating a simple example.   There is one hidden
point, however: there can be a difference between average band
frequency and average band-sharing frequency.

Suppose there are only two band positions, G and H, that have
different band frequencies, 1/2 and 1/4 respectively.   If both
bands appear in a crime stain, a random suspect will match only
one time in eight, so the correct likelihood ratio is 8.

The likelihood ratio computed by assuming the idealized model
will depend on how a value is chosen for the average band
frequency, and there are two possibilities.

The easier value to determine in practice is the average rate of
band sharing, which is equal to the band frequency when the band
frequency is constant.   To see what band sharing rate would be
observed, imagine a population of 1000 people.   Of these, 500
have a G band and 250 have an H band.   Hence if we pick a band
at random,

- 2/3 of the time we pick a G band, which is shared with 1/2 of the population;
- 1/3 of the time we pick an H band, which is shared with 1/4 of the population.

Therefore the average rate of band sharing would be

$$(2/3)(1/2) + (1/3)(1/4) = 5/12.$$

Using this figure, we would calculate a likelihood ratio of $(12/5)^2 = 6$ for matching two bands between stain and suspect, which is duly conservative compared to 8.

Alternatively, if we take the ideal model very seriously then we might imagine that we arrive at the correct average band frequency of 3/8 by using Hummel's method. In that case we would compute a likelihood ratio of $(8/3)^2 = 7$, still conservative.

For paternity evaluation purposes the situation is rather more complicated. Given the same example of two band positions, G and H, and assuming that the average band frequency, 3/8, is used for calculations according to the method of Evett et al and Hummel et al, the idealized assumptions result in a conservatively small likelihood ratio for some combinations of patterns, but an unfairly high number in other cases. For example, when the "incriminating" -++ pattern (no band in mother, band in child, band in man) occurs at the G position and not at the H position, the idealized number is unfair typically by 40%. Choosing the average band-share rate of 5/12 for band frequency reduces this particular over-estimate, but at the cost of unfairly exaggerating the evidentiary significance when child and man share non-band (+--, and the controversial --- case).

On the other hand, when -++ occurs at both loci the net effect is safely conservative. There is therefore a temptation to consider -++ patterns only. Also, by limiting analysis to that pattern one avoids the pitfall (alluded to by Evett et al, 1990) of needing an accurate value for band frequency; an overestimate of the band frequency is good enough to ensure a conservative likelihood ratio for the -++ pattern.

Independence of Bands

The most extreme example of interdependence would be two band positions that are always merely copies of one another. Clearly this would be a bad thing if ignored, resulting in a likelihood ratio that is too high by the square.

However, there are some surprises.

Imagine band positions, A and Z, that are 100% linked, but complementary. That is, considering the pair as a haplotype the only possibilities are A-Z+ and A+Z-. Suppose that these two haplotypes occur with equal frequency. As a measure of the effect of the linkage we can calculate the power of exclusion of this pair of systems compared with the power of exclusion of a similar but non-linked pair.

Position A excludes exactly when the mother has genotype A-A-, the child A-A+, and the tested man has A-A-, a 1/32 chance. Also, position Z excludes when the A locus genotypes are A+A+, A+A-, A+A+, which is an additional 1/32 chance, for a total exclusion probability of exactly 1/16. On the other hand, if A and Z were independent the combined exclusion probability would actually be a shade less -- $1/16-(1/32)^2$.

So lack of independence is not necessarily damning.

Nor is the example artificial. In fact, it is exactly a single locus with two equally frequent alleles, A and Z. Incidentally, if the bands are known to represent such a system, a further 1/8 of cases are exclusions: A-A- in the child with Z-Z- in the man, or the opposite (Jeff Morris, personal communication).

In order to investigate independence further, simulations were carried out with the aid of a computer. The idea is to create simulated data that violates the independence assumption, make calculations as if independence held, then see how far wrong the calculations are. Each simulation was a Monte Carlo construction of the following sort:

1. A value is chosen for N, the number of band positions.
2. A restricted set of permissible N-position haplotypes is chosen.
3. Mother-Child-Father true trios are generated using the haplotypes. False trios are generated by displacing the fathers to different cases.

This is a flexible scheme, as will appear. The analysis includes some of the following statistics:

4. For each false trio an "ideal" L value (=X/Y) is calculated by counting the incidence of each of the eight patterns ---, --+, ... and assuming the idealized model (i.e. using the Hummel/Evett formulae).
5. The average ideal L for false trios is computed.[1]
   As noted in Nijenhuis (1983), the average value of L for false trios is 1. If the average computed for the simulation is greater than 1, then L from the idealized model must on the average be unfair by that ratio.

---

[1] Equivalently, this number is the ratio of actual to predicted numbers of Random Men Not Excluded. The prediction is made by trusting the idealized L values and averaging 1/L among non-exclusion cases, per Nijenhuis (1983).

6. In some cases a "redundancy factor," f, was computed as follows: Let the ideal L values for the simulated false trios be denoted L_i. The factor f (usually f>1) is determined such that the average of the numbers $L_i^{1/f}$ is 1. This is a measure of the effective number of times the information at each band position is duplicated. Restated, a system with N bands and redundancy f is about equivalent in evidentiary power to an ideal system with N/f bands.

7. The true trio ideal L values are computed, then adjusted by taking the f-th root.

Simulation (1) has N=5 band positions, haplotypes +----, -+---, --+--, ---+-, ----+, thus modelling a locus with five alleles and allele frequency 0.2. Average ideal L for 2000 false trios was 1.15.

Simulation (2) models a locus with ten alleles, allele frequency 0.1. The average ideal L over 1000 false trios was 1.29.

Simulation (3) has N=10 and 55 haplotypes, namely those with only one or two +'s. This models two overlapping 10-allele loci. The average ideal L over 1000 false trios was 1.09.

For simulations (1)-(3), band position by position the ideal model L values are correct. However in multiplying them together statistical independence is incorrectly assumed, and that is why the average L values are a bit too large. That they are only a little too large suggests that allelism and overlap are not serious problems, and that it will be possible to determine compensating factors depending on N and on the band frequencies.

Simulation (4) has N=6 and only the two haplotypes ---+++ and +++---. Thus, band positions 1 and 4 are the "AZ" system described above, while the remaining band positions are redundant copies of these two informative ones. The simulation comprised 1667 false trios, with an average ideal L value of 1.9. The best fit for the redundancy factor f was 2.7, though the correct value is obviously 3. This simulation is included to indicate the limitation of the method for determining f.

Experiment (5) is a series of simulations designed to assess the impact of random linkage as N grows, and to overcome the difficulty of determining f accurately.

The series consists of simulations with N=3, 4, ... up to 31. For each simulation only 8 of the possible 2^N haplotypes are permitted. For N=3 these haplotypes are the complete set of possible combinations, so this simulation models complete independence. For each larger value of N each of the 3-haplotypes is augmented to length N by a random selection of + and -'s, as in Fig. 1. Since the entire haplotype is thus determined by the first three symbols, a naive hypothesis might be that the augmented haplotype is no more informative than when N=3. That is, one might predict that N/f=3. Such a view overlooks the situation illustrated in Fig. 2, where the phenotype at the bottom band position reveals information (an exclusion) not apparent from the first three band positions. In fact N/f gradually grows to about 8.

Experiment (6) is like (5), but intended to be more realistic by approximating an allele frequency of 0.2 rather than 0.5. In this case N/f grows to about 6, when N=20.

				+	+	+	+
-	-	+	+	-	+	+	+
+	+	-	+	+	+	-	-
-	+	-	-	+	-	-	+
h	i	j	k	l	m	n	o

haplotype

Figure 1
The haplotypes that were allowed for experiment (5), N=5. Each column is a haplotype; each row is a band position

	Mother	Child	Man
genotype	h j	j l	m n
phenotype	-	+	+
	+	+	+
	-	-	+
	+	+	+
>>>	-	+	-

Figure 2
A typical false trio in experiment (5), N=5. The haplotypes are from Fig. 1

Simulation (7) introduces a new idea of using the redundancy factor to reevaluate true trios. From 200 false trios using 64 random haplotypes with N=50 and allele frequency 0.2, f=1.96. Likelihood ratios were then calculated for 200 true trios assuming the ideal model. The geometric mean was 5900, and the largest was 230000000. When each was replaced by its 1/f power, the resulting collection had a geometric mean of 84 -- the sort of likelihood ratio that apparently follows even from assuming only a very small degree of independence.

This simulation seems to have the following interpretation: The haplotype information is highly redundant, equivalent of only 6 independent positions. Nonetheless, the phenotypic information is equivalent to that from 25 (50/1.96) independent positions.

Simulation (8) is designed to mimic the case data analyzed in Hummel et al, and to suggest some of the vast possibilities for analysis of such simulations. N=80, and 64 random haplotypes were selected with predominately -'s rather than +'s. From 125 Monte Carlo trios, the allele frequency was 0.054 and band frequency 0.104. Of the 125 false trios, 122 were excluded (not 99.9998% as predicted from the ideal L-values, but still pretty good), with 3.4±1.3 exclusions (-+- patterns) per trio. The true trios had a geometric mean ideal L value of 22000, reduced to 22 by taking the f=3.2 roots. The true trios had 3.8±1.4 -++ patterns per trio (compared to 1.3±0.8 for the false trios). The -++ contributions to the true trio ideal likelihood ratios account for about 1000 out of 22000.

Applying the maximum likelihood method of Hummel et al estimates N=69.9 and band frequency as 0.12, close to the Hummel case values. When these parameters are used to calculate ideal L values, the low N is safe because it results in underestimating the number of moderately paternity-indicative "---" patterns. Low maximum-likelihood estimates for N seem to be the rule. However, the overestimate for the band frequency inflates the evidentiary significance of most patterns. For example, the -++ pattern is thus counted with a likelihood ratio of 8.37, while it was actually observed only 7.54 times more frequently among the true trios than among the false trios.

Ambiguity, and Mutation

These problems contribute a significant share to the difficulty of analyzing multi-locus patterns and to their acceptability in forensics. The obvious approach is that they should included in the model. With regard to mutation this is often done already. As for questions of ambiguity, which means about the same as objectivity, it might be difficult but it can be done.

CONCLUSION

Linkage and independence are to some extent a bugbear. With 80 variable band positions there are 2^{80} possible haplotypes, all of which should exist assuming independence. But even a handful are enough to exclude nearly all non-fathers, and knowledge of their existence is enough to imply somewhat useful likelihood ratios for fathers.

Haplotypes and phenotypes are different things. Arguments and concerns about linkage, interdependence, and allelic association pertain mostly to haplotypes, and only indirectly to phenotypes. But measurements and observations are of phenotypes. That's why it is possible, and indeed turns out to be the case, that multi-locus measurements are not too tainted by haplotype interdependence.

These results herein are only an indication. It would be desirable to take some hard data that quantifies at least partial independence among some of the band positions, and build it into the simulations. It might turn out that a modest amount of independence is enough to justify very strong inferences from multi-locus probe data.

REFERENCES

Evett IW, Werrett DJ, Buckleton JS (1989) Paternity Calculations
    from DNA Multilocus Profiles. J Forens Sci Soc 29: 249-254
Fimmers R, Epplen JT, Schneider PM, Baur MP (1990) Likelihood
    Calculations in Paternity Testing on the Basis of DNA-Finger-
    prints. Advances in Forensic Haemogenetics 3: 14-16

Hummel K, Fukshansky N, Bär W, Zang K (1990) Biostatistical
  Approaches Using Minisatellite DNA Patterns in Paternity Cases
  (Mother-Child-Putative-father Trios).   Advances   in Forensic
  Haemogenetics 3: 17-19
Hummel K, Fukshansky N, Bär W (1990) Kinship Plausibilities from
  DNA Fingerprints. Advances in Forensic Haemogenetics 3: 20-22
Nijenhuis LE, A Critical Evaluation of Various Methods of
  Approaching Probability of Paternity (1983) Inclusion Probabil-
  ities in Parentage Testing, American Association of Blood Banks
  103-112

Comparison of Different Methods for the Calculation of Indices of Paternity

R. Fimmers*, P.M. Schneider**, M.P. Baur*

* Institute for Medical Statistics, University of Bonn, Sigmund-Freud-Str. 25, Germany

** Institut für Rechtsmedizin der Universität Mainz, am Pulverturm 3, Germany

INTRODUCTION

The qualitative decision about paternity in trio cases on the basis of DNA multilocus profiles is no problem. If there are more than 1 or 2 exclusion patterns (band present in child, which is neither present in mother or alleged father), the putative father has to be excluded. The problems arise, if, in the case of a non exclusion, one wants to quantify the evidence for paternity. Different statistics have been proposed for this purpose. This paper discusses three of these statistics and demonstrates their application to real data.

NUMBER OF INFORMATIVE BANDS

The simplest statistic is the number of informative bands, i.e. bands, which are present in the child and the alleged father, but not in the mother. Let b_i be the frequency of the i-th informative band for a given case, then

$$\prod_{i=1}^{k} b_i \tag{1}$$

is the chance of finding this set of bands in a random man (disregarding all other band positions) and

$$A = 1 - \prod_{i=1}^{k} b_i \tag{2}$$

is the exclusion chance for such a random man. The application of a conservative equal frequency b for all bands reduces 2 to

$$A = 1 - b^k \tag{3}$$

were k is the number of informative bands. The average posterior probability W assuming equal priors then is given by

$$\overline{W} = \frac{1}{1 + \frac{1-A}{1}} = \frac{1}{2 - A}. \tag{4}$$

Advances in Forensic Haemogenetics 4
Edited by Ch. Rittner and P. M. Schneider
© Springer-Verlag Berlin Heidelberg 1992

BAND SHARING

Band sharing is another straightforward measure of similarity between DNA multilocus profiles. It can be determined for any pair of individual band patterns, which normally should be placed in two adjacent lanes on the same blot. Let n_A and n_B be the number of bands in individual A and in individual B, and s_{AB} the number of bands shared between A and B.

From the simple question: "What is the probability, that B has a band, which is present in A", we get a natural definition of the band sharing rate

$$r_{AB}^* = \frac{s_{AB}}{n_A}. \tag{5}$$

This approach has the problem, that it is not symmetric in A and B (i.e. $r_{AB}^* \neq r_{BA}^*$), whenever $n_A \neq n_B$.

The most commonly used way to define band sharing is

$$\tilde{r}_{AB} = \frac{2 s_{AB}}{n_A + n_B}, \tag{6}$$

which of course is symmetric, but is biased to an underestimation of the band sharing rate, if the number of bands n_A and n_B are different.

An unbiased and symmetrical estimator of the band sharing rate is obtained by

$$r_{AB} = \frac{1}{2} \left(r_{AB}^* + r_{BA}^* \right) = \frac{s_{AB}}{2} \left(\frac{1}{n_A} + \frac{1}{n_B} \right), \tag{7}$$

the measure of band sharing, which will be used in the subsequent text.

Band sharing depends on the degree of relationship between the two individuals. Based on the kind of relationship and the expected band sharing between unrelated individuals, which stands for the chance of a random match, it is possible to calculate expected band sharing rates for all types of kinship. Honma et. al. [5] have given formulas for the most relevant types of kinship. For the parent child relationship the result was reformulated by Jeffreys et. al. [8] on the basis of band frequencies and transmission probabilities.

The grandparent grandchild and the uncle nephew cases seem to be wrong in the Honma paper. Describing the kinship in terms of the probabilities p_0, p_1 and p_2 of having 0, 1, or 2 alleles identical by descent, the expected band sharing rate can be calculated as ($a =$ allele frequency)

$$p_0(2a - a^2) + p_1 \frac{1 + a - a^2}{2 - a} + p_2. \tag{8}$$

For $p_0 = \frac{1}{2}, p_1 = \frac{1}{2}, p_2 = 0$ (grandparent-grandchild as well as uncle-nephew) this evaluates to

$$1 + 5a - 5a^2 + a^3, \tag{9}$$

deviating from Honma et. al.. Formula 8 can be applied for all kinds of kinship. For parent child we get ($p_0 = 0, p_1 = 1, p_2 = 0$)

$$\frac{1 + a - a^2}{2 - a}, \tag{10}$$

equivalent to Honma. Jeffreys et. al. give in this case the formula ($b =$ band frequency)

$$\frac{1}{b}(2b - 1 + \sqrt{1 - b}^3),\tag{11}$$

which is equivalent to formula 10 using the relation between band and allele frequency $b = a(2 - a)$. It has to be stressed, that the results are the same, though the approach by Jeffreys et. al. does not require the assumption of one locus with defined alleles producing the band, but works with band frequencies and transmission probabilities, which may be a more general approach.

LIKELIHOOD APPROACH

The method to quantify paternity, which is here called the likelihood approach, was proposed independently by Evett et. al. [1], Honma et. al. [4] and Hummel et. al. [6]. The main idea is to assume independence between the bands of a DNA multilocus profile. This allows to treat the band positions separately and to get an overall likelihood by multiplication. The assumption of independence is very strong. A genetic model for the band pattern, which leads to this independence, has to postulate, that the bands of a DNA multilocus profile are not allelic and that the loci are not linked. In practice, these requirements can only be fulfilled to a certain degree.

The special aspect of the Evett approach is, that he formulates the problem in terms of band frequencies and transmission probabilities. Therefore he needs no further assumptions except that independence between band position holds, and that bands are transmitted from parent to child with a certain probability (e.g. it does not bother how many loci are involved in the production of one band).

Honma et. al. [4] and Hummel et. al. [6] use a model, which seems formally more restrictive. They interpret the presence or absence of a band at a single position as coming from a diallelic locus with one recessive allele (no band). Consequently the calculation of likelihoods for the single band position is a standard procedure. The difference between Honma and Hummel is the question, which types of band pattern should be evaluated at the different band positions. The results are identical to the Evett approach. An additional assumption, which is not necessary, but often made, is to assume equal band or allele frequencies for all band positions. This may lead to wrong (anti conservative) results, if the overall estimation of the allele frequency is not chosen with caution.

For a usual trio case, with mother, child and alleged father and a fixed band position, the vector $(\cdot, \cdot, \cdot)$ will give the information, whether or not mother (first position), child (second position) and alleged father (third position) have a band at this position of their DNA profile. $+$ will indicate presence, $-$ will indicate absence of a band. E.g. $(-, +, +)$ means, that the mother has no band, but child and alleged father have a band at the position in question. Using this notation we have eight different types of band patterns which can occur in the different positions. Some of these are worth to be discussed in more detail.

Depending on whether the alleged father is excluded or not excluded the pattern $(-, +, -)$ can be designated as "exclusion" or as "mutation" band pattern. The qualitative decision about paternity can be based exclusively on this type of band pattern. The formal models, which are used here to calculate likelihoods, do not allow the occurrence of $(-, +, -)$ under the assumption of paternity.

In a case with one or two of these patterns, and the alleged father not excluded, it is necessary to include this information into the calculation of the likelihoods. Similar to the singlelocus case [3] one can use a kind of global mutation rate (the probability of the occurrence of $(-,+,-)$ patterns in the complete band pattern of a triplet). Together with the allele frequency a one can calculate an approximate paternity index of $\frac{\mu}{a}$ for the $(-,+,-)$ pattern.

The other important pattern with high information for paternity is $(-,+,+)$. Depending on the band frequency the evidence for paternity from this pattern is high in comparison to all other band patterns (except $(-,+,-)$). Honma et.al. [4] propose, to use this type of pattern only. The number of these "informative bands" can be regarded as an independent characteristic value for paternity (see above) and Honma's proposition leads to the above defined exclusion chance. The number of $(-,+,+)$ patterns is also the fundamental part of band sharing.

The most controversial pattern is $(-,-,-)$. This patterns, in contrast to all other patterns, are not defined by the occurrence of a band. Their number is gained by way of estimation of the potential number of band positions. Following Hummel [7], the effective number of bands N_{eff} can be estimated from the average number of bands per individual n and the average number of bands shared between pairs of two unrelated individuals s, as follows

$$N_{eff} = \frac{n^2}{s}. \tag{12}$$

A different way to define the number of $(-,-,-)$ patterns, is to define the number of band positions using a binning approach.

The question is, whether or not these patterns should be regarded as information about paternity and can be included into the calculation of the likelihoods? The strong independence assumptions, which had to be made (especially for the Hummel version) lead to a divergence between the model and the unknown genetic reality. The $(-,-,-)$ patterns can be regarded as an artifact introduced by the model. A meaningful approximation to the genetical background of a multilocus profile is to understand it as an overlay of an unknown number of singlelocus patterns. From this point of view there is no reason to assume information in positions without a band. A discussion about the usage of these patterns will always lead to a discussion, whether or not the assumptions of independence and multiple diallelic systems are appropriate. From a pure formal genetic point of view they are obviously not.

Nevertheless it is interesting to look at the empirical distribution of the resulting likelihood ratios in case of paternity and non paternity [2]. The $(-,-,-)$ patterns have to be judged according to their impact on the resulting likelihood values. Depending on the band frequencies the $(-,-,-)$ pattern suggests evidence for paternity, which increases exponentially with the number of postulated positions N_{eff}. The inclusion of this "information" into the calculation of overall likelihood will bias the result towards assuming paternity. Not to use the $(-,-,-)$ patterns is therefore conservative in the sense of the non excluded father. The effect of the use of the $(-,-,-)$ patterns will be demonstrated in the following application of the method to empirical data.

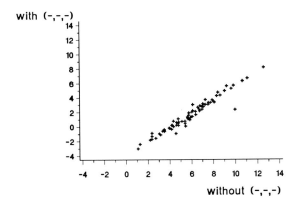

Figure 1: EM-values, with vs. without $(-,-,-)$ patterns

APPLICATION TO EMPIRICAL DATA

The objective of this paper is the comparison of different characteristics for paternity based on DNA multilocus profiles in their application to real data. The cases, which were used came from the MZ 1.3 study (see Schneider [9]). 76 Mother-child-alleged-father triplets were taken from the data of one participating laboratory. Paternity was confirmed by the results from blood-group, HLA and singlelocus DNA systems. The migration distances had been read to an accuracy of 0.5mm. Bands in adjacent lanes were regarded to come from equal sized fragment, if their running distances did not differ more than 0.5mm. An algorithm was used to correct for these differences. The numbers of the eight $+/-$ -patterns were counted for each of the 76 families. Based on this "$+/-$ -statistic" it was easily possible to calculate the paternity characteristics. For the application of the likelihood approach (incl. $(-,-,-)$) an overall allele frequency a and the effective number of bands were estimated as proposed by Hummel [7].

RESULTS

Figure 1 shows the comparison of the Essen-Möller-values (EM-values) with and without the $(-,-,-)$ combinations. The values from a more or less straight line, which shows, that the inclusion of $(-,-,-)$ does not give additional (different) information. The EM-values are shifted about 4 units towards assuming paternity, which means, that paternity indices are inflated by a factor of 10000.

Figures 2,3,4 show all bivariate plots for the number of $(-,+,+)$, band sharing and EM-values (without $(-,-,-)$). As expected from the theoretical considerations, the values are highly correlated. The correlation is smallest for band sharing and the number of $(-,+,+)$ patterns.

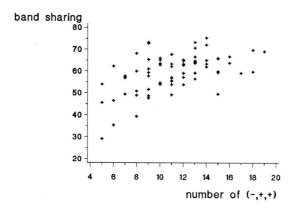

Figure 2: Band sharing vs. number of $(-,+,+)$ patterns

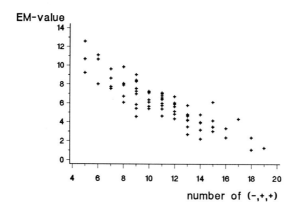

Figure 3: EM-values vs. number of $(-,+,+)$ patterns

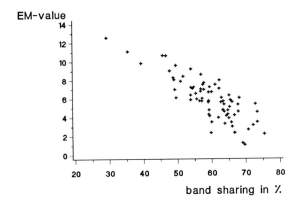

Figure 4: Band sharing vs. EM-values

DISCUSSION

The application of the three different paternity statistics for DNA multilocus profiles shows two important results. The inclusion of $(-,-,-)$ patterns into the calculation of likelihood values results in a systematical bias for likelihood ratios and EM-values. The interpretation for the $(-,-,-)$ patterns is questionable and may be only understood in connection with the assumptions of the "multiple diallelism model". The justification to chose this approach is its practicability and simplicity. Because of the strong anticonservative bias, which is introduced through the $(-,-,-)$ patterns, we strongly argue against this approach. The extension of this method to complex deficiency cases, which would be a standard procedure as in any other well defined Mendelian system, is not possible due to the strong impact of the false assumptions.

The comparison of the number of $(-,+,+)$ patterns, the band sharing rate and the EM-values showed that all three characteristics are highly correlated. Their informational contents is approximately the same. The larger difference between the band sharing and the number of $(-,+,+)$ patterns may be due to the fact, that band sharing also takes $(+,+,+)$ patterns into account and that the number of shared bands is put into relation to the total number of bands.

Nevertheless there is quite a large difference in the interpretation of the three statistics. Band sharing has expected values which depend on the degree of relation between the compared persons. High band sharing (above 50%) is information for a first degree relationship. Low band sharing is characteristic for unrelated individuals. The number of $(-,+,+)$ patterns can be transformed into an exclusion probability. The W-value (equivalent to the likelihood ratio and the EM-value) has the strongest interpretation as a Bayesian aposteriori probability for paternity. If one uses the W-value interpretation, one should be aware, that the resolution power of this statistic cannot be greater than for the band sharing rate, with all implications for the interpretation of the result.

References

[1] Evett IW, Werrett DJ, Buckleton JS (1989) Paternity calculation from DNA multi-locusprofiles. J Forens Sci Soc 29: 249-254

[2] Fimmers R, Epplen JT, Schneider PM, Baur MP (1989) Likelihood calculation in paternitytesting on the basis of DNA fingerprints. In: Polesky HF, Mayr WR (eds) Advances in forensic haemogenetics 3. Springer, Berlin Heidelberg New York, pp 14-16

[3] Fimmers R, Henke L, Henke J, Baur MP (1991) How to Deal with Mutations in DNA-Testing. This volume

[4] Honma M, Ishiyama I (1989) Probability of paternity in paternity testing using the DNA fingerprint procedure. Hum Hered 39:165-169

[5] Honma M, Ishiyama I (1990) Application of DNA fingerprinting to parentage and extended family relationship testing. Hum Hered 40:356-362

[6] Hummel K, Fukshanski N (1990) Biostatistical approaches using minisatelite DNA patterns in paternity cases (mother-child-putative father trios). In: Polesky HF, Mayr WR (eds) Advances in forensic haemogenetics 3. Springer, Berlin Heidelberg New York, pp 17-19

[7] Hummel K (1991) Biostatistische Auswertung von DNA-Bandenmustern in Fällen strittiger Identität und Blutsverwandtschaft. Klin Lab 37:252-258

[8] Jeffreys AJ, Turner M, Debenham P (1991) The efficiency of multilocus DNA finger-print probes for individualization and establishment of family relationships, determined from extensive casework. Am J Hum Genet 39: 11-24

[9] Schneider PM, Fimmers R, Bertrams J, Birkner P, Braunbeck K, Bulnheim U, Feu-erbach M, Henke L, Iten E, Osterhaus E, Prinz M, Simeoni E, Rittner C (1991) Biostatistical basis of individualization and segregation analysis using the multilocus DNA probe MZ 1.3: Results of a collaborative study. (submitted for publication)

How to Deal with Mutations in DNA-Testing

R. Fimmers*, L. Henke**, J. Henke***, M.P. Baur*

* Institute for Medical Statistics, University of Bonn, Sigmund-Freud-Str. 25, Germany

** Institut für Blugruppenforschung, Otto-Hahn Str. 39, Düsseldorf

*** Institut für Blugruppenforschung, Hohenzollernring 57, Köln

INTRODUCTION

Some of the DNA single locus polymorphisms, which are presently used in paternity testing have a comparably high mutation rate. Consequently changes in fragment size occur quite often, during the transmission from parent to child. An isolated event like this may not be interpreted as an exclusion, especially if the mutation rate for the system in question is high. In combination with other information from blood-group-, HLA- and DNA-systems one would like to include the evidence against paternity from a possible mutation into the global likelihood statement. This requires the ability to calculate likelihood values for "mutation" patterns. From the theoretical point of view this is no problem, as will be seen in the following text. The problem arises with the estimation of the parameters, which describe the mutational event. A more global approach has to be used.

CALCULATION OF LIKELIHOODS

Figure 1 presents a typical "exclusion" or "mutation" band pattern from an arbitrary DNA single locus system. To calculate the likelihood of this band pattern it is necessary to include the possibility of mutations into the formal genetic model. It will be assumed,

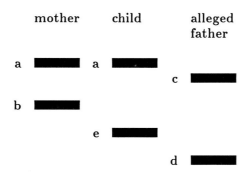

Figure 1: "Mutation" band pattern

that an allele x may change (its fragment size) to an allele y, while it is transmitted from parent to child. m_{xy} may denote the probability of such a mutational event. Including this possibility of change of fragment size, several explanations for the above band pattern in Fig. 1 possible under the assumption of paternity. One (unlikely) example is, that allele b is transmitted from the mother to the child and changes to allele e and that c is transmitted from the father to the child and changes into allele a. The probability of

Advances in Forensic Haemogenetics 4
Edited by Ch. Rittner and P. M. Schneider
© Springer-Verlag Berlin Heidelberg 1992

Table 1: Possible explanation of the band pattern

maternal band → filial band	paternal band → filial band	transmission probability
$a \longrightarrow a$	$c \longrightarrow e$	$\frac{1}{2} \cdot \frac{1}{2} m_{ce}$
$a \longrightarrow a$	$d \longrightarrow e$	$\frac{1}{2} \cdot \frac{1}{2} m_{de}$

this event is $\frac{1}{2} m_{be} \cdot \frac{1}{2} m_{ca}$. This event is very unlikely, because it requires two mutational events. If all explanations, which require more than one "mutation" are considered to be negligible, because of their low probability, only two possible explanations remain (Table 1). The likelihood for the band pattern, under the assumption of paternity, can therefore be calculated as

$$X = \underbrace{2f(a)f(b)}_{\text{mat. phenotype}} \cdot \underbrace{2f(c)f(d)}_{\text{pat. phenotype}} \cdot \underbrace{\frac{1}{2} \cdot \frac{1}{2}(m_{ce} + m_{de})}_{\text{transm. prob.}} \tag{1}$$

The likelihood under nonpaternity can be calculated as

$$Y = 2f(a)f(b) \cdot 2f(c)f(d) \cdot \left[f(e)\frac{1}{2}(1 + m_{ba})) + f(a)\frac{1}{2}(m_{ae} + m_{be}) \right] \tag{2}$$

$$\approx 2f(a)f(b) \cdot 2f(c)f(d) \cdot f(e) \cdot \frac{1}{2} \tag{3}$$

and consequently the likelihood ratio is

$$\frac{Y}{X} = \frac{2f(e)}{m_{ce} + m_{de}} \tag{4}$$

The problem with the application of this formula is, that the specific mutation rates m_{xy} cannot be estimated. They are by far smaller than the overall mutation rate and depend on the two fragment sizes. Small changes in the fragment size seem to be more likely than larger ones.

In order to evaluate this type of band pattern in terms of likelihood ratios, one has to choose a less specific model. A mutation rate, which can be estimated concerning a singlelocus DNA-system is the overall paternal mutation rate μ, which may differ from the maternal mutation rate. More precisely μ is the probability of the occurrence of a "mutation" band pattern under paternity. At this level only one information is drawn from the band pattern. Either the pattern is compatible with paternity or not. The frequencies of the alleles which are involved in a pattern are not taken into account. The resulting likelihoods are the same for all "mutation" band patterns for a given system.

Under nonpaternity the probability of a "mutation" band pattern is $1 - r$, where r is the probability of a (wrong) inclusion. r can be estimated from empirical data or calculated from the allele frequencies f.

$$r = \sum_{a \in \{alleles\}} f(a) \left[2f(a) - f(a)^2 \right] \tag{5}$$

The likelihood ratio, which can be calculated using μ and r is

$$\frac{Y}{X} = \frac{1 - r}{\mu}. \tag{6}$$

APPLICATION TO DATA

This method was applied to data for the probes MS1, MS31, MS43, G3, YNH24. The estimated paternal mutation rates and "wrong inclusion" probabilities are summarized in Table 2. MS1 has the highest paternal mutation rate, but the smallest number of "wrong"

Table 2: Estimation of μ and r, likelihood values

	μ		r		$\frac{Y}{X}$	EM	W
	n	%	n	%			
MS1	591	4.57	281	2.14	21.41	11.33	0.045
MS31	600	2.17	300	6.67	43.08	11.63	0.023
MS43	594	0.51	298	7.72	182.71	12.26	0.005
G3	589	0.51	276	3.26	189.93	12.28	0.005
YNH24	349	0.86	179	6.70	108.54	12.04	0.009

inclusions, which both may be related to a high degree of polymorphism.

The resulting likelihood values (likelihood ratio $\frac{Y}{X}$, EM-value and W-value) are also presented in Table 2. They depend mainly on the mutation rates. The influence of the "wrong inclusion" probability is low. Smaller mutation rates lead to higher likelihood ratios, that means higher evidence against paternity. A "mutation" band pattern for MS43 or G3 has a higher evidence against paternity than a similar pattern for MS1.

DISCUSSION

To be able to calculate likelihoods and likelihood ratios for "mutation" band patterns from DNA single locus polymorphisms requires to incorporate the possibility of mutations (fragment size changes) into the formal genetic model. This can only be done in a more global approach, where only a part of the available information is used. The resulting likelihoods are valid for all "mutation" patterns for a given system. The frequencies of the alleles or fragments which occur in the band pattern cannot be taken into account, unless more specific mutation rates can be estimated.

The resulting likelihood values make it possible, to combine the "mutation" information from a DNA single locus system with the evidence from other systems. A problem may be seen in the fact, that the available information cannot be used completely. A small change in the fragment size should be more likely than a large change. The evidence against paternity should be therefore different for different band patterns. The likelihood values, which are calculated here have to be regarded as a kind of average for the total system in question. They should be handled carefully, because they may over- or underinterpret the true evidence of paternity. To be conservative in the sense of the not excluded father, one should perhaps use low estimators (lower confidence limits) for the mutation rates and the probabilities of "wrong" inclusion.

The Relationship of the HLA Phenotype Frequency of the Alleged Father to the
Resulting Paternity Index in Caucasian Non-Exclusion Paternity Cases

R.H. Walker, A.B. Eisenbrey

William Beaumont Hospital, Royal Oak, MI, USA

INTRODUCTION

The system paternity index (PI) is derived from the phenotypes of the trio and
its value in non-exclusion cases is primarily determined by the gene frequency
of the paternal gene (obligatory gene) transmitted to the child. This study
was undertaken to determine: 1) The range of HLA phenotype frequencies
observed in our laboratory among non-excluded causasian alleged fathers, 2)
the distribution of the resulting paternity index values in these cases and 3)
the relationship of these two distributions to each other.

METHODS

Five hundred consecutive trio paternity cases involving causasians with non-
exclusions were reviewed to tabulate the HLA phenotype frequencies of the
alleged fathers and the resulting HLA paternity index values. The HLA
phenotype frequencies and PI values were derived using the Traver (1989)
computer program. Haplotype frequencies in the data base were those published
by Mickey et al. (1983) based on 5559 caucasian individuals from paternity
cases and the HLA A and B specificities recognized by the 1980
Histocompatibility Workshop. The laboratory was able to define 16 A locus and
28 B locus serological specificities which could yield over 45,000 possible
phenotypes.

RESULTS

Observed HLA phenotype frequencies ranged from 0.000002 (1 in 500,000) to
0.0094 (1 in 106) with a median of 0.00038 (1 in 2600) (Fig. 1). Observed HLA
PI values ranged from 1 to 1438 with a median of 27 (Fig. 2). Subpopulations
of the study group are shown in the table below.

Phenotype Frequencies	n	%	Median PI
>1 in 1,000	135	27	9
1 in 1,000 - 1 in 10,000	236	47	26
1 in 10,000 - 1 in 100,000	112	23	76
<1 in 100,000	17	3	175
	500	100	27

The distribution of the observed HLA phenotype frequencies, paternity index
values, and the relationship of these two distributions are displayed in
Figures 1,2, and 3, respectively.

Advances in Forensic Haemogenetics 4
Edited by Ch. Rittner and P. M. Schneider
© Springer-Verlag Berlin Heidelberg 1992

DISCUSSION

The biologic father, by definition, must share genetic markers with his child in all genetic systems. When they share an infrequent marker, the likelihood of paternity is greatly increased. In the HLA system, all genetic markers are infrequent, although there is a 4 log range of variance in the Class I gene frequencies. The HLA phenotype frequencies and the resulting PI values were negatively correlated ($r = -0.606$; $p \leq 0.00001$). Alleged fathers phenotype frequencies of <1 in 100,000 have PI values which are usually >100 (median 175) while alleged fathers phenotype frequenices of >1 in 1,000 have PI values <70 (median 9). Deviations from the usual reciprocal relationship occur when the alleged father has a phenotype of relatively moderate frequency in which instance he could transmit either a rare haplotype resulting in a high PI value or a more common haplotype resulting in a low PI. Therefore, the correlation in this mid-range (1 in 1,000 to 1 in 100,000) has little predictive value due to the broad distribution in the data about the least squares line of regression.

REFERENCES

Mickey MR, Tiwari J, Bond J, Gjertson D, Terasaki PI (1983) Paternity probability calculations for mixed races. In: Walker RH, (ed) Inclusion probabilities in parentage testing. Amer. Assoc. of Blood Banks, Arlington, p. 333-341

Traver M (1989) Paternity index calculations, version 8.0. Traver Paternity Software, Inc., Madison

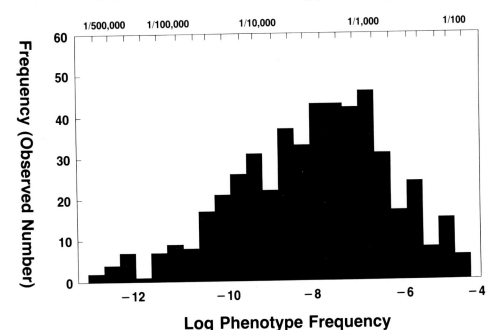

Fig. 1. Distribution of Phenotype Frequencies

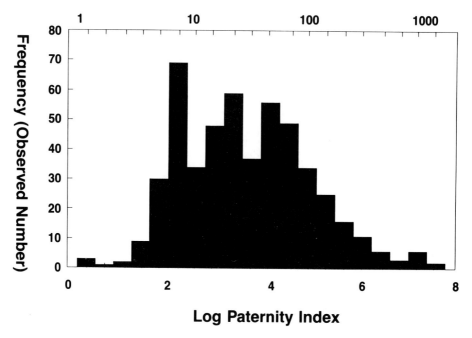

Fig. 2. Distribution of Paternity Index Values

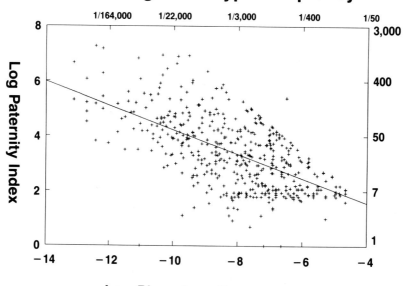

Log Phenotype Frequency
R − squared = .42

Fig. 3. Phenotype Frequency versus Paternity Index

DNASYS: A User-Friendly Computer Program for Evaluating Single Locus Probe Data in Forensic Casework

I.W. Evett, R. Pinchin and J. Scranage

The Forensic Science Service, Central Research and Support Establishment, Aldermaston, Reading, Berkshire, RG7 4PN, UK

INTRODUCTION

Match/binning is not an efficient method for evaluating single locus probe (SLP) data and there are several reasons why a Bayesian approach is preferable. See, for example, Evett et al. (1990), Berry (1991), Berry et al. (1991) and Evett et al. (1991).

We have been using Bayesian analysis, mainly as a research tool, in the Forensic Science Service (FSS) for over two years, but recently we have been able to develop a computer program known as DNASYS for use by forensic caseworkers. This will be made available worldwide in early 1992 through new marketing initiatives of the FSS.

In this note we briefly describe the method and give the results of just two of the many experiments we have carried out to test its robustness. We give an overview of DNASYS and of some of the support services which we will be able to provide for those who are interested in implementing the program for their own use.

METHOD

Whereas match/binning is a two stage process, it is much more sensible to evaluate evidence through a function which takes account of all of the relevant information in one step. This is the likelihood ratio (LR), which takes account of how close the measurements on the crime sample are to those on the suspect's sample and also of how rare or common those measurements are in the population of interest. Instead of a match function which switches from "match" to "non-match" at some arbitrary threshold it is a continuous function which is large when measurements are close, becoming progressively smaller as they become further apart. A critical feature of the rate at which the ratio falls off is an allowance for the correlation in band weight measurement errors - band shift. This increases discrimination and hence efficiency.

Values of the LR less than one support the hypothesis that crime and suspect samples come from different people. Values greater than one support the hypothesis that they came from the same person: the larger the ratio, the greater the support.

DATA

The following experiments were carried out on data for the probes MS1 and MS31 collected at the Metropolitan Police Forensic Science Laboratory (MPFSL) as

Advances in Forensic Haemogenetics 4
Edited by Ch. Rittner and P. M. Schneider
© Springer-Verlag Berlin Heidelberg 1992

described by Buffery et al. (1991). The reproducibility parameters (standard deviations and correlation coefficients) were estimated from duplicate profilings carried out by the MPFSL.

WITHIN-PERSON COMPARISONS

A total of 153 Caucasians had been profiled twice and we calculated the LR using the data from the two probes for each of the 153 pairs. Figure 1 is a histogram of the logarithm of the LR and the histogram intervals are labelled by their mid points; so 6.5, for example, corresponds to LR's from one million to ten million. Note that approximately 97% of the comparisons gave LR's in excess of 1000.

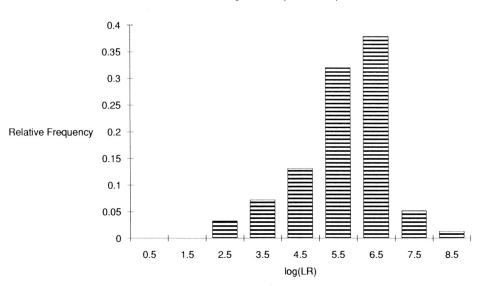

Fig.1. Within person comparisons

Of course, it is not sufficient to know that the method gives such high LR's when two samples from the same person are compared. We must also establish what can happen when samples from two different people are compared with each other.

BETWEEN-PERSON COMPARISONS

For this experiment we took a file of data on 1056 Caucasians and carried out all of the 557,040 between-person comparisons. The vast majority of these resulted in infinitesimal likelihood ratios but we are only concerned with those occasions when the LR exceeded one. These are summarised in Figure 2, again a histogram of the log of the LR.

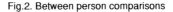

Fig.2. Between person comparisons

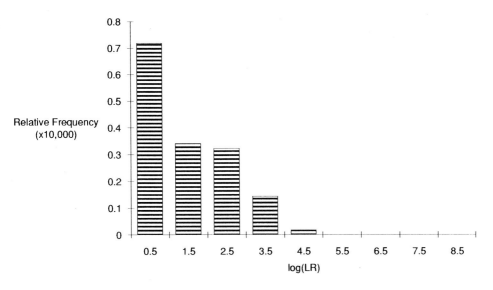

It is important to note that the vertical scale has been expanded by a factor
10,000 and to remember that this is the extreme right hand tail of the distribution.
The probability of incorrectly giving associative evidence is very small. Note,
in particular, that the chance of a LR in excess of 1000 is less than 1 in 56,000.
This is very conservative.

DNASYS

The program has been written in PASCAL to run on IBM PC's and clones. We have
placed particular emphasis on the user interface so the program is easy to use.
Data from up to four probes can be accommodated: we are aware that many
laboratories use more but, for crime work at least, there is little need to do
so given the statistical power of the method.

INTELLIGENCE SEARCHING

Several organisations have indicated an intention to maintain DNA databases on
known criminal offenders to assist in the solution of serious crimes. Databases
of unsolved sex crimes have considerable value because linking crimes provides
valuable information to investigators.

Retrieval from such databases by simple window searching is a clumsy and highly
inefficient procedure - particularly when the database is large. To ensure
successful retrieval of the correct entry the search window must be wide and this
means a substantial number of false hits - all of which need to be followed up
manually, costing time and money.

DNASYS has a search module which is much more efficient than window searching,
mainly because it takes account of the fact that measurement errors in the band
weights of one profile are highly correlated. Retrieval lists are much shorter
than from window searching and a further great advantage is that any hits are
ranked by the magnitude of the LR. This can save hours of manual checking.

FUTURE PLANS

Work is in hand to create a module for paternity analysis. Here, too, it is our aim to reduce the number of probes necessary to achieve good evidential results and also to create a good user interface. The effort that we devote to development of this module will be determined by the amount of interest that practitioners demonstrate. This conference is an excellent opportunity for us to gauge the level of that interest.

There is also scope for more advanced modules for dealing with mixed crime cases and for cases where relatives of the suspect may be suggested as hypothetical alternatives. Here again, the manpower which we devote to such developments will be determined by the level of interest.

The program clearly cannot run without databases and we are able to provide a service for converting users' databases to the correct format. We can also carry out analyses for determining standard deviations and correlation coefficients assuming that the users can provide suitable data.

We also have a suite of programs which we have used to test the robustness of our own procedures. We have studied, in particular, the robustness of the various independence assumptions which are much debated in the literature. We have also investigated the consequences of using non-representative databases and find that they have been exaggerated. In 1992 we will be making such analysis services available to other organisations on a consultancy basis.

CONCLUSION

The progress of DNA profiling has been hindered by poor quality statistical reasoning. Efficient statistical methods such as those embodied in DNASYS enable the real power of single locus profiling to be achieved. Good statistics mean that more information can safely be gleaned through the use of fewer probes: this saves time and it saves money.

REFERENCES

Berry DA (1991) Inferences using DNA profiling in forensic identification and paternity cases. Statistical Science. In press

Berry DA, Evett IW, Pinchin R (1991) Statistical inference in crime investigations using DNA profiling. Applied Statistics. In press

Buffery C, Burridge F, Greenhalgh M, Jones S, Willott G. Allele frequency distributions of four VNTR loci in the London area. Forensic Science International. In press

Evett IW, Werrett DJ, Pinchin R, Gill P (1990) Bayesian analysis of single locus DNA profiles. The International Symposium on Human Identificfation 1989. Promega, Madison, WI, USA

Evett IW, Scranage JK, Pinchin R (1991) An efficient statistical procedure for interpreting DNA single locus profiling data in crime cases. Journal of the Forensic Science Society. Submitted

SERIES SEXUAL CRIMES IDENTIFIED BY A DNA COMPUTERISED DATABASE

J.E. ALLARD

Metropolitan Police Forensic Science Laboratory
109 Lambeth Road, London SE1 7LP
United Kingdom

INTRODUCTION

The Metropolitan Police Forensic Science Laboratory has been recording DNA profiles on a computerised database since January 1990. This index contains profiles from personal samples and from unsolved cases where body fluid stains are thought to originate from the offender. At present there are approximately 2800 records from persons and 230 from unsolved cases - over 90% of the stains are semen from sexual assaults, the remainder include 12 bloodstains, mainly from murders, one saliva stain and one hair sample which the victim pulled from the offender.

When a profile is added to the database it is automatically compared against all existing records and any matches found are listed on a printout.

To date the index has made the first identification of series crime in five instances and added one case to each of three other series already known to the police. Additionally seven persons have been nominated for cases, three of whom were known serial offenders.

IDENTIFYING SERIES CRIME

The various police intelligence agencies and the Laboratory's own Sexual Assault Index record and compare modus operandi (MO) in order to identify and solve series crime. Unless an offender's behaviour is particularly unusual, such comparisons are generally limited to the local area. The DNA index is most successful in identifying links where the offender's behaviour is not distinctive, where behaviour changes between offences or where cases are separated by distance or time. The cases identified by our DNA index illustrate this:

1. One series where the first two offences, although similar in method, were two years apart.
2. One series where distance and behaviour separated cases.
3. Two series where the offender moved to another area and his MO was not distinctive enough to aid recognition of the case as part of the series.
4. Three series where the offender assaulted a completely different type of victim.
5. One series where one of the four cases lacked the particular idiosyncracy used to identify the offender.

Advances in Forensic Haemogenetics 4
Edited by Ch. Rittner and P. M. Schneider
© Springer-Verlag Berlin Heidelberg 1992

However the present lengthy technique of DNA profiling, together with heavy caseloads and hence backlogs, results in retrospective links, usually two to three months after the offence and sometimes as much as six months later.

The unequivocal identification of linked crimes by DNA profiling enables a study of the offender to be made. Details from several cases can be systematically analysed to build up a set of behavioural and physical characteristics which can be used to screen suspects and other potentially linked cases. This can act as a preliminary to producing a detailed "offender profile".

A CASE EXAMPLE

This series was first identified when a profile from a rape in 1989 was added to the DNA database. A match was found with another rape which had occurred almost two years previously. The two crimes were in the same locality and had a similar MO.

The police nominated several other cases which had similarities. DNA profiles were obtained from some of the cases,eliminating them from this series. However one proved to be part of a second series in the same area, as yet unresolved. Several suspects were also screened but no matches found and so the investigation was closed.

Eighteen months later the police recognised a third rape in the same area as being very similar in method to the first two cases. DNA profiling confirmed the link. A fourth case followed within three months. Later one robbery/indecent assault was thought to be by the same man, but lacked any DNA or other evidence for confirmation.

The crimes characteristically occurred late at night or early in the morning and all included theft of cash and/or jewellery. The offender was hooded or masked in three cases and had anal and/or vaginal intercourse from the rear in three cases.

This time the police decided to screen systematically all potential suspects in the local area. A study of the statements given by the four rape victims, together with the case circumstances, enabled an outline "offender profile" to be produced. This consisted of a weighted list of physical and behavioural characteristics to prioritise the suspects.

The close proximity of the offences suggested that the offender was a local man and most probably lived in the area central to the offences. Theft of valuables before the sexual assault in each of the cases suggested that he may have been a petty thief. He had an impersonal manner and his approach appeared to be criminally orientated rather than sexually orientated.

Such characteristics were rated by a points scheme, as shown below:

A.	Age 18-24 years	1 point
B.	Age 25-35 years	2
C.	Height 5'6" or over	2
D.	Previous conviction for theft and violence	3
E.	Previous conviction for theft, no violence	2
F.	Previous conviction for burglary	2
G.	Previous history of indecency	1
H.	Has had a custodial sentence	2
I.	Is unemployed	1
J.	Lives within half a mile of assaults	3
K.	Lives within one mile of assaults	2

The police used the weighted list together with their own intelligence records to nominate and prioritise possible suspects. They concentrated on those known for theft or theft together with sexual assault rather than those who were purely sexual offenders.

Approximately 300 samples were submitted to the Laboratory for screening. Fortunately conventional blood groups (ABO, Secretor and PGM) had been obtained from the seminal stains in the earlier cases, enabling rapid screening and exclusion of 90% of the suspects. The remaining suspects were checked by DNA profiling.

One of the samples submitted was found to match, giving an initial frequency of 1 in 3000 with the first probe (MS1). The full profile eventually provided a more definite identification. The man did fulfil several of the parameters suggested by the behavioural analysis, primarily that his home was central to the attacks and he had previous convictions for theft, burglary and violence but none for sexual assault.

CONCLUSION

The DNA index therefore provided the early recognition of this series. Other cases with similar MO could be unequivocally linked or rejected from the series by the DNA results, previously a rather uncertain issue for the investigator. DNA also allowed indisputable screening of suspects.

Most serial offenders do not travel great distances between their crimes and therefore local DNA indexes such as ours do operate effectively. However national or even international databases are required if we are to detect the serial offenders who are active in areas policed by different forces. The European DNA Profiling Group (EDNAP) has identified that the details of methodology are important for producing comparable results. In the United Kingdom it has been realised that at least two linking single locus probes are necessary for discriminatory results. Inter-laboratory databases can only operate if these are maintained.

EXPERIENCES WITH A COMPUTERISED DATABASE OF DNA PROFILES IN FORENSIC CASEWORK

M.J.Greenhalgh and J.E.Allard

Metropolitan Police Forensic Science Laboratory,
109 Lambeth Rd, London. SE1 7LP
United Kingdom

INTRODUCTION

 DNA profiling using single locus probes D1S7 (MS1),D7S21 (MS31), D12S11 (MS43A) and D2S44 (YNH24) has been used in casework at the Metropolitan Police Forensic Science Laboratory since November 1988. In this time approximately 1200 cases have been profiled including more than 2800 blood samples from different individuals. As the Laboratory had considerable experience in using computerised databases of conventional bloodgroups for intelligence purposes, it was a natural progression to continue this with DNA profiles. This was one of the factors that influenced our choice of single locus probes instead of a multi locus system as SLP results are relatively easy to store in numerical form and can be easily searched using a computerised database.

DESCRIPTION

 A set of autoradiographs from all four probes is prepared wherever possible and the bands in each track measured using a video scanner system developed at the Laboratory (Catterick and Russell 1991) which calculates the band weight values automatically. The results from all unsolved cases, which consist mostly of profiles from semen in sexual assaults, together with profiles from individuals are entered on the index. As each record is added it is automatically compared against all the others enabling links to be made between crimes committed by the same individual and also between crimes and possible suspects.

ARRANGEMENT OF THE INDEX

 The index is stored on a Prime 550 minicomputer in the form of a single file containing DNA records. Each record gives details of a single individual or crime stain. Fields within the record contain information such as name ,sex, racial type, gel reference of the original result and the band weights detected.

SEARCH WINDOW

 Since there is slight variability in the results obtained when a sample is repeatedly profiled it is not possible to search for direct matches between records as was the case with the index of conventional blood group results. Instead a search window approach has been adopted. The window is applied to each of the band values of the suspect profile and then any record with bands falling within the window is selected from the database. Absence of bands in either the suspect or searched record will not cause the record to be excluded. This is important as the situation can occur where a full profile is obtained from a suspect's blood sample and only a partial profile is obtained from the crime stain.

Advances in Forensic Haemogenetics 4
Edited by Ch. Rittner and P. M. Schneider
© Springer-Verlag Berlin Heidelberg 1992

The search window was initially set at +/- 10% of the band weight. This was an arbitrary decision and it was known from the data relating to the standard deviation of repeated samples that it was an extremely conservative value.It would include many profiles that were similar, rather than just exact matches, to avoid the possibility of missing a linked case or suspect.

As the index expanded the number of false matches that were produced, due to the large window, increased especially if a complete set of band sizes from four probes was not available.

The present window varies in size in a non-linear manner. An equation has been derived that calculates the molecular weight of points 1mm either side of the band position. These values together with an extra factor which ensures that they are conservative at all times now form the window. This has proved successful and it has reduced the number of false matches to a lower level.

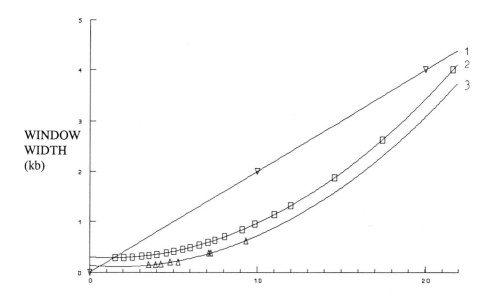

WINDOW WIDTH (kb)

MOLECULAR WEIGHT (kb)

Fig 1.   Plot of search window widths vs molecular weight

1) +/- 10% of band weight.
2) Present search window.
3) +/- 3 standard deviations obtained from genomic control (100 replicates).

The +/- 10% window can be seen to be excessively conservative in the low molecular weight regions.

RESULTS

The index has been fully operational since January 1990 and in that time has produced the following results:

Links between crime scenes (no suspect)	6
Links between crime scenes and suspect	7

All of these are links that would otherwise have escaped detection. Many other links between cases and suspects have been suggested by police officers or scientists who have seen similarities in modus operandi or the description of the suspect. These have later been confirmed by DNA profiling.

DISCUSSION

The ability to analyse data produced by a DNA profiling laboratory in this manner can be extremely rewarding. Without any additional DNA tests it is possible to detect unsolved series of crimes and nominate suspects to the police for unsolved crimes.

The DNA index program also produces population frequency data for 6 different racial groups. This automatic procedure has enabled us to build up one of the largest reference collections of DNA profiles in the world.

The legal and ethical status of such a system is likely to differ between countries. In The United Kingdom, data from DNA tests can be stored on computer providing it is on an officially registered system. However in cases where a match is obtained between an unsolved crime and a previous offender the police would normally have to obtain a fresh blood sample for comparison. Any reference to a suspects previous involvement in crimes (such as the presence of his profile on the index) could make the evidence inadmissible.

An index system restricts the freedom of a laboratory to make radical changes such as the use of different probes since much valuable information on previous offenders and crimes will become useless if those probes are no longer performed. As many of the criminals are recidivists it is vital that we are still able to recognise their profiles several years later when they are released from prison.

FUTURE DEVELOPMENTS

We are currently investigating the use of a more advanced computer search program that has been developed at CRSE Aldermaston which uses a Bayesian Likelihood Ratio method. Cooperation between the Metropolitan Police Laboratory and the other United Kingdom laboratories is already well under way to establish a national database.

It will also be necessary in the near future for bodies such as The European DNA Profiling Group (EDNAP) to develop a strategy for PCR technology in order that the compatibility that has been achieved with SLP methods is not to be lost when new techniques are introduced.

Reference: Catterick.T & Russell J.R.(1991). The development of a video scanner for forensic DNA autoradiographs.Lab Microcomputer 91.p105

4 Conventional Systems

4.1 General

Genetic and Molecular Aspects of the Human Red Cell Acid Phosphatase Polymorphism

J. Dissing

Institute of Forensic Genetics, University of Copenhagen,
Frederik den Femtes Vej 11, DK-2100 Copenhagen, Denmark

The red cell acid phosphatase polymorphism is a classical enzyme marker in paternity testing and blood stain analysis. It was discovered on the basis of its electrophoretic patterns (Hopkinson et al. 1963), but subsequently it was found to exhibit several other phenotypic characteristics such as differences in enzyme activity levels (Spencer et al. 1964), activity modulation by purines and pteridines (Mansfield and Sensabaugh 1978; Sensabaugh and Golden 1978; Mohrenweiser and Novotny 1982), phosphotransferase activity (Golden and Sensabaugh 1986), and stability (Luffman and Harris 1967). Another property is that each allele encodes two isozymes, f and s (Hopkinson et al. 1964). Recent results have provided new knowledge of the genetic and biochemical basis of this polymorphic system, and the objective of the present paper is to summarize these results.

Quantitation of the acid phosphatase isozymes using specific antibodies has shown that the allelic differences in the red cell enzyme activity levels (ACP1*C > ACP1*B > ACP1*A) is mainly the consequence of a similar allele dependent difference in enzyme protein level (Dissing 1987). It was further found that f and s isozymes are generated in allele specific ratios (f:s = 2:1, 4:1 and 1:4 for the ACP1*A, B and C alleles, respectively). The order of this allelic effect (B > A > C) is the same as that observed for activity modulation (Mansfield and Sensabaugh 1978; Sensabaugh and Golden 1978; Mohrenweiser and Novotny 1982). The three f and s isozyme pairs (Af/As, Bf/Bs and Cf/Cs) encoded by the ACP1*A, B and C alleles have been characterized and significant differences between f and s isozymes were observed in both enzymatic properties (Km, Ki, activity modulation, specific activity) and molecular properties (immunochemical properties, molecular size, stability) (Dissing 1986; Dissing and Svensmark 1990). In contrast the three genetically different f isozymes (Af, Bf, Cf) showed identical properties as did the three s isozymes. For example, f isozymes are inhibited with adenine and activated with hypoxanthine, whereas s isozymes are activated with adenine and insensitive towards hypoxanthine; this and the different f/s ratios account for the allelic differences in activity modulation. Similarly the higher stability of s isozymes relative to f isozymes explains earlier observations of a higher stability of the phenotypes BC and AC as compared to the phenotypes A, AB and B (Luffman and Harris 1967), the latter phenotypes having a higher f/s ratio.

Therefore, from a functional point of view the acid phosphatase system consists of only two different isozymes, f and s, the different proportion of which determine the properties of the various phenotypes. The different properties of f and s isozymes suggest that they serve different functions in the cell.

The amino acid sequence of the Af, As, Bf, Bs, Cf and Cs isozymes (Dissing et al. 1991; Dissing and Johnsen (unpublished results)) has recently been determined (fig. 1). All 6 isozymes consist of single peptide chains of equal length (157 residues). The most

Advances in Forensic Haemogenetics 4
Edited by Ch. Rittner and P. M. Schneider
© Springer-Verlag Berlin Heidelberg 1992

interesting finding is, however, that each **f/s** isozyme pair exhibits a substantial sequence difference in a specific region (40-73), despite being encoded by the same allele. This segment of 34 residues is identical for the three **f** isozymes and is also identical for the three **s** isozymes. The remaining four-fifths of the peptide chains of each isozyme pair are identical. Another finding is that the **Bf/Bs** and **Cf/Cs** isozyme pairs are identical, whereas the **Af/As** isozyme pair differs from these at residue 105, the neutral glutamine residue in the **B** and **C** isozymes being substituted with the basic arginine residue in the **A** isozymes. This explains the higher isoelectric points of the **A** isozymes relative to those of the **B** and **C** isozymes (Divall 1981).

The specific **f** and **s** sequence segments must necessarily account for the differences in catalytic and molecular properties of the **f** and **s** isozymes. The **s** specific sequence contains an extra basic residue (histidine 69) which explains the lesser anodal mobility of the **s** isozymes at acid pH values. The same histidine residue may also account for the higher Km values of **s** isozymes at acid pH values (Dissing and Svensmark 1990). The **f** specific sequence exhibits a lesser capacity for hydrophobic and a higher capacity for hydrophilic interaction than the **s** specific sequence. This may account for the lower stability of the **f** isozymes relative to the **s** isozymes.

As previously hyphotesized (Dissing and Sensabaugh 1987) it seems likely that the ACP1 locus is composed of at least 4 coding sequences, exons, interspersed with noncoding sequences, introns. These exons code for the N-terminal region (N), the f specific region (F), the **s** specific region (S) and the C-terminal region (C) of the isozymes, respectively. By alternative splicing of the primary RNA transcript two different mRNA molecules are generated from each allele, a f-mRNA and a s-mRNA, consisting of the N,F,C and the N,S,C exons, respectively.

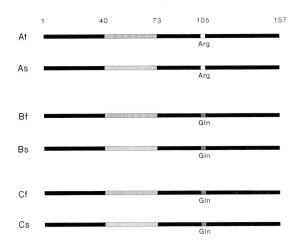

Fig. 1. Human red cell acid phosphatase: Schematic representation of the structure of the 6 common isozymes

The glutamine-arginine substitution at residue 105, which distinguish B and C isozymes from A isozymes, may be accounted for by a single base substitution in the respective codon. The ACP1*B and ACP1*C alleles encode, however, exactly the same isozymes, the only difference at the protein level being the f/s ratio. These two alleles may differ in the DNA sequence in a way that influences the splicing mechanism. It is apparent that an important question is how the allelic control of the f/s ratio is accompliced.

To further explore the ACP1 gene, the ACP1 locus is currently being sequenced, and preliminary results do indicate the existence of an intron between the N-coding region and the F-coding region (Dissing and Sensabaugh (unpublished results)).

References:

Dissing, J, Sensabaugh, GF (1987) Human Red Cell Acid Phosphatase (ACP1): Evidence for Differences in the Primary Structure of the Two Isozymes Encoded by the ACP1*B Allele. Biochem Genet 25: 919-927

Dissing, J, Svensmark, O (1990) Human Red Cell Acid Phosphatase: Purification and Properties of the A, B and C Isozymes. Biochim Biophys Acta 1041: 232-242

Dissing, J (1987) Immunochemical characterization of human red cell acid phosphatase isozymes. Biochem Genet 25: 901-918

Dissing, J (1986) Red cell acid phosphatase: only two different enzymes - the "slow" and the "fast" enzyme - determine different biochemical properties of the six common phenotypes. In: Brinkmann, B, Henningsen, K (eds) Advances in Forensic Haemogenetics, vol 1. Springer, Berlin Heidelberg New York, p 127-131

Dissing, J, Johnsen, AH, Sensabaugh, GF (1991) Human Red Cell Acid Phosphatase (ACP1): The Amino Acid Sequence of the Two Isozymes Bf and Bs Encoded by the ACP1*B allele. J Biol Chem 266: (in press)

Divall, GB (1981) Studies on the use of isoelectric focusing as a method of phenotyping erythrocyte acid phosphatase. Forensic Sci Int 18: 67-78

Golden, VL, Sensabaugh, GF (1986) Phenotypic variation in the phosphotransferase activity of human red cell acid phosphatase (ACP1). Hum Genet 72: 340-343

Hopkinson DA, Spencer N, Harris, H. (1963) Red cell acid phosphatase variants: a new human polymorphism. Nature 199: 969-971

Hopkinson, DA, Spencer, N, Harris, H (1964) Genetical studies on human red cell acid phosphatase. Am J Hum Genet 16: 141-154

Luffman, JE, Harris, H (1967) A comparison of some properties of human red cell acid phosphatase in different phenotypes. Ann Hum Genet 30: 387-400

Mansfield E, Sensabaugh GF (1978) Red cell acidphosphatase: modulation of activity by purines. in Brewer, G.J., (ed) The Red Cell, vol 4. Alan R. Liss, New York, p 233-249

Mohrenweiser, HW, Novotny, JE (1982) A low-activity variant of human erythrocyte acid phosphatase: Association with increased glutathione reductase activity. Am J Hum Genet 34: 425-433

Sensabaugh GF, Golden VL (1978) Phenotype dependence in the inhibition of red cell acid phosphatase (ACP) by folates. Am J Hum Genet 30: 553-560

Spencer N, Hopkinson DA, Harris H (1964) Quantitative differences and gene dosage in the human red cell acid phosphatase polymorphism. Nature 201: 299-300

A de novo Mutation in the Alpha-1-Antitrypsin Gene detected in a Case of disputed Paternity by DNA Sequence Analysis

S. Weidinger, J.-P. Faber [*], U. Bäcker [**], F. Schwarzfischer, and K. Olek [*]

Institut für Anthropologie u. Humangenetik der Universität München, Richard-Wagner-Str. 10/I, DW-8000 München 2, Federal Republic of Germany

INTRODUCTION

Alpha-1-antitrypsin (α1AT) is the major protease inhibitor (PI) in human plasma. It is a 52-kD glycoprotein which consists of a single polypeptide chain of 394 amino acids with three complex asparaginyl-linked carbohydrate chains (Carrell et al. 1982). The α1AT-gene comprises seven exons (three noncoding exons IA-C followed by four coding exons II-V) and six introns over 12.2 kb of chromosome 14q31-32.3 (Long et al. 1984; Brantly et al. 1988). Alpha-1-antitrypsin shows an extensive genetic variation. More than 75 PI variants have been identified by either isoelectric focusing of serum and/or sequence analysis. At the DNA level, mutations are known in all four coding exons.

MATERIALS and METHODS

Phenotyping by Isoelectric Focusing (IEF)

Blood samples from three individuals -the index case, mother and alleged father- were available for analysis. They were collected in plastic tubes containing K EDTA. Plasma was separated after centrifugation of whole blood and used without treatment. Phenotyping of α1AT was performed by IEF on 0.5 mm thin flat-bed polyacrylamide gels containing pharmalytes (pH range of 4.2-4.9) according to the method of Weidinger et al. (1985).

Haplotyping, PCR-Amplification and DNA-Sequencing

Genomic DNA was extracted from peripheral white blood cells by standard procedures. For haplotyping the DNA was digested with the appropriate restriction enzymes (Sst I, Ava II), electrophoresed in 1.0-1.8% agarose gels, and transferred to nitrocellulose membranes by Southern blotting. The α1AT specific genomic DNA probes used for detection of the restriction fragment length polymorphisms (RFLPs) and the hybridization protocol have been described elsewhere (Meisen et al. 1988).

---

[*] Institut für Klinische Biochemie der Universität Bonn, DW-5300 Bonn 1, FRG
[**] Blutspendedienst des BRK München, DW-8000 München 2, FRG

Advances in Forensic Haemogenetics 4
Edited by Ch. Rittner and P. M. Schneider
© Springer-Verlag Berlin Heidelberg 1992

HLA DQα typing was carried out using an AmpliType kit (Cetus). The D1S58 locus which contains a variable number of tandem repeats (VNTRs) was analyzed according to the method of Kasai et al. (1990).

Polymerase chain reaction (PCR)-amplification of all coding exons of the α1AT-gene was performed as reported previously (Faber et al. 1990). The PCR-products were directly sequenced using an automated fluorescent DNA sequencing method (McBride et al. 1989) and our standard protocol (Faber et al., submitted).

RESULTS and DISCUSSION

Analysis of alpha-1-antitrypsin by IEF revealed the subtype PI M1M2 in the mother and putative father. The one-year old child has clearly shown a variant in the so-called "P" range in addition to PI M1 (Fig. 1A). In comparison with standards the variant phenotype was classified as PI M1Pdonauwörth (abbreviated Pdon according to the PI nomenclature). All three individuals had α1AT-plasma concentrations in the normal range. Testing of the three individuals in 29 other genetic markers (8 blood group-, 12 serum protein-, and 9 enzyme systems) showed that the man could not be excluded from fatherhood. Adding the data for HLA-A, B, and C a strong evidence for paternity has been obtained. The PI data, however, were not compatible with paternity. Biostatistical evaluation of all serological markers (with the exception of PI) gave a paternity probability of W = 99.9972%. These serological data were confirmed by a DNA study.

First, restriction site variation in and around the α1AT-gene was studied by use of two different restriction enzymes and three different genomic DNA probes (1.17 kb and 4.6 kb 5'probes and a 6.5 kb 3'probe). The segregation pattern

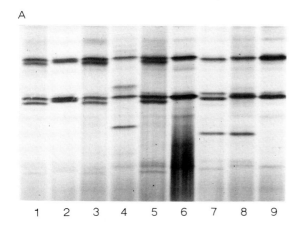
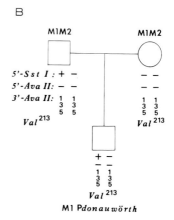

A

B

1   2   3   4   5   6   7   8   9

Fig. 1. (A) Demonstration of PI phenotypes as revealed by isoelectric focusing of serum and plasma samples in a polyacrylamide gel, pH range of 4.2-4.9. Lanes: (1) M1M2, (2) M1M3, (3) M1M2, mother, (4) M1Pdon, child, (5) M1M2, alleged father, (6) M1, (7) M3S, (8) M1S, and (9) M1. Anode is at the top. (B) Segregation of the DNA haplotypes in the case of paternity

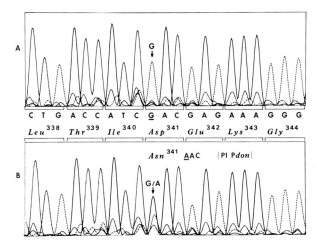

Fig. 2. Sequence analysis of the coding exons of α1AT-genes M1 and Pdon. A guanine (G) to adenine (A) transition causes an amino acid substitution of Asn341(AAC) for Asp341(GAC) in the gene Pdonauwörth

of the DNA haplotypes was compatible with paternity (Fig. 1B). Secondly, analysis of the polymorphic HLA DQα locus was performed. The alleged father and the child were both determined to be DQα type 1.1, 3, and the mother was determined to be type 3, 4 (Fig. not shown). These typing data are also compatible with paternity. Additional evidence in favor of paternity of the alleged father has been obtained by investigation the D1S58 VNTR-locus. To determine the precise nature of the discrepancy within the PI system, we have conducted automated direct sequencing of the childs α1AT-genes. Sequence analysis of all coding exons of the childs Pdon gene has shown a point mutation in exon V which causes an amino acid substitution of Asn341(AAC) for Asp341 (GAC) (Fig. 2). This mutation was not found after testing both parental DNAs, thus confirming a de novo mutation in the childs α1AT-gene.

REFERENCES

Brantly M, Nukiwa T, Crystal RG (1988) Am J Med 84: 13-26
Carrell RW, Jeppsson J-O, Laurell C-B, Brennan SO, Owen MC, Vaughan L, Boswell DR (1982) Nature 298: 329-334
Faber J-P, Weidinger S, Olek K (1990) Am J Hum Genet 46: 1158-1162
Kasai K, Nakamura Y, White R (1990) J Forensic Sciences 35: 1196-1200
Long GL, Chandra T, Woo SLC, Davie EW, Kurachi K (1984) Biochemistry 23: 4828-4837
McBride LJ, Koepf SM, Gibbs RA, Salser W, Mayrand PE, Hunkapiller MW, Kronick MN (1989) Clin Chem 35: 2196-2201
Meisen C, Higuchi M, Bräutigam S, Driesel AJ, Blandfort M, Olek K (1988) Hum Genet 79: 190-192
Weidinger S, Jahn W, Cujnik F, Schwarzfischer F (1985) Hum Genet 71: 27-29

ISOELECTRIC FOCUSING OF INTER-ALPHA-TRYPSIN INHIBITOR (ITI)

C Luckenbach*, J Kömpf*, A Amorim**, J Rocha**, A Trein*

* Inst.Anthropologie und Humangenetik 7400 Tübingen F.R.Germany

**Inst.Antropologia, Univ.Porto, 4000 Porto, Portugal

INTRODUCTION

The genetic polymorphism of human plasma inter-alpha-trypsin inhibitor (ITI), a serine protease inhibitor, was first described by Vogt and Cleve (1990). Both precise subunit composition and chromosomal assignment of the corresponding locus remain under investigation (Schreitmüller et al., 1987, Luckenbach et al., 1991). In this work we present formal and population genetics results obtained in families from SW Germany and NW Portugal.

MATERIAL AND METHODS

Blood samples were obtained by venipuncture and EDTA plasmas stored at -20°C until use. Sample treatment and phenotyping were performed as previously described (Luckenbach et al, 1991).

RESULTS AND DISCUSSION

Phenotypes of ITI are shown in Fig.1; nomenclature was made according to Vogt and Cleve (1990). Banding patterns (a main band for homozygotes and two for heterozygotes) in non-denaturing conditions are consistent with a monomeric protein. However, given the presence of additional weaker bands and the possibility of loose association between monomeres, we can not rule out more complex quaternary structures, as suggested by Schreitmüller et al.(1987)

In Tables 1 and 2 we show the mating type distribution found in SW Germany and NW Portugal. Both distributions agree well with Hardy-Weinberg expectations. They clearly support both qualitatively and quantitatively the formal hypothesis for ITI: an autosomal locus with two common codominant alleles (ITI*1, ITI*2) and a rare one, also codominant (ITI*3). No evidence of silent genes was found.

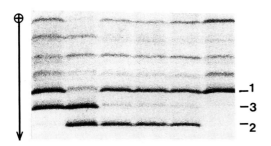

Fig.1. ITI phenotypes. From left to right: 3-1; 3-2; 2-1; 2-1; 2-1 and 1

Advances in Forensic Haemogenetics 4
Edited by Ch. Rittner and P. M. Schneider
© Springer-Verlag Berlin Heidelberg 1992

TABLE 1. ITI segregation analysis. Families from SW Germany

mating type	no families	offspring phenotypes					Allele frequencies
		1	2-1	3-1	2	3-2	
1 x 1	39	103					ITI*1 0.607
	32.38						ITI*2 0.388
1 x 2-1	75	91	101				ITI*3 0.005
	82.85	96.0	96.0				
1 x 3-1	2	3		3			
	1.12	3.0		3.0			
1 x 2	32		105				
	26.50						
2-1x 2-1	47	43	72		28		
	52.99	35.75	71.50		35.75		
2-1x 2	34		51		50		
	33.90		50.5		50.5		
2-1x 3-2	1		0	1	0	2	
	0.91		0.75	0.75	0.75	0.75	
2 x 2	7				17		
	5.42						
2 x 3-2	2				4	3	
	0.29				3.5	3.5	
Others	0						
	2.64						
Total	239	240	329	4	99	5	

TABLE 2. ITI segregation analysis. Families from NW Portugal

mating type	no families	offspring phenotypes			Allele frequencies
		1	2-1	2	
1 x 1	2	8			ITI*1 0.552
	2.69				ITI*2 0.448
1 x 2-1	10	12	16		
	8.73	14.0	14.0		
1 x 2	3		9		
	3.55				
2-1x 2-1	8	9	7	2	
	7.10	4.5	9.0	4.5	
2-1x 2	4		7	3	
	5.77		5.0	5.0	
2 x 2	2			5	
	1.17				
Total	29	29	39	10	

REFERENCES

Schreitmüller T, Hochstrasser K, Reisinger PWM, Wachter E, Gebhard W (1987) cDNA cloning of human inter-alpha-trypsin inhibitor discloses three different proteins. Biol Chem Hoppe Seyler 368: 963-970

Luckenbach C, Kömpf J, Ritter H (1991). Genetic polymorphism of inter-alpha-trypsin-inhibitor (ITI): formal genetics and linkage analysis. Hum Genet 87: 89-90

Vogt U, Cleve H (1990) A "new" genetic polymorphism of a human serum protein: inter-alpha-trypsin inhibitor. Hum Genet 84: 151-154

ACKNOWLEDGEMENTS: This research was partially supported by DAAD.

HUMAN ZN-ALPHA 2-GLYCOPROTEIN PHENOTYPING IN SEVERAL POPULATIONS

N.Nakayashiki, I.Yuasa*, K.Umetsu**, K.Suenaga*, K.Omoto***, T.Ishida***, S.Misawa**** and S.Katsura

      Department of Legal Medicine, Iwate Medical University, Morioka,
      Japan
*   Department of Legal Medicine, Tottri University, Yonago, Japan
**   Department of Forensic Medicine, Yamagata University, Yamagata,
      Japan
***   Department of Anthropology, University of Tokyo, Tokyo, Japan
**** Department of Legal Medicine, University of Tsukuba, Ibaraki,
      Japan

Human Zn-alpha 2-glycoprotein (ZAG) is widely distributed in various body fluids such as plasma, semen, sweat, saliva, urine and tear, however, the biological function is still unknown. Lately, by means of isoelectric focusing (IEF) followed by immunoblotting, the genetic variation of plasma ZAG has been reported (Kamboh and Ferrell 1986; Nakayashiki and Katsura 1989; Ding et al. 1990). In this study, five new ZAG alleles and the distribution of ZAG alleles in the Japanese, Korean, Philippine, Thai, Brazilian Indian and Papua New Guinean popuations will be reported.

MATERIALS AND METHODS

Plasma or serum samples were obtained from following populations: 2180 Japanese composing of 182 Ainu individuals from Hokkaido, 1080 individuals from Iwate prefecture, 554 from Yamaguchi prefecture and 364 from Okinawa prefecture; 554 Koreans from Seoul city; 115 Philippines of 69 from Kadaklan and 46 from Bagbag village of Luzon island; 218 Thai from Tha-Keow-Pleuk village; 398 Brazilian Indians composing of three tribes, 205 from Pacaás Novos, 77 from Urubu-Kaapor and 116 from Parakanã; 52 Papua New Guineans from Lae city.

ZAG phenotyping for native and desialized samples were performed mostly according to the previous description (Nakayashiki and Katsura 1989). When separator IEF (SIEF) was applied to asialo ZAG typing, 1% HEPES was added to the IEF gel and the focusing time was prolonged.

RESULTS AND DISCUSSION

Figure 1 and 2 show eleven IEF phenotypes of native and asialo ZAG in plasma, respectively. Although the genetic background could not be examined, five new ZAG bands produced by ZAG*6 to ZAG*10, which tentatively named, were observed. The sequence of asialo ZAG band mobilities in IEF gel was as follows: ZAG 10 (pI about 5)→2→5→1 (common band, pI 5.15)→7→6→3→4→9→8 (pI about 5.3) in increasing order of pI.

Advances in Forensic Haemogenetics 4
Edited by Ch. Rittner and P. M. Schneider
© Springer-Verlag Berlin Heidelberg 1992

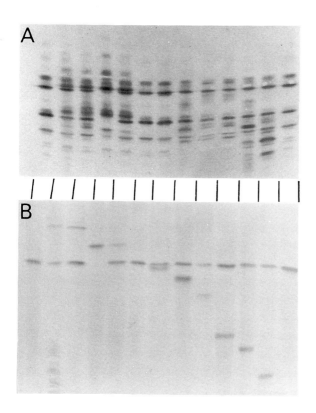

Fig. 1. Different phenotypes of plasma ZAG analyzed by immunoblotting after polyacrylamide gel IEF of native samples (A) and after SIEF of desialized samples (B). Anode at top. From left to right:ZAG 1, 10-1, 2-1, 5, 5-1, 1, 7-1, 6-1, 3-1, 4-1, 9-1, 8-1, 1

Table 1. Distribution of ZAG phenotypes in twelve populations

Population	n	Phenotype, n										
		1	2-1	3-1	4-1	5	5-1	6-1	7-1	8-1	9-1	10-1
JAPANESE com.	2180	2148	16	3	1	1	9	1			1	
Ainu (Hokkaido)	182	182										
Iwate	1080	1062	4	3	1	1	7	1			1	
Yamaguchi	554	543	9				2					
Okinawa	364	361	3									
KOREAN	525	517		4			2		1	1		
PHILIPPINE com.	115	115										
Kadaklan	69	69										
Bagbag	46	46										
THAI	218	217				1						
BRAZILIAN INDIAN com.	398	398										
Pacaás Novos	205	205										
Urubu-Kaapor	77	77										
Parakanã	116	116										
PAPUA NEW GUINEAN	52	47										5
Total	3488	3442	16	7	1	1	12	1	1	1	1	5

com., combined

Table 2. ZAG allele frequencies in different populations

Population	n	ZAG*1	ZAG*2	ZAG*3	ZAG*4	ZAG*5	ZAG*6	ZAG*7	ZAG*8	ZAG*9	ZAG*10	Others	References
JAPANESE													
Ainu	182	1.0000											This study
Iwate	1224	.9935	.0025	.0016	.0004	.0020							Reference 1
Iwate	1080	.9912	.0019	.0014	.0005	.0042	.0005			.0005			This study
Yamaguchi	554	.9901	.0081			.0018							This study
Okinawa	364	.9959	.0041										This study
CHINESE													
Shenyang	390	.9962				.0038							Reference 2
Kaohsiung	200	1.0000											Reference 2
KOREAN													
Cheju	350	.9929		.0071									Reference 2
Seoul	523	.9971		.0029									Reference 2
Seoul	525	.9923		.0038		.0019		.0010	.0010				This study
PHILIPPINE com.	115	1.0000											This study
THAI	218	.9977				.0023							This study
BRAZILIAN INDIAN com.	398	1.0000											This study
PAPUA NEW GUINEAN	52	.9519									.0481		This study
AMERICAN (The United States)													
Black	111	.9955										.0045[a]	Reference 3
Caucasian	228	1.0000											Reference 3
Eskimo	106	1.0000											Reference 3

a, not identified
Reference: 1, Nakayashiki and Katsura 1989; 2, Ding et al. 1990; 3, Kamboh and Ferrell 1986

Table 1 shows the distribution of ZAG phenotypes observed in this study and Table 2 summarizes the ZAG allele frequencies in the different populations up to now. In all of the populations, ZAG*1 was a predominant allele and the other alleles were seen less than polymorphic frequency (0.01) except for ZAG*10 (0.0481).

Ding et al. (1990) suggested the characteristic presence of ZAG*3 for the Koreans and ZAG*5 for the Chinese. We could not clarify this, however, the restricted distribution of some ZAG alleles might be possible, e.g., ZAG*2 for the Japanese and ZAG*10 for the Papua New Guineans. In addition, some ZAG alleles, e.g., the ZAG*10 in the Papua New Guinean population, might be distributed as a polymorphic marker. Therefore, further studies on ZAG phenotyping in various populations are necessary, to reveal its usefulness with regard to a genetic information in both fields of anthropology and forensic science.

We wish to express our gratitude to Prof. Francisco M. Salzano (Rio Grande) for the permission of ZAG phenotyping on his samples.

REFERENCES

Ding M, Umetsu K, Nakayashiki N, Choi WY, Jia J, Suzuki T (1990) Distribution of human Zn-alpha-2-glycoprotein types in Chinese and Korean populations. Hum Hered 40:311-312
Kamboh MI, Ferrell RE (1986) Genetic studies of low-abundance human plasma proteins. I. Microheterogeneity of Zinc-α2-glycoprotein in biological fluids. Biochem Genet 24:849-857
Nakayashiki N, Katsura S (1989) Four variants of human plasma Zn-α_2-glycoprotein (ZAG) in the Japanese population. Hum Genet 82:293-295

Comparative Typing of Orosomucoid Variants and Proposal for a New Nomenclature

I. Yuasa, S. Weidinger*, and K. Umetsu**

Department of Legal Medicine, Tottori University School of Medicine, 683 Yonago, Japan
* Institut für Anthropologie und Humangenetik der Universität München, D-8000 München, FRG
** Department of Forensic Medicine, Yamagata University School of Medicine, 990-23 Yamagata, Japan

INTRODUCTION

There are two forms of orosomucoid (ORM) in the sera of most individuals. The ORM1 and ORM2 phenotypes are encoded by two separate but closely linked loci on the long arm of chromosome 9. Duplications and non-expressions are observed in some populations. The ORM system is very complicated and its nomenclature is very confusing. This paper presents a proposal for a new nomenclature of all ORM variants found in different populations hitherto.

MATERIALS AND METHODS

Serum and plasma samples were desialylated with 4-fold volumes of neuraminidase (1U/ml, Sigma, pH 5.5) overnight at room temperature.

ORM phenotypes were classified by three different techniques of isoelectic focusing (IEF) using horizontal flat-bed polyacrylamide gels containing additives such as Triton X-100 and/or glycerol (Yuasa et al. 1987, 1888, 1990).

ORM bands obtained by immunoprinting were assigned to either ORM1 or ORM2 locus according to visual difference in their intensity. ORM1 bands are more intense than ORM2 bands.

RESULTS AND DISCUSSION

In honor of the first genetic study by Johnson et al. (1969), we maintain the notations ORM1*F and ORM1*S for the two common alleles at ORM1 locus. The ORM1*F is divided into two common subtype alleles, ORM1*F1 and ORM1*F2. For the common allele at ORM2 locus, the designation of ORM2*M is recommended.

As shown in Table 1, ORM variants were classified into 49

Advances in Forensic Haemogenetics 4
Edited by Ch. Rittner and P. M. Schneider
© Springer-Verlag Berlin Heidelberg 1992

different variants. The new nomenclature was designated alphanumerically on the basis of relative mobilities observed by IEF in the presence of Triton X-100 and glycerol (Yuasa et al. 1987).

The ORM system is expressed by a total of 57 different ORM alleles including duplicated and non-expressed alleles at the two highly polymorphic loci. Escallon et al. (1987) described a few variants at ORM2 locus in American Blacks. Unfortunately, the serum samples were not available. It is probable that a number of new additional variants are disclosed, particularly by studying of populations other than Europeans and East Asians.

REFERENCES

Escallon MH, Ferrell RE, Kamboh MI (1987) Genetic studies of low-abundance human plasma proteins. Evidence for a second orosomucoid structural locus expressed in plasma. Am J Hum Genet 41:418–427

Johnson AM, Schmid K, Alper CA (1969) Inheritance of human α_1-acid glycoprotein (orosomucoid) variants. J Clin Invest 48:2293–2299

Yuasa I, Suenaga K, Umetsu K, Ito K, Robinet-Levy M (1987) Orosomucoid (ORM) typing by isoelectric focusing evidence for gene duplication of ORM1 and genetic polymorphism of ORM2. Hum Genet 77:255–258

Yuasa I, Umetsu K, Suenaga K (1988) Orosomucoid (ORM) typing by isoelectric focusing: evidence for an additional duplicated ORM1 locus haplotype and close linkage of two loci. Am J Hum Genet 43:165–169

Yuasa I, Umetsu K, Nakayashiki N, Tamaki N, Shiono H, Okada K (1990) Orosomucoid (ORM) typing by isoelectric focusing: an improved method for ORM1 subtyping and the reactivity of anti-human ORM antibodies with animal ORM. In: Nagano T (ed) Proc Int Symp Advances in Legal Medicine. pp. 447–449

Table 1. List of compared ORM variants and proposal for new nomenclature

ORM1

New nomenclature	Old nomenclature: Geographic or ethnic origin of samples	References
‡ ORM1*A4	ORM1*7	Japanese, Taiwanese — Umetsu et al., 1988
‡ –	ORM1*A2	German — Weidinger (unpublished)
–	ORM1*A1	German — Weidinger (unpublished)
‡ ORM1*A3	ORM1*18	Japanese — Yuasa (unpublished)
ORM1*A2	ORM1*16	Paraguayan — Umetsu et al., 1989
ORM1*A1	ORM1*10	French — Yuasa (unpublished)

ORM2

New nomenclature	Old nomenclature: Geographic or ethnic origin of samples	References
‡ ORM2*L9	ORM2*14	Japanese — Yuasa et al., 1990b
ORM2*L8	ORM2*21	Sri Lankan — Umetsu et al., 1989
ORM2*L7	ORM2*4	Japanese — Yuasa et al., 1987
‡ ORM2*L6	ORM2*ThS	German — Weidinger (unpublished)
‡ ‡ ORM2*L5	ORM2*2	Japanese — Yuasa et al., 1987
ORM2*L4	ORM2*22	Sri Lankan — Umetsu et al., 1989
ORM2*L3	ORM2*20	Chinese — Umetsu (unpublished)

#	ORM1	ORM1	Population	Reference		#	ORM2	ORM2	Population	Reference
	ORM1*F2	ORM1*3	French, Nepalese	Yuasa et al., 1986			ORM2*L2	ORM2*13	German	Umetsu et al., 1989
##	-	ORM1*F2	German	Weidinger et al., 1987			ORM2*L1	ORM2*8	Taiwanese	Umetsu et al., 1988
##	ORM1*F1	ORM1*1	Japanese	Umetsu et al., 1985		##	ORM2*M	ORM2*1	French, Nepalese	Yuasa et al., 1986
##		ORM1*F1	German	Weidinger et al., 1987			ORM2*H1	ORM2*A	German	Weidinger et al., 1987
	ORM1*B1	ORM1*12	New Zealander	Yuasa (unpublished)		##	ORM2*H2	ORM2*18	Japanese	Yuasa et al., 1990a
	ORM1*B2	ORM1*F4	Swiss	Eap et al., 1988 and 1989			-	ORM2*3	Japanese	Yuasa et al., 1987
	ORM1*B3	ORM1*8	Japanese, Taiwanese	Umetsu et al., 1988		##	-	ORM2*v1	Japanese	Tsuge et al., 1987
##		ORM1*4	Japanese	Yuasa et al., 1987		##	-	ORM2*DR	German	Weidinger (unpublished)
	ORM1*B4	ORM1*V1	Japanese	Tsuge et al., 1987			ORM2*H3	ORM2*10	Japanese	Umetsu et al., 1988
##		ORM1*11	New Zealander	Yuasa (unpublished)			ORM2*H4	ORM2*AD	French	Duche (unpublished)
	ORM1*B5	ORM1*17	Chinese	Yuasa (unpublished)			ORM2*H5	ORM2*11	French	Yuasa (unpublished)
	ORM1*B6	ORM1*NW	German	Weidinger (unpublished)			-	ORM2*C1	Swiss	Eap (unpublished)
	ORM1*B7	ORM1*F3	Swiss	Eap et al., 1988		##	ORM2*H6	ORM2*5	Japanese	Yuasa et al., 1987
	ORM1*B8	ORM1*RJ	German	Weidinger (unpublished)			ORM2*H7	ORM2*16	Japanese	Fukuma et al., 1990
##		ORM1*5	Japanese	Yuasa et al., 1990b			ORM2*H8	ORM2*12	French	Yuasa (unpublished)
	ORM1*B9	ORM1*14	German	Umetsu et al., 1989		##	ORM2*H9	ORM2*9	Japanese	Yuasa et al., 1990b
	ORM1*B10	ORM1*2	Japanese	Umetsu et al., 1985			ORM2*H10	ORM2*B2	German	Weidinger et al., 1987
	ORM1*S	ORM1*S	German	Weidinger et al., 1987			ORM2*H11	ORM2*B3	German	Weidinger (unpublished)
##		ORM1*VU	German	Weidinger (unpublished)		##	ORM2*H12	ORM2*17	Japanese	Fukuma et al., 1990
	ORM1*C1	ORM1*S1	German	Weidinger et al., 1987			-	ORM2*17	Lebanese	Yuasa et al., 1990
	ORM1*C2	ORM1*S1	French	Yuasa (unpublished)			ORM2*H13	ORM2*1D	Lebanese	Duche (unpublished)
	ORM1*C3	ORM1*9	German	Weidinger (unpublished)			ORM2*H14	ORM2*7	Japanese	Yuasa et al., 1988
##		ORM1*S2	Swiss	Eap et al., 1988			ORM2*H15	ORM2*19	Japanese	Yuasa et al., 1990a
	ORM1*C4	ORM2*B1	German	Weidinger (unpublished)			ORM2*H16	ORM2*15	Japanese	Yuasa et al., 1990b
	ORM1*C5	ORM1*SJ	Japanese	Yuasa et al., 1988		##	ORM2*H17	ORM2*HG	Libanese	Weidinger (unpublished)
	ORM1*C6	ORM1*6	Libanese	Weidinger (unpublished)		##	ORM2*H19	ORM2*6	Japanese	Yuasa et al., 1987
##	ORM1*C7	ORM1*HG	Japanese	Tsuge et al., 1987		##	-	ORM2*v4	Japanese	Tsuge et al., 1987
		ORM1*V2					-	ORM2*Xo	Vietnamese	Duche (unpublished)
							-	ORM2*PFT	German	Weidinger (unpublished)

Duplicated alleles

#	ORM1	ORM1	Population	Reference		#	ORM2	ORM2	Population	Reference
##	ORM1*dF1S	ORM1*2·1	Japanese	Yuasa et al., 1987		##	ORM2*dH16H18	ORM2*DaS	German	Weidinger (unpublished)
##	ORM1*dB9S	ORM1*5·2	Japanese	Yuasa et al., 1988						
##		ORM1*BA	Argentina	Weidinger (unpublished)						

Null allele

#	ORM1	ORM1	Population	Reference		#	ORM2	ORM2	Population	Reference
##	ORM1*Q0	ORM1*Q0	Japanese	Yuasa et al., 1990b		##	ORM2*Q0	ORM2*Q0	Japanese	Tsuge et al., 1987
##	-	ORM1*Q0	German	Kasulke and Weidinger, 1990			-	ORM2*Q0	Japanese	Umetsu et al., 1988
						##	-	ORM2*Q0	Japanese	Yuasa et al., 1990b

indicates that family data were available.

Intragenic Recombination within the Alpha-1-Antitrypsin Locus

G. Wetterling

Institute of Forensic Serology, University Hospital, S-581 85 Linköping,
Sweden

INTRODUCTION

The alpha-1-antitrypsin (Pi) system displays more than 60 alleles. The M
allele is the most frequent with a frequency of 0.9463 in a Swedish
population (Hjalmarsson 1988). More unusual alleles are the S, Z and F
alleles. Furthermore, the M allele can be split into the suballeles M1,
M2, M3 and M4. The amino acid sequences have been determined by DNA
sequencing and the following genetic model for the Pi M suballeles has
been suggested (Long 1984; Nukiwa 1988; Crystal 1989; Graham 1990).

Allele	Codons/amino acids at positions 101	376	Frequency
M1	Arg CGT	Glu GAA	0.6894
M2	His CAT	Asp GAC	0.1649
M3	Arg CGT	Asp GAC	0.0904
M4	His CAT	Glu GAA	0.0179

The nucleotide substitutions are underlined. The gene frequencies are
according to Weidinger (1982).

MATERIAL and METHODS

Blood samples from 1048 families involved in paternity cases in Sweden
have been subtyped for the Pi M alleles by isoelectric focusing
(Hjalmarsson 1988). The Pi M3 and M4 alleles were not separated due to
very small differences in charge.

Advances in Forensic Haemogenetics 4
Edited by Ch. Rittner and P. M. Schneider
© Springer-Verlag Berlin Heidelberg 1992

RESULTS and DISCUSSION

A mother-child exclusion which could not be explained by the presence of a silent allele was observed in the alpha-1-antitrypsin system (Pi). The mother was typed Pi M1,M2, the child Pi M3 and the father Pi M3,S. In addition to the Pi M system the family members have been typed for all genetic markers available at the institute, including HLA and DNA. The results have been verified after resampling. The probability of maternity is 0.992.

Table 1. Phenotypes of the family

Marker	Mother	Child	Father
ABO	B	O	O
MNSs	MS	MNS	NSs
Rh	CDe	CDe	CcDe
Fy	b	ab	a
Kk	k	k	k
Gm	-1.-2	1.-2	1.2
Hp	2,1	1	2,1
Gc	2,1S	1F,1S	1F,1S
Pi	M2,M1	M3	M3,S
Tf	2,1	2,1	1
F13B	1	2,1	2,1
PGM	a1	a1	a3,a1
EAP	BA	BA	BA
GLO	2	2,1	1
EsD	1	1	2,1
HLA	A2,28;B15,35	Aw19,28;B12,15	A9,w19;B12,27
D2S44	4.11,3.35	4.13,3.36	4.11,3,76

The most plausible explanation to the observed mother-child exclusion is an intragenic recombination in the oogenesis.

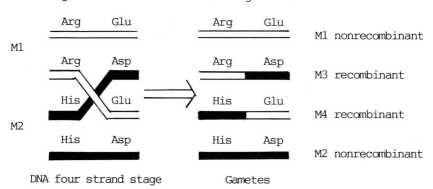

Fig. 1. Recombination scheme. Obviously the child Pi M3 has inherited the M3 (or M4) allele from the Pi M1,M2 mother after a crossover event in the meiosis. As can be seen in the figure new recombinants are only possible when all four amino acids are different, hence only by persons who belong

to the phenotypes Pi M1,M2 and M3,M4. Due to the difficulties in separating the M3 and M4 allele the genotype M3,M4 is defined as M3 by most investigators.

A possible sequence for the recombination events within the Pi M system is:

	point mut.		point mut.		crossover	
1. M1	$\longrightarrow$	M3	2. M1 $\longrightarrow$ M4		3. M3,M4 $\longrightarrow$ M2	

Table 2. Parent-child pairs where a recombination may cause false exclusion (M3 includes M4)

Mother or Father	Child
M1,M2	M1,M3
	M3
	M2,M3
M3(M3,M4)	M1
	M1,M2
	M2

Another recombination within the Pi gene has been described by Bender et al. 1991 due to a crossover in the spermatogenesis.

Intragenic recombination within other genetic markers has earlier only been observed within the PGM 1 gene (Wetterling 1990). In these systems, as well as in others, the risk of false exclusions in paternity cases must be considered, when the alleles include amino acid substitutions at several different sites, distant enough to allow a crossover event.

REFERENCES

Bender K, Kasulke D, Mayerova A, Hummel K, Weidinger S, Epplen JT, Wienker TF (1991) New mutation versus exclusion at the alpha-1-antitrypsin locus: a multifaceted approach in a problematical paternity case. Hum Hered 41:1-11

Crystal RG (1989) The alpha-antitrypsin gene and its deficiency states. Trends Genet 5:411-417

Graham A, Hayes K, Wiedinger S, Newton CR, Markham AF (1990) Characterisation of the alpha-1-antitrypsin M3 gene, a normal variant. Hum Genet 85:381-382

Hjalmarsson K (1988) Distribution of alpha-1-antitrypsin phenotypes in Sweden. Hum Hered 38:27-30

Long GL, Chandra T, Woo SLC, Davie EW, Kurachi K (1984) Complete sequence of the cDNA for human alpha-1-antitrypsin and the gene for the S variant. Biochemistry 23:4828-4837

Nukiwa T, Brantly ML, Ogushi F, Fells GA, Crystal RG (1988) Characterization of the gene and protein of the common alpha-1-antitrypsin normal M2 allele. Am J Hum Genet 43:322-330

Weidinger S, Cleve H, Patutschick (1982) Alpha-1-antitrypsin: evidence for a fourth Pi M allele. Distribution of the PiM subtypes in southern Germany. Z Rechtsmed 88:203-211

Wetterling G (1990) Intragenic recombination within the PGM1 locus. In Polesky HF, Mayr WR (eds) Advances in Forensic Haemogenetics 3. Springer, Berlin Heidelberg, p 218

4.2 Methodology

Blotting Techniques for the Detection of Protein Polymorphisms in Stains

S. Rand

Institut für Rechtsmedizin der Westf. Wilhelms-Universität, Münster, von Esmarch-Str. 86, D-4400 Münster, FRG

INTRODUCTION

The aim of this paper is to give a review of the methods available for the detection of protein polymorphisms in stains. The characteristics of the various blotting methods are described as a guide to selection of the most suitable for the protein under investigation. With this in mind the paper has been subtitled "The successful blot - luck or judgement?". Most problems, which occur are due to human error and can be avoided if proper care is taken. However to identify the cause of a particular problem background knowledge and experience is essential. The various stages involved are discussed here in detail.

IMMUNOCHEMOPHORESIS:

Blotting is only one of the essential stages in the complete process for detection of protein polymorphisms, which has come to be known as immunochemophoresis (Rand et al 1989). The individual stages are shown in Figure 1.

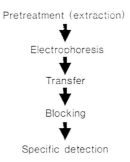

Fig.1: Stages involved in immunochemophoresis

Pretreatment (extraction)
↓
Electrophoresis
↓
Transfer
↓
Blocking
↓
Specific detection

Pretreatment:

During stain formation and/or storage proteins can undergo changes which then require some form of pretreatment before successful typing can be carried out. The pretreatment stage can be combined with the extraction of the protein from the stain. Two important factors are:

- Cleavage of sialic acid residues (e.g. N-acetylneuraminic acid: NANA) where the unequal loss of NANA moieties leads to inhomogeneities in the protein molecules. The action of neuraminidase strips the NANA-residues leaving only the protein backbone.
- The reductive cleavage of internal disulphide bonds of the protein which can be oxidised during stain formation to form complexes within the same molecule or with other proteins or fragments of proteins.

Pretreatment methods for some important proteins are listed in Rand (1990).

Advances in Forensic Haemogenetics 4
Edited by Ch. Rittner and P. M. Schneider
© Springer-Verlag Berlin Heidelberg 1992

Electrophoresis:
Separation of the protein subtypes can be carried out in a variety of gels, but the most commonly used are agarose and polyacrylamide. The modifications for each particular system are too numerous to list here and the reader is advised to read Spielmann and Kühnl (1982), Gaensslen (1983) and Rand (1990) for further details.

BLOTTING:
The blotting technique was first described by Southern (1975) for the transfer of DNA molecules and became known as "Southern Blotting". Subsequent modifications for use with other molecules were also geographically named. The term "Northern Blotting" was used for transfer of RNA (Alwine et al 1977), "Western Blotting" for proteins (Burnette 1981) and last but not least a variation called "Eastern Blotting" (Reinhart and Malamud 1982) also for proteins. There are 4 basic types of blotting mechanism.

Diffusion blotting:
This is the simplest form of blotting. The transfer relies solely on diffusion of the proteins from the gel to the membrane (Bowen et al 1980). Transfer can be carried out unidirectionally by placing a membrane directly on the gel without removing the gel from the glass backing plate. Filters paper are then placed on the membrane and covered by protective foil and small weight.

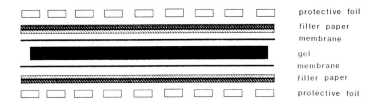

Fig.2: Construction of diffusion blotting

The method is simple but relatively inefficient (ca. 50% transfer) and many hours are required for adequate transfer. The advantage of this method lies in research in the form of bidirectional blotting whereby two identical copies can be obtained by placing a membrane on either side of the gel. However the disadvantages of this method do not make it suitable for stain work.

Capillary blotting:
Capillary blotting, first described by Southern (1975), is more efficient and less time consuming than simple diffusion blotting. Transfer of protein molecules is enhanced by the capillary flow of buffer which passes from the reservoir through the gel to the membrane carrying the molecules along the capillary gradient (Fig.3).

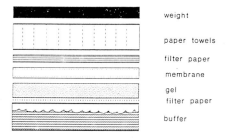

Fig.3: Construction of capillary blotting

Vacuum blotting:
In order to increase the flow of buffer through the gel to the membrane, vacuum blotting has been suggested as a more efficient alternative (Peferoen et al 1985). Although an increased flow rate is achieved the method has not found wide acceptance because the apparatus is more difficult to operate. The set up is essentially the same as capillary blotting except that a vacuum apparatus is placed on top of the membrane.

Electroblotting:
The concept of electroblotting was first introduced by Towbin et al (1979) and the protein molecules are transferred from the gel to the membrane due to a field gradient set up between 2 electrodes. There are 2 main versions of electroblotting. The first method described was vertical electroblotting (Fig. 4) in which the gel and transfer matrix (membrane) were placed in an electrophoresis tank between two electrodes and submerged in buffer.

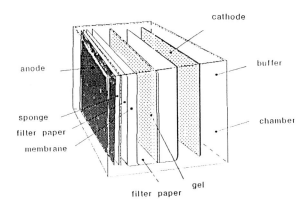

Fig.4: Construction of tank electroblotting

Due to problems of handling the gels had to be relatively stable and this method is not suitable for the more modern ultrathin polyacrylamide gels. A more recent innovation is shown in Fig. 6, the semi-dry electroblotting method. Blotting is carried out in a horizontal system using graphite electrodes (Kyhse-Andersen 1984). A "transunit pack" consists of filter paper moistened with the anodic and cathodic buffers placed on either side of the gel and membrane (Fig.5).

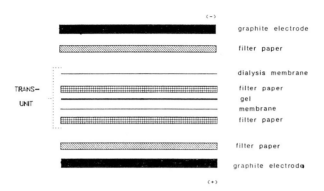

Fig.5: Construction of semi dry electroblot

Transfer is extremely efficient and vitually 100% transfer can be achieved within one hour. The method is also suitable for ultrathin polyacrylamide gels. By placing the membrane directly on the electrophoresis gel and topped by a light weight the gel can then be carefully pealed away from the glass backing plate together with the membrane and placed on the filter paper which has been soaked in the appropriate buffer. The use of block graphite electrodes also ensures the homogenous transfer of proteins across the whole of the gel. Many transunit packs can also be assembled together enabling multiple transfer to be carried out simultaneously. This is by far the most efficient method for transfer of proteins and has also become the most widely used.

Dot blot:
In this method the substance under investigation is spotted directly onto the membrane. It is suitable for use with soluble blood group substances or DNA typing but not for the detection of protein subtypes. The subsequent stages involved are however similar to those described here.

Advantages of blotting:
The new generation of detection methods are multistage procedures involving extensive washing and incubation stages. It is therefore necessary to transfer the electrophoretically separated proteins from the gels to a stable and flexible matrix (membrane). This allows ease of handling and provides a permanent record of the results. Because the proteins are dis-tributed throughout the thickness of the gel the transfer to the surface of a membrane will cause a concentration effect and an increase in sensitivity. Multiple probings with different detection techniques can be carried out on one membrane either by stripping the previous antibody from the membrane or by subsequent incubation using different antibody-substrate combinations (Steffen and Linck 1989). While multiple immunoblots are theoretically possible there are few systems in the forensic repertoire which can be combined giving optimal separation for each system and this is not generally recommended for stain work.

Because of the increase in sensitivity the antibody solutions can be used in a very diluted form (e.g. 1:500 or 1:1000) resulting in a substantial reduction in cost (for details see Rand 1990).

Blotting efficiency:
The efficiency of the blotting procedure is dependent on a variety of factors. The most important ones are listed below:
Gel: - Agarose gel has large pore sizes which allow freedom of flow for all molecules independent of their size and can be used in combination with diffusion blotting. The very small pore sizes in polyacrylamide gels lead to unequal and therefore selective transfer of different protein bands when relying only on diffsion blotting. An active mechanism of transfer such as capillary blotting or the much more efficient electroblotting is not subject to such limiting factors and both are suitable for use with polyacrylamide gels.

Membrane: - The binding capacity of the transfer matrix (membrane) and the mechanism of binding play a very important role in blotting. The appropriate membrane must be selected depending on the characteristics of the protein under investigation (Table I).

Membranes	Binding mechanism	Efficiency (μg/cm^2)
Nitrocellulose	hydrophobic	80
Nylon	electrostatic	480
DBM/DBT	covalent	10-20
DEAE	ionic	115
Teflon		
Polybrene		
Activated glass fibre		
CNBr		

Table I: Membranes used for protein blotting

The type of transfer apparatus used is not the only important criteria for achieving optimal transfer. Another important factor is the elution efficiency of the particular protein from the gel to the membrane. This is mainly influenced by the acrylamide concentration, the degree of crosslinking in the gel, the ionic strength and pH of the buffers used. The addition of other reagents to the gel or transfer buffer may also affect the quality of transfer. Methanol for example decreases the elution efficiency because the proteins will - to some extent - be denatured but increases the binding capacity of nitrocellulose membranes. The inclusion of SDS and urea in gels necessitates the use of alternative blotting conditions (for details see reviews by Beisiegel 1986; Gershoni and Palade 1983). The size and charge of a particular protein molecule will also play an important role. Large proteins - ie greater than 100 000 Daltons - are particularly susceptible to the factors described above but as most of the proteins investigated in forensic work are smaller this is usually not a great problem.

Blocking:

In order to prevent non-specific binding of antibodies to the membrane it is necessary to block the unoccupied binding sites after blotting (quenching) using a neutral substance. The blocking agent used depends on the type of membrane and the protein under investigation. There is no general rule as to which should be used for which protein and the various alternatives must be tested for each particular system. Some of the more common blocking agents are listed in Table II. Factors which must be borne in mind when selecting a blocking agent are:

- No crossreaction should occur with any of the antibodies used in subsequent stages.
- Care must also be taken when using non-ionic detergents because they can cause dissociation and subsequent elution of proteins from nitrocellulose membranes (Stott 1989).

-	BSA	5	%
-	Tween 20	0.05	%
-	Gelatine	0.25	%
-	Serum	10	%
-	Casein	1	%
-	Bactogelatin	0.1	%

Table II: List of some common blocking reagents

DETECTION METHODS:

A variety of methods are available for the localization and visualization of proteins once they have been fixed on the membrane, but can be divided into 3 categories:

Unspecific Staining:

General protein stains such as Coomassie Blue or Amido Black can be used to localize proteins. Although this is the most simple method it is also the most insensitive, is non-specific and it can sometimes be difficult to identify the protein in question. The sensitivity and specificity can be improved by including incubation with a specific antibody by immuno-fixation. The so called immunofixation is still relatively insensitive. The use of silver staining (see Carracedo et al 1983) greatly improves sensitivity but the lack of specificity and high background are disadvantageous.

Direct labeling:

Specific labeling of the protein can be achieved by incubating the membrane with a specific antibody to which a label or enzyme has been incorporated. However the antibody will bind to the antigen site on a one-to-one basis so that although specificity has been achieved sensitivity depends on the amount of label. The most common enzyme/label combinations are listed in Table III.

Indirect labeling:

For this method the first (primary) antibody is directed against the specific ligand or antigen. The membrane is then incubated with a secondary labeled antibody directed against the Fc part of the primary antibody. Alternatively a third bridging antibody can be incorporated in the reaction between the primary and secondary antibodies as was initially proposed by Steinberger et al (1970).

- Radiolabeling
- Biotin-Avidin
- Biotin-Streptavidin
- Alk. phosphatase
- Peroxidase
- Immunogold + Silver enhancer
- Chemiluminescense

Tab.III: Common labels and enzymes used for detection of proteins

By the use of indirect labeling the sensitivitiy of the method can be increased multifold because the ratio of antigen sites to label is no longer on a one-to-one basis.

Many labeling methods can be used to detect proteins. The most common detection systems are listed here:

Radiolabeling:
This has not found wide acceptance for protein blotting mainly due to precautions which are neccessary for handling radioactivity. No great advantage in sensitivity is observed and relatively long exposure times are necessary.

Enzyme conjugated probes:
Enzyme conjugated antibodies are the most commonly used method for detection of proteins. The enzyme must be subsequently incubated with a chromogenic substrate which is converted to an insoluble coloured precipitate at the site of activity. The 2 enzymes in common use are horseradish peroxidase and alkaline phosphatase which can be combined with a wide variety of substrates; the main ones are listed in Table IV.

Peroxidase	- 4-Chloro-1-naphthol
	- Diaminobenzidine
	- o-Dianisidin
	- Luminol/luciferin
	- Dioxetane
	- 3-Amino-9-ethyl carbazole
Alk. phosphatase	- 5-Bromo-4-chloro-3-indolylphosphate
	- Nitro blue tetrazolium
	- ß-Naphthyl phosphate

Tab.IV: Possible combinations of enzyme/substrate labeling systems

There are two modifications of this method which should be mentioned.
As an alternative to the chromogenic substrate it is possible to combine the peroxidase-conjugated antibody with luminol. The substrate is oxidised to a chemiluminescent product which reacts in the form of emission of light photons, and can then be detected by exposing the membrane to an X-ray film. This method has only recently been developed but would appear to offer many advantages including increased sensitivity, easier handling and extremely short incubation times.

The second alternative is the inclusion of a biotin/avidin or streptavidin complex as a bridging molecule. The most common method is the use of a biotinylated secondary antibody and avidin or streptavidin complexed with a biotinylated enzyme. This method exploits the very high affinity of biotin for multiple binding sites avidin and streptavidin and leads to a "christmas tree" effect and a multifold increase in senstivity.

The labeling of antibodies with colloidal gold with or without the addition of a silver staining method is claimed to be very sensitive. As little as 50 pg of antigenic protein can be detected but as yet this method has not been widely used for protein detection.

Flurescence labeling of antibodies has also been proposed but has not found wide acceptance probably due to its relative insensitivity. A more detailed review of the various methods is given by Stott (1989).

SUMMARY

Protein blotting has become a commonly used application in the repertoire of forensic stain investigations. A variety of methods including different stain extraction procedures, protein pretreatments, blotting techniques and detection methods have been developed, so that the user must select the optimal and most suitable method for detecting each particular protein.

LITERATURE:

1. Alwine J.C., Kemp D.J.; Stark G.R. (1977): Method for detection of specific RNA's in agarose gels by transfer to diazobenzyloxymethyl - paper and hybridization with DNA probes. Proc. Natl. Acad. Sci USA 74: 5350 - 5354

2. Beisiegel U. (1986): Protein blotting. Electrophoresis 7: 1 - 18

3. Bowen B., Steinberg J., Laemmli U.K., Weintraub H. (1980): The determination of DNA-binding proteins by protein blotting. Nucleic Acids Res. 8: 1 - 20

4. Burnette W.N. (1981): "Western blotting" Electrophoretic transfer of proteins from SDS - polyacrylamide gels to unmodified nitrocellulose and radiographic detection with antibody and radioiodinated protein A. Anal. biochem. 112: 195 - 203

5. Carracedo A., Concheiro L., Requena I., Lopez-Rivadulla M. (1983): A silver staining method for the detection of polymorphic proteins in minute bloodstains after iso-electric focusing. Forensic Sci. Int 23: 241 - 248

6. Gaensslen R.E. (1983): Sourcebook in forensic serology, immunology and biochemistry. National Institute of Justice, US Government Printing Office, Washington DC

7. Gershoni J.M., Palade G.E. (1983): Protein blotting: principles and applications. Anal. Biochem. 131: 1 - 15

8. Kyhse-Anderson J. (1984): Electroblotting of multiple gels: a simple apparatus without buffer tank for rapid transfer of proteins from polyacrylamide to nitrocellulose. J. Biochem. Biophys. Methods 10: 203 - 209

9. Peferoen M., Huybrecths R., DeLoof A. (1982): Vacuumblotting: a new and efficient transfer of proteins from sodium dodecyl sulphate-polyacrylamide gels to nitrocellulose. FEBS Lett 145: 369 - 372

10. Rand S. (1990): Individualisierung der biologischen Spur durch Analyse der Proteinpolymorphismen. Inaug. Diss. Münster

11. Reinhart M.P., Malamud D. (1982): Protein transfer from isoelectric focusing gels: the native blot. Anal Biochem. 123: 229 - 235

12. Spielmann W., Kühnl P. (1982): Blutgruppenkunde, Georg Thieme Verlag, Stuttgart, New York

13. Southern EM (1975): Detection of specific sequences among DNA fragments separated by gel electrophoresis. J. Mol. Biol 98: 503 - 517

14. Steffen W., Linck R.W. (1989): Multiple immunoblot: a sensitive technique to stain proteins and detect multiple antigens on a single two dimensional replica. Electrophoresis 10: 714 - 718

15. Steinberger L. A., Hardy P. H. Jr., Cuculis J. J., Meyer H. G. (1970): The unlabeled antibody enzyme method of immunohistochemistry. Preparation and properties of soluble antigen-antibody complex (horseradish peroxidase-antihorseradish peroxidase) and its use in identification of spirochetes. J. Histochem. Cytochem. 18: 315 - 333

16. Stott D.I. (1989): Immunoblotting and dot blotting. J. Immunol. Methods 119: 153 - 187

17. Towbin H., Staehlin T., Gordon J (1979): Electrophoretic transfer of proteins from polyacrylamide gels to nitrocellulose sheets: procedure and some applications. Proc. Natl. Acad. Sci. USA 76: 4350 - 4354

TWO–DIMENSIONAL ISOELECTRIC FOCUSING ANALYSIS OF RARE AND SILENT ESTERASE D TYPES. DESCRIPTION OF A NEW ESD VARIANT PHENOTYPE

A. Alonso*, S. Weidinger**, G. Visedo***, M. Sancho*, J. Fernandez-piqueras***

(*)Instituto Nacional de Toxicologia. Madrid. Spain
(**)Institut für Anthropologie und Humangenetik, Universität München, FRG
(***) Departamento de Biologia, Universidad Autonoma de Madrid, Spain

INTRODUCTION

We have recently shown that the analysis of ESD phenotypes by one-dimensional isoelectric focusing (1-D IEF) under reducing and mild denaturing conditions offers high resolution in the separation of the different ESD allele products (Alonso et al. 1991).Furthermore a new two-dimensional isoelectric focusing method (2-D IEF) has been described that permitted the identification of the ESD subunits from the homodimeric and heterodimeric forms of five common ESD phenotypes.

In this report, we analyzed three ESD variant phenotypes (ESD 7-1, ESD 7-2, and a new ESD 1-VAR phenotype observed in a Spanish population) as well as two heterozygous phenotypes of a silent allele (ESD 1-QO and ESD 2-QO, found in a case of disputed paternity) by 1-D IEF under reducing conditions or under reducing and mild denaturing conditions and by 2-D IEF.

MATERIALS AND METHODS

One-dimensional separations as well as the first dimensional separation of the 2-D IEF method were carried out by IEF under reducing conditions(50mM DTT) or under reducing and mild denaturing conditions (50mM DTT and 1.5M urea) using a narrow pH gradient (Pharmalyte 4.5-5.4) in combination with two separators (HEPES and ACES). The second-dimensional separation was performed by focusing the first-dimensional ESD bands under denaturing conditions (9M urea) with a wide pH gradient (4-10.5), according to the method of Alonso et al. (1991).

RESULTS AND DISCUSSION

Figures 1a and 1b show the band pattern of different rare and silent ESD types (ESD7-1, ESD7-2, ESD1-VAR, ESD1-QO and ESD2-QO) analyzed by 1-D IEF under reducing conditions or under reducing and mild denaturing conditions, respectively. As previously described, the presence of low urea concentrations in the gel induces an inversion in the relative mobility of the ESD1 and ESD2 allele products. A similar inversion in the relative mobility of the ESD7-1 and ESD7-2 bands was observed in this study. Furthermore, figures 1a, 1b, and 1c show the 1-D IEF pattern of a "new" ESD1-VAR phenotype found in a Spanish population. The new variant which was tentatively named ESD1-Gijon (ESD1-Gij) is characterized by a very cathodal pattern. For identification it was necessary to use a broader pH gradient (a mixture of Pharmalyte 4-6.5 and Pharmalyte 4.5-5.4)(fig. 1c). Unfortunately, it was not possible to confirm the inheritance of this rare variant by family studies.

Advances in Forensic Haemogenetics 4
Edited by Ch. Rittner and P. M. Schneider
© Springer-Verlag Berlin Heidelberg 1992

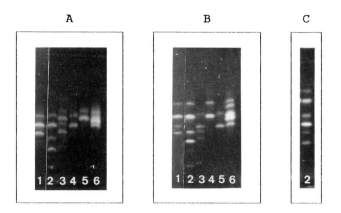

Fig.1. Rare and silent ESD types analyzed by 1-D IEF under reducing conditions. A: in the absence of urea, B and C: in the presence of 1.5 M urea. Samples: 1: ESD7-1, 2: ESD1-Gij, 3: ESD7-2, 4: ESD1-QO, 5: ESD2-QO, and 6: ESD2-1

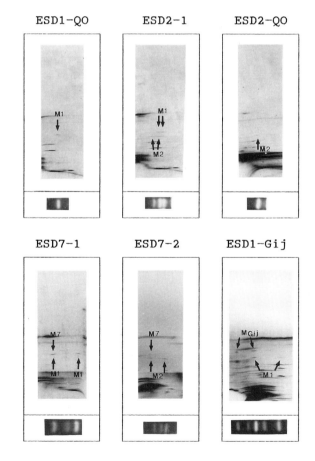

Fig.2. 2-D IEF analysis of silent and rare ESD types followed by silver staining. ESD monomers (M) are indicated with arrows

We have also analyzed rare and silent ESD phenotypes by a recently developed 2-D IEF procedure that consist of a first-dimensional separation of the different ESD dimeric forms by IEF under reducing and mild denaturing conditions using a narrow pH gradient capable of producing high resolution ESD bands, followed by a second-dimensional separation under denaturing conditions with a wide pH gradient. In this way we can correlate the focusing pattern of the dimeric ESD forms with the focusing pattern of its dissociated subunits. Figure 2 shows the result of these 2-D IEF analysis.

The 2-D IEF pattern of the ESD1-QO and ESD2-QO phenotypes were characterized by the presence of the monomeric band M1 (corresponding to the ESD1 one-dimensional dimeric band) and the monomeric band M2 (corresponding to the ESD2 one-dimensional dimeric band), respectively. No additional bands could be observed. This result allowed to rule out the possibility that the ESD*QO allele was a mutation that produced a polypeptide chain which was able to form dimers without enzymatic activity. The two remaining possibilities that explain the existence of a ESD*QO allele (a mutation that produces a polypeptide chain that is unable to form dimers or a mutation that leads to a lack of polypeptide product) could be distinguished by another two-dimensional electrophoretic analysis (Kondo et al. 1984).

The 2-D IEF analysis of the ESD7-1 and ESD7-2 phenotypes has permitted the identification of the ESD7 monomer (M7) as a band with similar isoelectric point found for ESD M1. This result suggest that the ESD*7 allele shows a neutral mutation that can be recognized by 1-D IEF because of a conformational change in the dimeric structure of the protein. It was also shown that the more cathodal one-dimensional bands of these phenotypes are heterodimeric forms composed of the M1 and M7 (ESD7-1 phenotype) or the M2 and M7 (ESD7-2 phenotype) monomers. We assume that cathodal to these heterodimeric forms is probably focusing the H 7-7 homodimeric form (Weidinger and Henke. 1988). However, this band has not been visualized in this study. Possibly there was a dissociation of the H 7-7 homodimeric form into its monomers by ageing.

Finally, the 2-D IEF analysis of the rare ESD1-Gij phenotype has permitted the identification of the ESD Gij monomer (M Gij) with a mobility cathodal to the M1 monomer. In addition the homodimeric (H Gij-Gij and H 1-1) and the heterodimeric forms (HE 1-Gij) of this phenotype, could be identified.

REFERENCES

Alonso A, Visedo G, Sancho M, Fernandez-Piqueras J (1991) Identification of human esterase D subunits from the homodimeric and heterodimeric forms of five phenotypes by a new two-dimensional isoelectric focusing method. Electrophoresis 12: 348- 351

Kondo I, Yamamoto T, Yamakawa K, Harada S, Oishi H, Nishigaki I, Hamaguchi H (1984) Genetic analysis of human lymphocyte proteins by two-dimensional gel electrphoresis: VI. Identification of esterase D in the two-dimensional gel electrophoresis pattern of cellular proteins. Hum. Genet. 66: 248-251

Weidinger S, Henke J (1988) Two new esterase D (ESD) variants revealed by isoelectric focusing in agarose gel. Electrophoresis 9: 429-432

A SIMPLE TECHNIQUE FOR THE DETERMINATION OF GGTP TYPES

M. Oya, Y. Kimura, N. Komatsu and A. Kido

Department of Legal Medicine, Yamanashi Medical University
Yamanashi-ken, Japan

Introduction

Human seminal plasma contains a high enzyme activity of gamma-glutamyl transpeptidase (GGTP, EC 2.3.2.2) (Rosalki and Rowe 1973). Abe and Hiraiwa (1986) discovered polymorphism of seminal GGTP by means of slab-disc electrophoresis. We describe a simple procedure for phenotyping seminal GGTP using starch gel electrophoresis.

Materials and Methods

Ejaculates were obtained from 350 male volunteers living in Yamanashi Prefecture, a central part of Japan. Semen samples were absorbed onto 3 x 8 mm filter paper strips (Whatman No. 3, Maidstone, UK) and inserted in the slots of the gel 4 cm from the cathode.

Horizontal starch gel electrophoresis was performed by the method of Poulik (1957) using 10 % hydrolyzed starch (Biotest-AG, Frankfurt, FRG) on 150 x 150 x 4 mm gel plates. Electrophoresis was carried out at a constant current of 20 mA for 3.5 h at 4°C.

After run, the gel was horizontally sliced and covered with a 15 x 15 cm sheet of filter paper (Whatman No. 3) soaked in 15 ml 0.1 M glycylglycine containing 150 mg L-gamma-glutamyl-p-diethylaminoanilide dihydrochloride and 30 mg α-naphthol (prepare freshly and adjust to pH 8.6 with 2 N sodium hydroxide) for 3 h at 37°C. In order to avoid dessication the gel plate was wrapped with a sheet of thin plastic film. After incubation, the filter paper was removed and the gel treated with 0.2 % periodic acid for 5 min. The GGTP patterns appeared as blue bands.

Advances in Forensic Haemogenetics 4
Edited by Ch. Rittner and P. M. Schneider
© Springer-Verlag Berlin Heidelberg 1992

Results and Discussion

Figure 1 shows three GGTP types (GGTP 1, 2-1 and 2) obtained by the present starch gel electrophoretic technique. GGTP 1 and GGTP 2 exhibited one major band with different electrophoretic mobility, each sometimes being accompanied with an additional minor band. GGTP 2-1 consisted of two bands: anodal one corresponded to the GGTP 1 band and cathodal one to the GGTP 2 band.

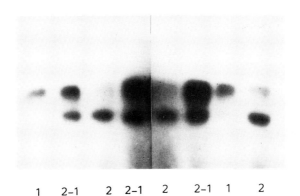

1 2-1   2 2-1   2   2-1 1   2

Fig. 1. Electrophoretic pattern of
seminal GGTP types.
The anode is at the top

The results for the distribution are given in Table 1. The population data fitted the Hardy-Weinberg law. The GGTP*1 frequency in our population sample (0.616) is considerably high as compared with that observed by Abe and Hiraiwa (0.446).

Table 1. Distribution of GGTP types in a Japanese population

Phenotype	No. observed	(%)	No. expected
1	129	(36.9)	132.8
2-1	173	(49.4)	165.5
2	48	(13.7)	51.6
Total	350	(100.0)	350.0

Allelle frequencies: GGTP*1 = 0.616, GGTP*2 = 0.384
χ^2 = 0.73, d.f. = 1, 0.50 > P > 0.30

The present method is simple and rapid and will therefore have broad application to further forensic, anthropological and population studies.

References

Rosalki SB, Rowe JA (1973) Gamma-glutamyl-transpeptidase activity of human seminal fluid. Lancet 1: 323-324

Abe S, Hiraiwa K (1986) Polymorphism of seminal γ-glutamyl transpeptidase. Forensic Sci Int 32: 29-32

Poulik MD (1957) Starch gel electrophoresis in a discontinuous system of buffers. Nature 180: 1477-1479

New Variation in Low-Sulfur Keratins Detected by Hybrid Isoelectric Focusing (HIEF)

M. S. Rodriguez-Calvo, I. Muñoz, A. Carracedo

Institute of Legal Medicine. University of Santiago de Compostela. Galicia. Spain

INTRODUCTION

Variability in non-carboxymethylated keratins by IEF in the presence of 6M urea, 1.5% Nonidet P40 and correlation with SDS-PAGE patterns has been recently demonstrated (Rodriguez-Calvo et al. 1990). Using the IEF technique, the variability could only be detected by the silver staining method, nevertheless with SDS-PAGE the patterns could be seen after Coomassie staining, so variability in other parts of the gels with higher concentration of proteins should exist. Further investigation on the variability of hair keratins applying HIEF in various pH ranges is reported.

MATERIAL AND METHODS

Treatment of samples

1. Washing: Petroleum ether (X3), ethanol (X2) and distilled water (X2)
2. Drying
3. Cutting into small pieces
4. Extraction: according to Marshall and Gillespie (1982) but without carboxymethylation (Carracedo et al. 1985).
3 cm of hair/15 µl of solution: 0.05M TRIS, 0.05M DTT and 8M urea (pH 9.3).

HIEF procedure

1. Formation of IPGs: according to Bjellqvist et al. (1982) (260x100x0.5mm)

Table 1.- Composition of the acidic and basic components of the gradient mixer

Components	Acidic (dense) solution	Basic (light) solution
Immobiline volumes	see Table 2	see Table 2
Acrylamide (29.1%) + bis-acrylamide (0.9%)	1.25	1.25
Glycerol 87%	2.10	0.00
H_2O	X	Y
Total volume	7.50	7.50
TEMED (10 ml%)	0.01	0 01
Ammonium persulfate (10g%)	0.01	0.01

Advances in Forensic Haemogenetics 4
Edited by Ch. Rittner and P. M. Schneider
© Springer-Verlag Berlin Heidelberg 1992

Table 2.- Specific 0.2M Immobiline volumes (µl)

pH range	Immobiline(pK)	Acidic sol.	Basic sol.
4.7-5.6	3.6	252.90	--
	4.6	313.15	431.50
	6.2	431.50	431.50
	9.3	5.25	52.50
4-6	3.6	284.50	195
	4.6	49.50	260.50
	6.2	219.50	138
	9.3	--	361

2. HIEF

- Polimerization: 15 min at room temperature + 1 h at 50°C
- Washing: 6x10 min with distilled water
         1x30 min with 2% Glycerol
- Drying
- Rehydratation (mold method): at least 3 h
  *IPG 4.7-5.6 with1.5% Ampholine 4-6, 6M urea,
                1.5% Nonidet P40 and 0.05M DTT
  *IPG 4-6 with 1% Ampholine 4-6, 6M urea,
                1.5% Nonidet P40 and 0.05M DTT

3. Running conditions

- 7W, 4mA, 3000V, for 5 h at 14°C
- Electrode solutions: 10mM NaOH for the cathode and 10mM glutamic acid
for the anode
- Sample application: 0.5x0.5 with Whatman 3 MM, in the cathode.

3. Staining

Silver staining method according to Carracedo et al. (1983).

RESULTS AND DISCUSSION

IEF patterns of non-carboxymethylated keratins in the pH range 2.5-8,
with 6M urea and 1.5% Nonidet P40 (Fig. 1) has been recently demonstrated
(Rodriguez-Calvo et al. 1990).

Additional variation was explored with HIEF in various pH ranges: first in
a wide pH range to determine the pI of interest, then in a narrow pH to
analyze the variability.

With this technique, bands are sharper and more clearly defined so the
interpretation of the patterns is easier. The different keratin phenotypes
were clearly distinguished in the pH range 4.7-5.6 (Fig. 2) and their
correlation with the variability previously described by IEF has been
proved. The reproductibility and insensitivity of salts makes HIEF the
method of choice for the study of the keratins in areas of the gel with
high concentration of proteins.

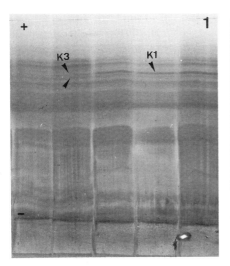 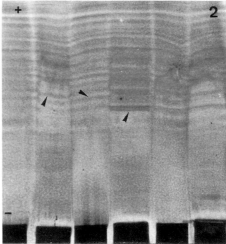

Fig. 1: IEF keratin patterns (T=4.65%; C=3.2%; pH 2.5-8) in the presence of 6M urea and 1.5% NP40

Fig. 2: Variability of hair keratins detected by HIEF (pH range 4.7-5.6)

ACKNOWLEGEMENTS

This study was supported by grants from Ministerio de Educación y Ciencia (CICYT PA86-0453) and Xunta de Galicia (XUGA 8420689).

REFERENCES

Bjellqvist, B.; Ek, K.; Righetti, P.G.; Gianazza, E.; Görg, A.; Postel, W. Isolectric focusing in immobilized pH gradients: principle, methodology and some applications. J. Biochem. Biophys. Methods 6:317-339 (1982)

Carracedo, A.; Concheiro, L.; Requena, I. The isoelectric focusing of keratins in hair followed by silver staining. For. Sci. Int. 29:83-89 (1985)

Carracedo, A.; Concheiro, L.; Requena, I.; López-Rivadulla, M. A silver staining method for the detection of polymorphic proteins in minute bloodstains after isoelectric focusing. For. Sci. Int. 23:241-248 (1983)

Marshall, R.C.; Gillespie, J.M. Comparison of samples of human hair by two-dimensional electrophoresis. J. For. Sci. Soc. 22:377-385 (1982)

Rodriguez-Calvo, M.S.; Carracedo, A.; Lareu, M.V.; Concheiro, L. Correlation between IEF and SDS-PAGE phenotypes of keratins. 12nd International Meeting of Forensic Sciences. Adelaide.1990

The Influence of Infused Erythrocytes on the Detection of Individual Membrane-, Enzyme- and DNA- Systems

W. Huckenbeck[**], B. Mainzer[*], P. Lipfert[*], H. Müller[**] , A. Wehr[**], V. Stancu[**]

Institute of Legal Medicine[**] and Institute of Anaesthesiology[*]
Heinrich-Heine-University Düsseldorf, FRG

SUMMARY

We report on a case of affiliation. The putative father has passed away before a blood sample having been taken . Serological examinations were complicated by the fact that the patient had been infused with concentrates of erythrocytes. In such cases not only the red cell markers but also DNA bands can be falsified. Most likely the use of single locus probes and determination of plasma protein polymorphisms may lead to conclusive results.

INTRODUCTION

In rarer cases of affiliation or identification serological examinations have to be taken on blood samples from individuals having been treated with blood transfusions. It is known that in such cases serological markers can be falsified (1,2,3,4). Usually the results can be verified by a second blood test (three months later). If the patient has passed away in the meantime such control examination is not possible. Determination of plasma protein polymorphisms and DNA fingerprinting promise the most meaningful results. But DNA patterns can also be falsified. Dependend on cleansing the donor's blood concentrates of erythrocytes can contain white blood cells.

MATERIAL & METHODS

Blood samples were taken from patients which had to undergo an operation with expected higher loss of blood. Sampling was carried out just before and immediately after operation. The in-vitro experiments were carried out on pints of stored blood.

CASUISTIC

A four-year-old girl wanted to be accepted as illegitimate child of a sixty-year-old man who had died some days before. Blood sampling was carried out in the cemetery. The corpse had attained an advanced status of putrefaction. Samples could be taken from the heart blood. It was known that the putative father had been treated with 27 concentrates of red cells over a period of two weeks. 20 conventional serological markers could be determined, biostatistical evaluation of them all led to W = 72.33 % (likelihood in accordance to Hummel). Separate evaluation of the not affected markers (ABO, Gm, Km, PI, D) resulted in W = 72,95 %. DNA fingerprinting was carried out with the single locus probes MS 43, 3'HVR, G3 and YNH 24. The definite results (no additional bands) led to likelihood of more than 99.9 %.

RESULTS AND DISCUSSION

Depending on the number of infusions and intervals of blood extraction pints of stored blood can influence serological examinations on the patients blood. For the examiner it is important to know what kind of stored blood had been infused. Today concentrates of red cells are prefered (except: heart-lung machine etc.!). Therefore plasma protein polymorphisms can unambigously be interpreted in such instances. Due to importance of compatibility the donor's red cell antigens have to agree with the patient's blood on ABO-, Kell-, Duffy-

Advances in Forensic Haemogenetics 4
Edited by Ch. Rittner and P. M. Schneider
© Springer-Verlag Berlin Heidelberg 1992

and Rhesus– (at least: D) system. The remaining red cell antigens and the iso enzymes have to be carefully interpreted. On what scale the serological blood pucture can change is shown in table 1. The five patients were treated with 2-24 transfusions and 0-5 additional markers were detected after operation. The number of alterations is surely dependend on frequency of the marker concerned. For example: patient 2 (frequency of the marker combination : 1 in 19267) can have alterations less likely than patient 4 (1 in 27780). The frequency of the marker M is about 80%. There is a good chance to get an additional marker M (patient 2) because most of the donors show this mark.

Conclusive evidential value is expected from genetic fingerprinting. But concentrated erythrocytes can contain white cells and therefore foreign DNA. Washed and unwashed concentrates are available. Furthermore the anaesthetist himself can carry out a bedside filtration on unwashed red cells. The content of DNA in unwashed concentrates seems to be relatively comparable to native blood (presumable above 50%). Fig.1 shows a titration mixture of native blood and concentrated red cells. Using multilocus probes it may become difficult to identify additional foreign bands. The same titration mixture is shown in fig.2. Using singlelocus probes the examiner can detect additional bands (except : homozygous) In practice he will recognize the foreign bands by different density, especially because of rarer use of unwashed concentrates.

Furthermore the survival time of foreign white cells is of importance. To our estimation it may be short. Examinations on these problems and the effect of bedside filtration of unwashed concentrates are already under way. We will report on the results as soon as possible.

CONCLUSIONS

In cases of blood transfusion it is of importance to know what kind and what number of transfusions has been carried out. Typing of plasma protein polymorphisms and the tranfusion-relevant red cell markers is a useful examination. Concentrates of erythrocytes (mostly used kind of transfusion) can contain DNA. Therefore one should give singlelocus probes preference. Foreign DNA bands can be detected considerably easier. However in practice this phenomen will take a secondary role. The chance of identical DNA bands is small. Foreign DNA will result in smear only. Principally the medical file has to be requested. Interpretation of the symptoms can be useful (immune reactions, neoformation of red and white cells).

marker	patient 0 14 r.c.c.		patient 1 21 r.c.c. 3 p.		patient 2 2 r.c.c.		patient 3 4 r.c.c.		patient 4 7 r.c.c.	
	ante	post	ante	post	ante	post	ante	post	ante	post
ABO	A1	A1A2	B	B	A1	A1	0	0	B	B
MNSs	Ns	MNSs	MNSs	MNSs	MSs	MNSs	MNSs	MNSs	MNSs	MNSs
Rhesus	CcDEe	CcDEe	cDEe	CcDEe	cDEe	CcDEe	CcDe	CcDe	CcDEe	CcDEe
Kell	K-	K-	K-	K-	K+	K+	K-	K-	K-	K-
Duffy	a+b-	a+b+	a+b+	a+b+	a-b+	a+b+	a-b+	a+b+	a+b+	a+b+
P	P-	P+	P+	P+	P+	P+	P+	P+	P+	P+
Kidd	a+b+	a+b+	a+b-	a+b+	a+b+	a+b+	a-b+	a+b+	a+b+	a+b+
Lutheran	a+	a+	a-	a-	a-	a-	a-	a-	a-	a-
Colton	b-	b-	b-	b-	b-	b-	b-	b-	b+	b+

r.c.c.: red cell concentrate   p: pints of stored native blood

TAB.1 ALTERATIONS OF RED CELL MARKERS BY TRANSFUSION

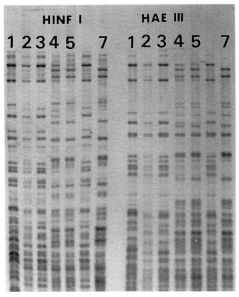

FIG.1 ALTERATION OF DNA BANDS BY
TRANSFUSION – IN VITRO EX-
PERIMENTS , MZ 1.3
Left to right;
Blood : red cell concentrate
Lane 1: 10 to 0
Lane 2: 9 to 1
Lane 3: 7 to 3
Lane 4: 5 to 5
Lane 5: 3 to 7
Lane 7: 0 to 10

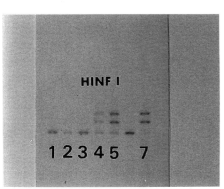

FIG.2 ALTERATION OF DNA BANDS BY
TRANSFUSION – IN VITRO EX-
PERIMENTS , NICE MS43 A
Left to right;
Blood : red cell concentrate
Lane 1: 10 to 0
Lane 2: 9 to 1
Lane 3: 7 to 3
Lane 4: 5 to 5
Lane 5: 3 to 7
Lane 7: 0 to 10

REFERENCES

1) Keil, W., Ishiyama, I., Prokop, O., Geserick, G. (1983)
Die MCAR zur Beurteilung von letalen Transfusionszwischenfällen im ABO-
Blutgruppensystem. In: Barz,J., Bösche, J., Frohberg, H., Joachim, H., Käppner,
R., Mattern, R. (eds) Fortschritte der Rechtsmedizin, Festschrift für Georg
Schmidt. Springer Verlag, Berlin Heidelberg New York: 399–404

2) Myhre, A.B (1980)
Fatalities from Blood Transfusion. JAMA 244 : 1333–1335

3) Pedal, I., Madea, B., Oehmichen, M. (1986)
Immuncytochemische Identifizierung ABO-inkompatibler Erythrocyten nach einem
tödlichen Transfusionszwischenfall. Z.Rechtsmed. 97: 269–276

4) Pineda,A.A., Brizica, S.M., Taswell, H.F. (1978)
Hemolytic Transfusion reaction. Recent experience in a large blood bank. Mayo
Clin.Proc. 53: 378–390

SERUM PROTEIN TYPING/-SUBTYPING by IEF in PAG

G. Geserick, H. Schröder, A. Correns, P. Otremba and H. Waltz

Institute for Forensic Medicine, Humboldt-University, Hannoversche Str. 06, O-1040 Berlin, FRG

INTRODUCTION

For several years we've been gathering experiences in the disengagement of serumprotein-polymorphisms using isoelectrofocusing (IEF). This is mainly due to the systems BF, GC, HP, PI, PLG and TF. During the recent years we raised the efficiency of several methods by modifying them, for instance for the BF-subtypes. Moreover we gathered during the recent years experiences in the forensic use of focusing A2HS, F13A, F13B and ORM1 too.
In the following the most important technical processes used for the optimal visualization of the systems are surveyed.

MATERIAL AND METHOD

With the exception of F13A, where plasma or thrombozyte-lysates are applied, in all systems serum has been used for the identification of the types.
Table 1 lists the necessary details concerning the ampholytes (all from LKB, only A2HS and ORM1 from PHARMACIA) and the electrolyte-solutions.
In Table 2 the most important details of sample-application, focusing and immunofixation are enlistet.

The following methods are to be pointed out:
1. We prefer polyacrylamide gel (PAG) in all systems.
2. Besides PLG, F13B and ORM1 we suggest also for the BF-subtypes a pre-treatment with neuramidase. This results in an outstanding distinctiveness of the subtypes BF FA and FB (SIEMENS 1989).
3. As Table 2 shows, the protein strings of the systems BF, PLG, F13B, ORM1, A2HS and F13A are very good detected through immunofixation.
In detail, a diluted (BF, ORM1, A2HS) or non-diluted (PLG, F13B, F13A) antiserum is directly put on the surface of the gel immediately after the separation and allowed to react for 15 to 60 minutes.
The figures 1 to 3 demonstrate the quality of the sucessful separations.
All the systems mentioned can be used efficiently for the descent identification. They provide the chance to exclude paternity between 14% (F13A) and more than 30% (GC-, PI-, HP-subtypes).

The frequencies of alleles had been observed:
A2HS: 1 = 0,6598, 2 = 0,3392, 3 = 0,0010 (N = 513)
ORM1: F1 = 0,5770, F2 = 0,0196, S = 0,4021, S1 = 0,0013 (n = 383)
F13B: 1 = 0,7750, 2 = 0,0872, 3 = 0,1339, 4 = 0,0027, 6 = 0,0009 (n = 560)
F13A: 1 = 0,7998, 2 = 0,1977, Var. = 0,0025 (n = 607)

Advances in Forensic Haemogenetics 4
Edited by Ch. Rittner and P. M. Schneider
© Springer-Verlag Berlin Heidelberg 1992

According to our experiences which coincide with them of other researchers, the following systems are especially appropriate to investigate blood stains: GC, A2HS, ORM1.
The other systems are also considered useful, though we look upon this from a critical point of view. That only does not apply to the HP-subtypes. Using preparation of haptoglobin-protein by immunoprecipitation good detection of types from blood stains is possible (DIMO-SIMONIN et al. 1990, SCHERZ et al. 1990, see also CORRENS et al. in this issue).

Table 1

IEF in PAG[1]

System	Ampholyte		Anolyt		Catholyt		Neuraminidase[2]
BF	4 - 6 5 - 8 3,5-10	0,5 ml 0,4 ml 0,1 ml	H_3PO_4 0,5 M Glutamic acid 0,1M		NaOH 0,2 M		+
PLG	3,5-10 6 - 8 7 - 9	0,4 ml 0,3 ml 0,3 ml	H_3PO_4 0,5 M		NaOH 0,5 M		+
F13B	3,5-10 4-6,5 5 - 7	0,1 ml 0,6 ml 0,8 ml	H_3PO_4 0,5 M		NaOH 0,5 M		+
ORM1	4,2-4,9 4,5-5,4	0,8 ml 0,2 ml	Glutamic- 0,04 M acid		NaOH 0,1 M		+
A2HS	4,2-4,9 4 -6,5	0,9 ml 0,1 ml	Glutamic- 0,04 M acid		NaOH 0,1 M		-
F13A	3,5-10 4 -6,5 5 - 7	0,1 ml 0,6 ml 0,8 ml	H_3PO_4 0,5 M		NaOH 0,5 M		-

------
[1] PAG T = 5 % C = 3 %
[2] SIGMA V 50 µl Serum + 10 µl NANA'se (= 0,1 U), 3 h, 37° C

Table 2

System	Sample- Application	Focusing	Immunofixation
BF	3x5 mm cathod. 30 min.	1 h prefoc. 4 h focusing 1600 V, 10 mA, 10W	Anti-BF ATAB 1:2 dil. 30 min
PLG	3x5 mm anod. 30 min.	1 h prefoc. 4 h focusing 1600 V, 10 mA, 10W	Anti-PLG goat self made undiluted, 15 min
F13B	13x5 mm anod. 60 min.	1 h prefoc. 4 h focusing 1600 V, 10 mA, 10W	Anti-F13B-S BEHRING undiluted 60 min.
ORM1	3x5 mm cathod. 30min/Se+NANASe 1:15 dil.	3 h focusing 2000 V, 15 mA, 20W	Anti-ORM ATAB 1 : 15 dil. 15 min.
A2HS	3x5 mm cathod. 30 min. Serum 1:4 diluted	1 h prefoc. 4 h foc. 1600 V, 10 mA, 10W	Anti-A2HS ATAB 1 : 4 dil. 30 min.
F13A	5x5 mm cathod. 60 min. Thrombozyte-Lysat or Plasma	1 h prefoc. 4 h foc. 1600 V, 10 mA, 10 W	Anti-F13A BEHRING undiluted 60 min.

----
* Antiserum was poured directly on the gel

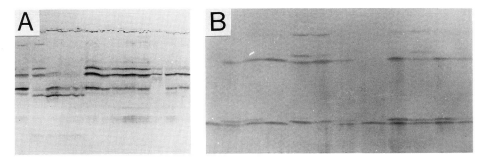

Fig. 1A. BF-phenotypes (nativ). From left to right: S; FASO,7;
   SSO,7; SSO,7; SSO,7; FAS; FBS; FAS; FAS; FAS; FA; FBS; FBS;
Fig. 1B. BF-phenotypes (NANA'se). From left to right: S; FBS; FBS;
   FBS; FA; FA; FBS; S; FAS; FAS; FBS; FBS. The anode is at the top

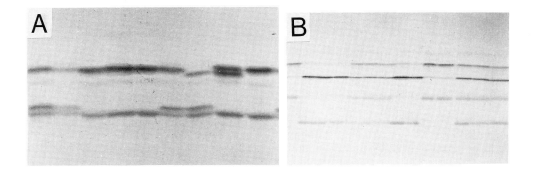

Fig. 2A. ORM1-phenotypes. From left to right: F1S; F1S; F1; F1; F1;
   F1S; F2S; F1F2; F1.
Fig. 2B. PLG-phenotypes. From left to right: A; B; B; B; AB; AB; AB;
   B; B; A; A; AB; AB; AB. The anode is at the top

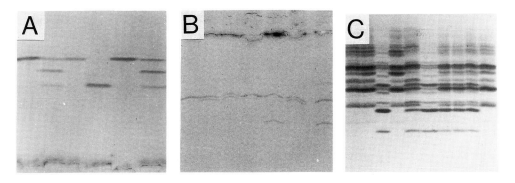

Fig. 3A. F13A-phenotypes. From left to right: 1; 1-2; 1; 2; 1; 1-2.
Fig. 3B. F13B-phenotypes. From left to right: 1; 1-2; 1-2; 1; 1-3;
   1-2; 1-3.
Fig. 3C. A2HS-phenotypes. From left to right: 1; 1; 2; 1; 1-2; 2;
   1-2; 1-2; 1-2; 1. The anode is at the top

DOT BLOT IMMUNOASSAY FOR DETECTION OF HLA ANTIGENS IN FORENSIC STAINS

D V RAO & V K KASHYAP*

Central Forensic Science Laboratory
Ramanthapur, Hyderabad 500 013
A. P.   India

ABSTRACT

A new highly sensitive and specific microplate based dot blot immunoassay for detection of HLA antigens in blood and stains is reported. The unique feature of this assay is that the final result is unambiguous since it is a distinct colour reaction. The assay has been used in detection of antigens in fresh and old blood stains with equal success.

INTRODUCTION

Polymorphism of HLA has been widely exploited in organ transplantation and forensic analysis (Berah et al 1970; Newall 1979). Several modified cytotoxicity tests and enzyme immunoassays for detection of HLA antigens in forensic samples have been reported (Newall 1981; Nelson et al 1983; Rittner and Waiyawath 1975 and Bishara et al 1983). Most of these methods either lack the required accuracy or they are too complex to be used routinely. We have developed a highly sensitive and specific microplate dot blot immunoassay (MDBI) for typing HLA in blood and its stains for individualisation, initially using a panel of antisera of high specificity to HLA-A1, A2, A11, A24, A28, B7, B8, Bw52, DR2, DR7 and DR8.

MATERIALS AND METHODS

Sample Preparation and Plan of Study

Blood samples from the volunteers were collected and their HLA phenotypes were ascertained by standard microcytotoxicity test and stains of the same were prepared on cloth. Each stain of the size of 0.5 cm   was extracted in 1.0ml of PBS containing 0.1% of Tween20. The extract (50ul) was then used to detect HLA antigens. The extract was serially diluted from 1:100 to 1:1400 to test the sensitivity of the method. To know the applicability of the assay to old samples, the stains were stored both at room temperature and at 4°C for a period

* Author for correspondence to

Advances in Forensic Haemogenetics 4
Edited by Ch. Rittner and P. M. Schneider
© Springer-Verlag Berlin Heidelberg 1992

of 12 months and tested at the end of every 3rd month. 50 unknown blood stains from old case samples were tested to evaluate its suitabilty actual forensic analysis. Double-blind experiments were repeated to further confirm the results.

Microplate Dot Blot Immunoassay (MDBI)

Blood/stain extracts were loaded on nitrocellulose membrane (NC) using a dot blot apparatus. Discs (3mm dia.) were punched, placed in the wells of microplate and incubated with 200ul of 3% H_2O_2 for 30 min at room temperature to inhibit the endogenous peroxidase. The wells and the discs were blocked twice, first by incubating with 200ul of 2% BSA at 37°C for one hour and secondly with 100ul of 1:500 dilution of antihuman globulins for another hour at 37°C. Wells were washed with phosphate buffer with Tween20 (PBST). 100ul of 1:100 diluted different HLA antisera were placed in their respective wells. The plate was covered with parafilm and incubated for an hour at 37°C. The wells were washed with PBST. In each well 100ul of 1:500 diluted antihuman IgG-peroxidase conjugate was added and incubated for 2 hours at 37°C and washed with PBST. 100ul of substrate mixture containing 0.1% 4-chloronaphthol and 0.002% H O in PBS was placed in each well. Development of purple colour on NC discs within 30 min indicated positive reaction.

RESULTS AND DISCUSSION

Figure 1 shows the result of HLA antigens detection in one of the stains. HLA antigens even in 1000 times diluted extract were accurately detected. The stains stored for a year at 4°C as well as room temperature were correctly typed except 4% of 9 and 12 month old stains stored at room temperature (Table 1). Antigens in 90% of random case samples were successfully identified by MDBI.

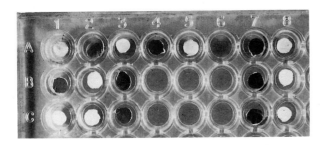

Fig. 1. Photograph showing positive (black) and negative (white) reactions to different HLA antigens obtained in MDBI. Tests performed in wells for different antigens are as follows : A row : 1) A1; (2) A2; (3) A11; (4) A24; (5) A28. B row : 1)B7; (2)B8; (3)Bw52. C row : 1)DR2; (2)DR7; (3)DR8. Column 7 and 8 represent positive and negative controls

Table 1. Effect of storage on the detectability of HLA antigens

Period of Storage	Samples tested	No. of correctly typed stain (%)	
		Stored at room temp	Stored at 4°C
One week	50	100	100
3 months	50	100	100
6 months	50	100	100
9 months	50	96	100
12 months	50	96	100

MDBI combines the best of both micro ELISA and dot blot assay. NC discs hold larger quantity of antigen which enhances the assay's detectability and the end result is a permanent colour reaction on the NC disc. Simultaneous processing of several samples in MDBI using very small volumes of reagents is inherited from micro ELISA. Treatment of sample discs with H_2O_2 eliminate the endogeneous peroxidase interference. False positive reactions initially obtained due to the presence of endogenous immunoglobulins in stain extract has been effectively overcome by introducing a second blocking step with unlabellled antihuman IgG. The criteria for selection of antisera panel in MDBI is the availability of high specificity antisera and their prevelance in Indian population. Enzyme amplification and high quantity of target antigen on disc are the reasons for better sensitivity. Storage studies suggest that the HLA antigens are relatively stable and are best preserved at 4°C. Disintegration of antigen due to microbial contamination and aging may be the reason for marginal decline in detection of some of the experimentally stored and forensic samples. Absence of corresponding antigens tested for in the sample may be the other reason for failure in the detection of 10% of forensic samples. MDBI is highly suitable for forensic and clinical diagnosis of HLA antigens.

REFERENCES

Berah M, Hors J, and Dausset J (1970) A study of HLA antigens in human organs. Transplantation 9, 185-192

Bishara A, Brautbar C, and Bonavida B (1983) Enzyme linked immunosorbent assay for HLA determination on fresh and dried lymphocytes. J Immunol Method 62:265-271

Nelson MS, Turner LL and Reisner EG (1983) A feasibility study of human leucocyte antigen (HLA) typing for dried bloodstains J Forens Sci 28:608-614

Newall PJ (1979) The identification of HLA-A2 and HLA-B5 antigens in dried bloodstains. Can Soc Forens Sci J 12:1-16

Newall PJ (1981) The identification of HLA-A9 in dried stains of blood and body secretions. Can Soc Forens Sci J 14:104-112

Rittner C and Waiyawuth V (1975) HLA typing in dried blood stains. II comperative studies on microcytotoxicity and microcomplement fixation tests. J Immunogenet 2:211-222

The use of microtiter techniques for the determination of red
blood cell phenotypes in paternity testing

D. Mayr, W.R. Mayr

Institut für Transfusionsmedizin, Klinikum der RWTH,
Pauwelsstraße 30, D-5100 Aachen, FRG

INTRODUCTION

The use of standard slide or tube techniques for the
determination of red blood cell phenotypes is rather
cumbersome and requires a large amount of work which can be
the reason of clerical errors. In order to avoid these
problems, microtiter techniques have been included in our
routine paternity tests for the definition of alloantigens of
the erythrocyte membrane. The comparison of the results
obtained by the microtiter methods and standard techniques is
shown in this report.

MATERIAL AND METHODS

Erythrocytes: the red cells to be tested originated from
individuals involved in paternity investigations (mothers,
children and putative fathers)

Microtiter techniques:
1. For the definition of Rh (C, c, C^w, D, E, e), Ss, K (K,
k), Fy (Fy^a, Fy^b), Jk (Jk^a, Jk^b), Lu (Lu^a, Lu^b), Co^b, and Xg^a
the commercially available solid phase immunoassay Capture-
R^{TM} (Immucor, Norcross, GA/USA) which is performed in
microtiter trays (Plapp et al. 1984) has been used according
to the manufacturer's specifications with human IgG
alloantisera,
2. For the definition of ABO (with A subgroups), MNS, P_1, Le
(Le^a, Le^b) and Jk (Jk^a, Jk^b) a liquid-phase microplate method
has been used. One drop (50 µl) of a 2% erythrocyte
suspension in isotonic saline was mixed with 1 drop (50 µl)
monoclonal antibody (for ABO, MN, Le and Jk), alloantiserum
(S), xenoantiserum (P_1) or lectin (A subgroups) in U-shaped
polystyrol microtiter plates (Greiner #650101,
Nürtingen/FRG); after an incubation of 20 - 30 minutes at
22°C, the trays were centrifuged for 1 minute at 110 x g
(BCSH Blood Transfusion Task Force and BBTS Working Group
1990).

Advances in Forensic Haemogenetics 4
Edited by Ch. Rittner and P. M. Schneider
© Springer-Verlag Berlin Heidelberg 1992

RESULTS AND DISCUSSION

1. Solid phase immunoassay Capture-R[TM]
Approximately 2000 samples have been tested in this technique
for Fy, Jk, Lu and Co[b]; the number of tested samples for Ss,
Rh, K and Xg[a] are 1200, 200, 150 and 300, respectively. Due
to the higher sensitivity of this system for the detection of
IgG alloantisera (in comparison to the standard tube
techniques with or without indirect anti-humanglobulin-test),
it was necessary to dilute the alloantisera used. The
dilutions ranged between 1:20 and 1:2 (1:20 - 1:15 for Rh
antisera, 1:4 for anti-S, -s, -K, -k, -Fy, -Jk and 1:2 for
anti-Lu, -Co[b] and -Xg[a]). The optimal dilution of the
alloantisera had to be determined in a preliminary titration
of the reagents against the erythrocytes of a heterozygous
donor. In all the tests, 14 discrepancies (< 0.1%) in
comparison to the standard tube or slide tests were observed.
These differences were mainly due to the higher sensitivity
of the Capture-R[TM] technique (Mayr et al. 1989) which gave
for instance a much better definition of Fy[x] than the
conventional tube tests (3 cases). The higher sensitivity of
Capture-R[TM], however, also produced some false positive
reactions with antisera containing extraantibodies which did
not react in the standard tube test.

2. Liquid-phase microtiter tests
The number of samples tested for ABO, MNS, P₁ and Jk was 500;
100 samples were tested for Le. All reagents were used in the
same dilution as in the conventional slide or tube tests.
The phenotyping of ABO (with A subgroups), MNS, P₁ and Jk
also showed a perfect concordance with the results of the
standard tests (no discrepancies). The monoclonal antibodies
(of different origin) used for the definition of the Le
phenotypes did not give clear-cut results, so that the typing
for Le has been discontinued for the moment.

The microplate assays offer several advantages: by using
Capture-R[TM], it is possible to perform the tests in a much
shorter time (96 reactions in approximately 40 minutes) and
the alloantisera can be diluted between 1:20 and 1:2 thus
decreasing the costs for these reagents. An analogous saving
of time is observed for the liquid-phase technique.
The handling of microtiter trays is much easier than the
handling of a large number of tubes and slides; furthermore,
all microtiter methods can be rather easily automatized.
The microtiter trays can be stored for a longer period of
time, so that all readings can be checked independently by
another investigator.
A drawback of the microtiter techniques, however, is the fact
that not all reagents working in conventional tests can be
employed in these methods; before using them, the sera have
to be reevaluated in the relevant microplate technique.
Nevertheless, the advantages prompted us to include
microplate techniques in our routine paternity testing; in
practice, one series of tests is performed in the
conventional tube and slide methods and, for confirmation,
the above-mentioned microtiter techniques are used in the
second series of phenotypings.

REFERENCES

BCSH Blood Transfusion Task Force and BBTS Working Group
(1990)
   Guidelines for microplate techniques in liquid-phase blood
   grouping and antibody screening. Clin lab Haemat 12:437-460
Mayr WR, Gassner H, Kempkes A, Mayr D, Goertz-Kaiser B (1989)
   Erste Erfahrungen mit einem Festphasen-Immunassay für
   erythrozytäre IgG-Antikörper. Lab med 13:6-7
Plapp FV, Sinor LT, Rachel JM, Beck ML, Coenen WM, Bayer WL
(1984)
   A solid phase antibody screen. Am J Clin Pathol 82:719-721

D^u detection by an automated direct agglutination method that equals detection by indirect antiglobulin test

J. Obst

Abbott GmbH Diagnostika, Max-Planck-Ring 2, 6200 Wiesbaden, Germany

INTRODUCTION

Since D^u was described by STRATTON in 1946 as a "new" Rh system antigen, there has been an ongoing scientific debate about the necessity of testing for D^u.

Furthermore D^u detection is dependent on methods and reagents used (e.g. polyclonal vs monoclonal) as there is no clinical significance of immunogenicity of D^u.

We describe a novel agglutination method (ABT) that is at least comparable to IAT, easier to perform and more sensitive.

MATERIALS AND METHODS

We used commercial polyclonal anti-D reagents as well as Rh controls diluted in 3% BSA for IAT testing and antibody diluent for ABT.

Bromelin 0.15% in NaCl/Tween diluent was used for the dilution of donor red cells.

74 EDTA anticoagulated donor samples were initially tested on the Dynatech Microbank System and found to be non-reactive. These samples were tested by a manual indirect antiglobulin method demonstrating a range of 1-3 + reactivity. For the ABT method 60 µl of 1:50 diluted anti-D or Rh control was added to the test wells of a flat bottom 96 well microtiter tray as well as 60 µl of 0.15% Bromelin in NaCl/Tween 20 was added to primary and secondary dilution wells. 70 µl packed cells were added to the primary dilution wells and diluted in several steps with Bromelin solution.

The ABT was performed after addition of sample and reagents. The procedure includes automatic tilting of the tray back and forth as it moves down the track.

---

*   Footnote
    Abbreviations: IAT = indirect antiglobulintest
                       ABT = automated Bi-directional tilt

Advances in Forensic Haemogenetics 4
Edited by Ch. Rittner and P. M. Schneider
© Springer-Verlag Berlin Heidelberg 1992

Fig. 1. AGGLUTINATION ASSAY PROCESSING

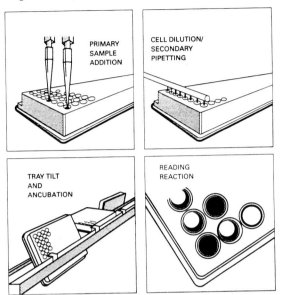

With this process no centrifugation is required. After the tray
proceeds through the series of tilts, any positive reactions will
result in a very distinct crescent shaped agglutinate. An agglutination reader at the end of the track then detects either the presence or absence of the crescent.

RESULTS

Table 1 shows the results of a comparison of 74 D^u samples as endpoint result for ABT and IAT. Results demonstrate that anti-D can
be diluted to a greater extent in the ABT method than IAT.

Table 1. ENDPOINT COMPARISON STUDY - ANALYSIS OF 74 D^u SAMPLES

ABT Endpoint	No. of Samples Tested	IAT Endpoint (Range)
100	1	50
200	2	50 - 100
400	15	12.5 - 100
800	26	50 - 400
1600	21	25 - 400
3200	7	200 - 800
6400	1	200
12,800	1	400

Similar population distributions are demonstrated with both common
D and D^u phenotypes. (Table 2.)

Table 2. POPULATION DISTRIBUTION COMMON D AND D^U PHENOTYPES

	D POSITIVE	D^U POSITIVE	D NEGATIVE
MEAN	250,214	216,202	6799
S. D.	33,350	31,090	1517
% CV	13.3	14.4	22.3
MINIMUM	146,113	125,009	4508
MAXIMUM	314,919	283,606	9645
NUMBER	119	74	40

D mosaics from all categories were also tested to assess specificity when using diluted anti-D in the system. The results indicate
that all categories of the D mosaic were detected. (Table 3.)

Table 3. D MOSAIC TESTING

CATEGORY	ABT COUNT
RYR	3857
D II	213868
D III	222892
D III	234337
D IV	235818
D V	232502
D VI	197741
D VI	235152
D VI	200803
D VI	198566
D VI	198235
D VI	255213

SUMMARY

The studies suggest that the ABT method requires less antibody than
the manual IAT method to provide D^U detection.
When performing testing with anti-D, no confirmation of D negative
results is required.
There is no problem with false positives with the ABT system, as
evidenced by performance with D negative samples.
The D mosaic testing indicates that there is no loss in
specificity by diluting the anti-D.

REFERENCES

Contreras M, Knight RC (1991) Controversies in transfusion medicine
    Testing for D^U: CON Transfusion 31: 270-272
Lynen R, Gallasch E, Tiede G, Neumeyer H (1990) Benignes Auto-Anti-D
    nach Transfusion von Rh-positivem Blut bei einem Patienten mit dem
    Rh-Faktor D^U. Ärztl. Lab 36: 12-17
Stratton F, (1946) New Rh allelomorph. Nature 158:25-6
Stroup M (1991) Controversies in transfusion medicine Testing for
    D^U: Pro Transfusion 31: 273-276

Absorption-Elution Test for ABO-Determination of Secretor and Nonsecretor Saliva Stains

J. Bolt, J. Lötterle

Institute of Forensic Medicine, Friedrich Alexander University,
8520 Erlangen FRG

Introduction

During the last years sensitive elution tests have been described for the ABO-determination of saliva stains of nonsecretors (LINCOLN 1988, RABL et al. 1990). The object of the present study was to determine the ABO blood group in saliva stains of practical cases and compare the results of the usual inhibition test with those of the absorption-elution test.

Materials and Methods

100 saliva stains of practical cases were tested. The distribution of the ABO-blood groups was as follows:

$$A_1: 35, \quad A_2: 4, \quad B: 14, \quad O: 39, \quad A_1B: 6, \quad A_2B: 2$$

Inhibition Test

Equal volumes of saliva stain and anti-AB-Serum (titer of 16) were mixt and left at 4 °C overnight, after which two drops from each tube were titrated using isotonic saline as diluent. Equal volumes of appropiate A_1- or B-indicator cells were added to each tube. The tests were macroscopically read for agglutination after incubation at room temperature for 15 min. The same test was done with Ulex europaeus (titer of 16) using O indicator cells. Results obtained from the stain were compared with those of the unstained material. Reduction in titer of at least three dilutions was necessary to demonstrate the presence of blood group substance.

Absorption-Elution Test

The test was carried out according to the method of KIND and CLEEVELY (1969) with minor changes. An appropiate portion of stain was extracted in a known volume of 5% aqueous ammonia. Aliquots of the extracts were spotted on glass slides, which were left to dry at room temperature. Drops ($\pm 30 \ \mu l$) of undiluted anti-A- and anti-B-sera were added to each slide and carefully spread to cover the area of the dried extract. Absorption took place overnight at 4°C in a humid chamber. The slides were then carefully rinsed with ice-cold isotonic saline for a period of about 30 seconds. Fresh indicator cells were used in a concentration of 0.5% and immediately covered with a coverslide. Elution took place for 15 min at a temperature of 56°C in a suitable moist chamber. After elution the slides were kept at room temperature and were

Advances in Forensic Haemogenetics 4
Edited by Ch. Rittner and P. M. Schneider
© Springer-Verlag Berlin Heidelberg 1992

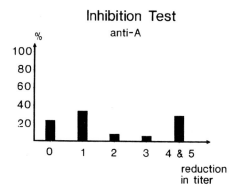

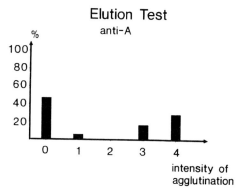

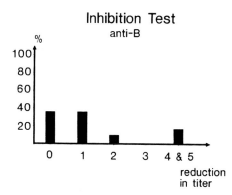

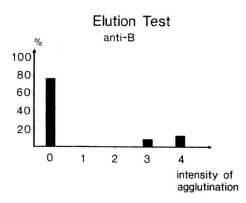

1b

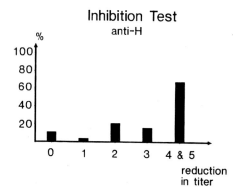

1a

Fig 1a, 1b

1a Results with anti-AB and Ulex
europaeus (inhibition test)

1b Results with anti-A and anti-B
(elution test)

read under microscope (100 X) within a time period of 10-20 min after completion of the elution procedure. Results were read from negative to 4+.

Some experiments were performed with an anti-H (Ulex europaeus) and O-indicator cells, but reliable reactions could not always be obtained.

Results

The results of anti-A- and anti-B-serum of all saliva stains with the inhibition and the absorption-elution test are shown in Fig. 1a and 1b. Furthermore the results with Ulex europaeus are given for the inhibition test. The inhibition test showed much more "weak" reactions (reduction of 2 titers) than the elution test, which gave in nearly every case clear cut results.

In agreement with the standards in our laboratory, it was established that the saliva stain belonged to a secretor of the concerned blood group when a reduction in titer of 3 or more grades was detected in the inhibition test.

The results show, that with the inhibition test seven A-nonsecretors, four B-nonsecretors, five AB-nonsecretors and fifteen O-nonsecretors were detected. With the absorption-elution-test the ABO-blood group of these 16 A-, AB- or B-nonsecretors could, with one exeption (A-nonsecretor in ABO-elution test 2+), correctly be determined. False positive results were not found.

Discussion

The successful grouping of the A- and B-antigens in the saliva stains shows the high sensitivity of the method. The results of this study are in good agreement with the findings of RABL et al. (1990), who were successful in typing A- and B-nonsecretor saliva stains with a method similar to that used in our labaratory. In agreement to our results, RABL et al. were not successful in grouping O-nonsecretor saliva stains, as in some cases they obtained only negative or weak reactions with Ulex europaeus.

The absorption-elution test is now used in routine cases for ABO-grouping of cigarette ends in our laboratory. In most of these cases the antigens A and B of nonsecretor smokers are detectable, whereas the absorption test gives negative results. The elution test described in this paper can be recommended as a supplementary method, when the absorption test is performed without conclusive results. With this method the saliva stains with an age of up to several months could be successfully typed, as the Type I antigens of the ABO-system, present in body fluids, remain stable for quite a long time. The test needs only minute amounts of saliva stain.

Literature

KIND SS, CLEEVELY RM (1969) The Use of Ammoniacal Bloodstain Extracts in ABO Groupings. J For Sci Soc 9: 131-134

LINCOLN PJ (1988) Blood Groups in forensic Science. In: Blood Group Serology, Boorman KE, Dodd BE, Lincoln PJ (Eds), Churchill Livingstone, Edinburgh London Melbourne New York

RABL W, AMBACH E, TRIBUTSCH W (1990) Schnellbestimmung der ABO-Gruppe aus Speichelspuren. Ärztl Lab 36: 124-126

Determination of ORM Phenotypes using gels PRECOTES 4-6[R] and PhastSystem[TM]

M. De La Iglesia, A. Gremo, M.A. Martínez-Aguilera, J.M. Ruíz De La Cuesta

Department of Legal Medicine, pab. 7
Complutense University
28040-Madrid, Spain

INTRODUCTION

Miniaturized IEF gels, run and stained with PhastSystem offer a number of
advantages over conventional procedures. Two gels (24 samples) can be run
simultaneously in the Separation Unit and two others gels can be stained
in the Development Unit at same time. The system is better for proteins
needing immuofixation, because only a minimal amount of expensive antisera
is needed.

In this paper we describe l optimal program for separation of ORM patterns
using miniaturized polyacrylamide gels PRECOTES 4-6 (Boheringer Ingelheim).
This method has potential advantages not only in paternity cases but also
in criminal investigations (e.g. typing a very minute bloodstains).

MATERIALS AND METHODS

Polyacrylamide gels PRECOTES 4-6 (Boheringer Ingelheim) were used. The gel
is cut as a minigel size (5 x 5 cm) and pretreated before IEF with a Solution mixture of Servalyt 4-6 (Serva) and Nonidet P-40 (LKB).

The sera samples were diluted in Neuraminidase (type V, Sigma) and distilled water, and incubation 24 h at 4ºC (overnigth).

ORM phenotypes were carried out in Microprocessor PhastSystem (Pharmacia)
using our IEF method file. Visualization of results was accomplished by
Immuonofixation using anti-ORM (1:1 v/v), incubated 30 minutes at 37ºC
in humid chamber and washing with distilled water for 24 h. The day after
was staining into the Development Unit with CBB staining techinique.

Equipment: Microprocessor PhastSystem[TM]

Minigel: PRECOTES 4-6 (Boheringer Ingelheim)
           cutting slabs for aprppiate size (5 x 5 cm).

Pretreatment minigel: Solution:
                        Sacarose .... 0.6 g
                        Nonidet P-40 (20%) .... 0.25 ml
                        Servalyt 4-6 (Serva) .... 1 ml
                        Deionized water .... 5 ml
Place minigel in a chamber and immerse minigel in this solution 1 h at RT

Advances in Forensic Haemogenetics 4
Edited by Ch. Rittner and P. M. Schneider
© Springer-Verlag Berlin Heidelberg 1992

<u>Pretreatment Samples</u>: Plasme .... 10 μl
                              Neuraminidase 2% .... 80 μl
                              Distilled water .... 80 μl
incubated 24 h at 4ºC.

<u>Sample Application</u>: Applicator 8/ 0.5 (cathode)

<u>METHOD FOR IEF PROGRAM PHASTSYSTEM</u> :

Sample appl.	down	at	1.2		0 vh
Sample appl.	up	at	1.2		20 vh
Extra alarm	to sound	at	1.1		70 vh
Sep. 1.1	2000V	10.0mA	2.0w	15ºC	75 vh
Sep. 1.2	2000V	5.0mA	1.5w	15ºC	20 vh
Sep. 1.3	2000V	25.0mA	4.0w	15ºC	600 vh

<u>METHOD FOR COOMASSIE BLUE STAINING</u>:

Dev. 1.1	IN=1	OUT=1	t=5 min.	T=20ºC
Dev. 1.2	IN=2	OUT=0	t=5 min.	T=50ºC
Dev. 1.3	IN=3	OUT=0	t=15 min.	T=50ºC
Dev. 1.4	IN=2	OUT=0	t=5 min.	T=30ºC

<u>Immunofixation</u>: anti-ORM diluted 1:1 with 0.9% saline
                  Directly on the minigel (2 cm anodal) and cover it
                  Place minigel in a humid chamber for 30 min at 37ºC
                  Rinse minigel in 0.9% saline for 1 day at RT
                  Staining into de Development Unit with CBB R-250

<u>Visualization Patterns</u>: ORM (FF, SS, FS)

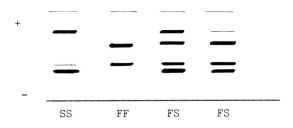

DISCUSSION

Figure 1 shows the separation of patterns ORM clearly delineated on the minigel. An increase in distance between the cathodal and anodal ORM-bands using narrow ranfe (pH 4-6) and soaked it in solution of pretreatment was observed. The advantages of our improved method being good identification bands, less expensive, fast and easy to work with make this technique and desirable for routine paternity and forensic casework. The disadvantages are no differentiation between phenotypes F_1 and F_2. Further studies with our method migth solve this question.

REFERENCES

Carracedo a, et al. (1990) Fast IEF of somr Polymorphic Proteins and Enzymes in Bloodstains using the PhastSystem. In: Advances in Forensic Haemogenetics 3. Springer-Verlag, Berlin-New York, p 251

Montiel MD, Carracedo A, et al. (1988) Comparison between Isoelectric Focusing Methods for the Detection of Orosomocoid Phenotypes. Electrophoresis 9: 268-272

ACKNOWLEDGMENTS

I would like to extend my thanks to the Professors and Scientists of this Department of Legal Medicine (Complutense University, Madrid, Spain) for training since many years ago. Specially thanks to Dr. Ana Gremo and Dr. José María Ruíz De La Cuesta (personal note from Dr. M. De La Iglesia).

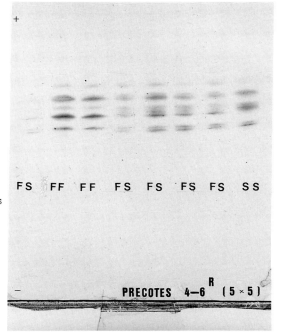

Fig. 1:   ORM Patterns bands
           & PhastSystem

Fast Determination of TF Phenotypes Using Minigel Gradient 4-6.5
Modificated

M. De La Iglesia, M.A. Martínez-Aguilera, A. Gremo, J.M. Ruíz De La Cuesta

Department of Legal Medicine, pab. 7
Complutense University
28040-Madrid, Spain

INTRODUCTION

Application of minigels and PhastSystem to obtain phenotyping results from
blood samples in TF system was proposed by several authors recently. Miniaturized gels disposables commercially offer a number of advantages (no
preparation casting gel), but no usually good resolution pattern bands.
Microprcessor PhastSystem offer potential advantages in routine testing:
faster separations are possible, 24 samples can be run simultaneously (two
minigels), while two others minigels can be stained at the same time.

In this paper we propose a technique wich proved to be reproducible, fast
and easy to perform in routine TF C testing (C_1, C_2, C_3). Advantages and
disadvantages of the method are discussed.

MATERIALS AND METHODS

Conventional minigels gradient 4-6.5 (PhastGel 4-6.5, Pharmacia) and Microprocessor PhastSystem were used. After IEF procedures, a pretreatment of
the minigel with a mixture of Servalyt 5-7 (Serva) and Nonidet P-40 (LKB)
solution was done.

The sera samples were pretreated with Ferrous Ammonium Sulphate solution
and incubated 3 h at 37ºC. TF phenotypes were carried out in Microprocessor PhastSystem using our IEF program method file. Visualization of results
are not needing immunofixation and can be stained in th Development Unit
with Coomassie Brilliant Blue (CBB R-250) staining technique.

Equipment: Microprocessor PhastSystem[TM]

Minigel: PhastGel 4-6.5 (Pharmacia)

Pretreatment Minigel: Solution composed by:
                      Sacarose .... 0.6 g
                      Nonidet P-40 (20%) .... 0.25 ml
                      Servalyt 5-7 (Serva)............... 1 ml
                      Deionized water .... 5 ml
     Place minigel in a chamber and immerse minigel in this solution 1 h at RT

Pretreatment samples: sera .... 10 µl (1:3)
                      Ferrous Ammonium Sulphate (0.3% w/v)..30 µl

in incubation 3h at 37ºC

Advances in Forensic Haemogenetics 4
Edited by Ch. Rittner and P. M. Schneider
© Springer-Verlag Berlin Heidelberg 1992

<u>Samples Application</u>: Applicator 8/1.0 or 12/1.0 (cathode).

<u>METHOD FOR IEF PROGRAM PHASTSYSTEM</u>:

Sample	appl.	down at	1.2				0	vh
Sample	appl.	up at	1.3				0	vh
Extra	alarm	to sound at	1.4				73	vh
Sep.	1.1	2000V	2.0mA	3.5w	15ºC		75	vh
Sep.	1.2	2000V	2.0mA	3.5w	15ºC		20	vh
Sep.	1.3	2000V	2.0mA	3.5w	15ºC		700	vh

<u>METHOD FOR COOMASSIE BLUE STAINING</u>:

Dev.	1.1	IN=1	OUT=1	t=5 min	T=20ºC
Dev.	1.2	IN=2	OUT=0	t=5 min	T=50ºC
Dev.	1.3	IN=3	OUT=0	t=15 min	T=50ºC
Dev.	1.4	IN=2	OUT=0	t=5 min	T=30ºC

<u>Visualization Patterns</u>: TF C (C_1, C_2, C_3)

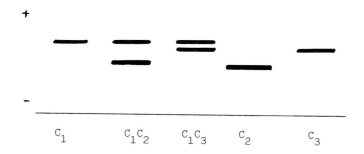

DISCUSSION

Figure 1 shows the separation of several TF C phenotypes. Immerse minigel
in a Solution composed with Servalyt 5-7 and Nonidet P-40 offer results
comparable to those described using IEF gel with chemicals spacers. An increase in distance between the cathodal and anodal bands for the minigels
using pretreatment solution was observed, specially for detection TF C_3
band.

The advantages of this technique being less expensive, fast procedure, good results and easy to work with make this improved method, highly desirable for routine paternity, population genetics, significant associations with diseases, and forensic practice.

REFERENCES

Carracedo A, and cols. (1990) Fast IEF of some Polymorphic Proteins and Enzymes in Bloodstains Using the PhastSystem. In: Advances in Forensic Haemogenetics 3. Springer-Verlag, Berlin-New york, p 251

Gill P, and cols. (1984) Separation of some Polymorphic Protein Systems of Forensic Significance by Isoelectric Focusing with Separators. Electrophoresis ´84: 94-97

Kamboh MI, Ferrell RE (1987) Human Transferrin Polymorphism. Hum. Hered. 37: 65-81

Pascali V, Ranalletta D (1982) Improved Typing of Human Serum Transferrin by Isoelectric Focusing on Ultrathin Layer Polyacrylamide Slab Gels. Hum. Genet. 61: 39-41

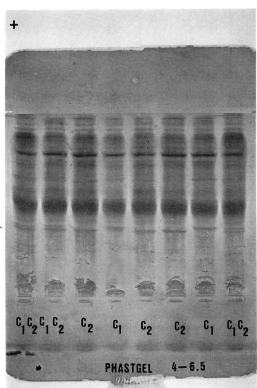

FIG. 1: TF C Patterns bands and PhastSystem

THE USE OF MICROTITER PLATES AND THE APPARATUS DYNATECH FOR
AUTOMATION OF THE ROUTINE DETERMINATION OF ABO-GROUP FROM BODY
FLUIDS (OR STAINS) AND HAIR

P. Makovec, M. Laupy, M. Brezina

Institute of Criminalistic
182 00 PRAGUE 82, P.O.Box 16, CZECHOSLOVAKIA

Introduction

        The routine analysis of ABO-groups continues to be one
of the basic method of forensic serology examination but there
exists a variety of used modifications. We describe a method with
modified DYNATECH apparatus for time and material saving
examination of large series of samples by absorption-elution and
absorption-inhibition methods.

Absorption-elution method

        The important part of the method is perfect washing of
superfluous diagnostic antiserum from cotton segments soaked by
the examined biological material. This time consuming part was
solved by means apparatus ULTRAWASH II with interchangeable head
with 96 pairs of aspirating and dispensing jets. For washing of
segments it is necessary to cover aspirating jets by suitable net
(100 um). There is possible to program number of washing cycles,
the intensity of aspiration and infusion and the amount of
washing fluid.

        The pressured segments of hair (apr. 5 - 8 mm) are
collected (2 - 3 pieces together) by celluloid partially
dissolved by acetone on apex.

        One of the advantages of this modification is the fact
that the samples remain from the very beginning (ensuring of
traces) to the end of operation (evaluation of agglutination) in
the same wells of microtiter plate and the danger of mistaking
of samples is reduced.

        After releasing of the thermolabile binding of absorbed
antibodies in the elution part of the method (20 minutes - 56°C)
the cotton segments are removed and the suspension of testing
erythrocytes is dropped to eluate. The agglutination is read
after centrifugation.

        In regard to the individual character of traces it is
not possible to use the shaker but to resuspend agglutinates
individually in each well of microplate under direct control by
stereomicroscope. The agglutinates are resuspended by air flow
directed to the individual wells.

Absorption-inhibition method

        The use of connected apparatus AUTODILUTER II and
dispenser SRD II (modern version AUTODILUTER III and SRD III)

allows a fast and exact dilution of tested sera to desired degree of dilution. The transport and mixing of sera in dilution rows of microplate is provided by means of Takatsy crowns (25 and 50 ul). It is possible to choose the volume of dispensed buffered saline so that agglutination in dilution row of tested serum continually decreased from +++ to -.

Unlike the absorption-elution method shaker can be used to resuspendation of agglutinates.

The evaluation of agglutination by apparatus MR 7000

The former reader MR 700 valued agglutination measuring the optical density in the centre of well after slopping whole apparatus.

Modern type MR 7000 with agglutination program cartridge can evaluate as many as 32 values of optical density measured in diameter of each well on microplate. The obtained data are processed in four parameters A, B, C and D, which can form any equation or rule. The producer recommends for evaluation of agglutinates the equation A x B or A x B / C. We prefer the evaluation of parameter B after determination of suitable limits.

The results are printed in symbols +, ? and -. The apparatus MR 7000 is equipped by time-programmed shaker (0 - 59 sec.).

The microtiter plate is moved on on unclosed line and this allows the addition other apparatus. DYNATECH offers the temperate store and washing units. This set can be used as completely automatized equipment, where microplate with samples is moved on among apparatus, that provide the examination and printing documentation. The recommended connection of MR 7000 to PC enlarge the possibility of intervention to the programmes and documentation of results.

PI, C2, GC, ATIII, PLG Typing in Bloodstains by Hybrid Isoelectric Focusing (HIEF)

I. Muñoz; A. Carracedo; L. Concheiro; V.L. Pascali*

Institute of Legal Medicine, Santiago de Compostela, Galicia, Spain

INTRODUCTION

Immobilized pH gradients (IPG) show a number of advantages over IEF with carrier ampholytes (CA). Its power of resolution is 10 times greater, any pH gradient can be created, sample of up to 10 times greater can be loaded and cathodic drift is eliminated (Righetti et al. 1988). Nevertheless, previous experience with immobilized pH gradients gels has shown them to be insensitive compared to Ampholine gels (Altland et al. 1986).This is a great inconvenience for the detection of polymorphism in minute seminal and bloodstains. Incorporating CA into IPG gels (HIEF) produces improvement of sensitivity because the CA improves the conductivity and prevents the precipitation of protein before separation can be achieved (Altland et al. 1987).

Protein markers *alpha 1-antitrypsine (PI), plasminogen (PLG), Group Specific Component (GC), antithrombine III* (ATIII) and *complement component C2* (C2) are analyzed in series of bloodstains to determinate the usefulness of the hybrid isoelectric focusing (HIEF) for typing electrophoretic markers for forensic material.

MATERIAL AND METHODS

Samples: 30 µL bloodstains (2 weeks old) on cotton cloth.
Bloodstain extraction: 30 uL 0,05 M DTT and doubling dilutions were prepared.
Samples treatment: 10 uL bloodstain extracts were treated with neuraminidase (1 units/mL) for at least 12 h at 4 °C for PLG and ATIII typing.
HIEF: *IPG* gels were cast according to Bjellqvist et al. (1982) on a GelBond PAG films with a gel dimensions of 260 x 100 x 0.5 mm.

FORMATION OF IMMOBILIZED pH GRADIENTS

Composition of the acidic and basic components of the gradient mixer (see * for specific *immobilines* volumes)

Basic light	mL	Acidic dense	mL
Acrylamide (29.1%) + bis-acrylamide (0.9%)	1.25	Acrylamide + bis-acrylamide 1.25	
Glycerol 87%	0.00	Glycerol	2.10
H2O	X	H2O	Y
Total volume	7.5	Total volume	7.50
TEMED (10 mL%)	0.01	TEMED	0.01
Ammonium persulfate (10 g%)	0.01	Ammonium perfulfate	0.01

*Institute of Legal Medicine, Universita Cattolica del S. Cuore, Roma, Italy

* VOLUME (ul) 0.2 M *IMMOBILINE* pK

pK		Acidic dense solut				Basic light solution		
	3.6	4.6	6.2	9.3	3.6	4.6	6.2	9.3
pH 4.1-5.1		356.5		88.5		401.5		329.5
pH 4.2-4.8		377		121.5		373		292
pH 4.5-5.4		367.6		174.3		566.5		510.5
pH 5.7-6.7	299		377.5		80.5		372.5	
pH 5.4-6.4	449.5		508.5		121		314	
pH 5.5-6.5	387.5		451.5		104.5		384	

HIEF GEL CASTING

Polymerization: 15 min room temperature + 1h 50 °C

Washing: 6 x 10 min with distilled water + 1 x 30 min with 2% Glycerol

Drying

Rehydration (mold method) more than 1 h
IPG 4.1-5.1 :2% Ampholine pH 4-6
IPG 4.2-4.8: 2% Ampholine pH 4-6
IPG 4.5-5.4: 1.5% Pharmalyte pH 4.5-5.4
IPG 5.7-6.7: 2% Ampholine pH 5-7
IPG 5.4-6.4: 1% Ampholine pH 5-7
IPG 5.5-6.5: 1% Ampholine pH 5-7

RUNNING CONDITIONS AND STAINING METHODS

Electrode solutions: + 10 mM glutamic acid. - 10 mM NaOH

Sample application: cathode (PI, GC, ATIII, C2), anode (PLG)

Focusing conditions:
   HIEF 4.2-4.8: 7 W, 4 mA, 3500 V for 5 h
   HIEF 4.5-5.4: 7 W, 4 mA, 3500 V for 3 h
   HIEF 4.1-5.1; 5.7-6.7; 5.5-6.5 and 5.4-6.4: 7 W, 4 mA, 3000 V for 3 h

Coomassie Brilliant Blue R-250 for PI, fixation with Sulfosalicylic acid and stained with Coomassie Brilliant Blue R-250 and immunoprinting with cellulose acetate strips soaked with monospecific *GC*-antiserum and stained with Coomassie Brilliant Blue R-250 [5] for GC, immunofixation with specific antisera and stained with CBB R-250 or silver staining methods for PLG, ATIII and C2.

RESULTS AND DISCUSSION

   PIM subtypes obtained with *HIEF* are much more distinguishable by IPGs than by IEF with CA, since the pH range can be considerably reduced. Furthermore, bands are sharper and straighter using *IPGs*, particularly with contaminated bloodstains. Other additional advantages are that *IPGs* are not sensitive to salts, and much more sample can be loaded in *IPGs*. *IPGs* gave good results to the final extract solution of) 1:64 when 10 uL were loaded on the sample paper (equivalent   to   0.15   uL   of liquid blood). The sensitivity is similar to IEF with conventional CA and superior to IPG gels without rehydration with CA. This may be due to the solubilizing properties of CA. Although the pH range 4.2-4.8 improved the resolution of PI M subtypes, some PI variants can be lost, and so we usually use, for routine case work, a pH range 4.1-5.1, which partially covers all variants, allowing a clear identification of subtypes Pi M1, M2, M3, and M5.

GC subtypes are much better distinguishable by *HIEF* than by IEF with CA since pH range can be considerably reduced. Bands are sharper and straighter using *HIEF* particularly with contaminated bloodstains. *HIEF* gave good results to the final extract solution of 1:32.

PLG phenotypes are observed by *HIEF* only after immunofixation and CBB or silver staining methods, bands are sharper compared with IEF with CA, and *HIEF* improved the resolution of PLG patterns.

The use of immunofixation and silver staining methods following *HIEF* means that ATIII phenotypes can be detected in 5 uL of two week-old bloodstains extracted with distilled water without concentration procedures.

For C2, only 3 day-old bloodstains can be detected due to activation but phenotypes are clearly distinguished in more recent bloodstains and *HIEF* gave good results to the final extract solution of 1:8 when 10 uL were loaded on the paper.

In conclusion we recommend the routine use of *HIEF* for the detection of these proteins and enzymes on forensic casework because it is clearly the method of choice for the detection of these polymorphic proteins in bloodstains since phenotypes are better distinguished, much more sample can be loaded, bands are straighter and sharper (even with contaminants) and the sensitivity is similar to IEF with CA.

REFERENCES

Altland K, Eckardstein A, Banzhoff A, Wagner M, Rossmann U (1987) Hybrid isoelectric focusing: Adsorption of proteins onto immobilized pH gradient matrices and desorption by carrier ampholytes. Electrophoresis 8:52-62

Altland K, Hackler R, Rossmann U (1986) Avoiding liquid exudation on the surface of rehydrated gels used for hybrid isoelectric focusing in carrier ampholyte supplemented immobilized pH gradients. Electrophoresis 7:251-259

Bjellqvist B, Ek K, Righetti PG, Gianazza E, Görg A, Westermeier R, Postel W (1982) Isoelectric focusing in immobilized pH gradients: Principle. methodology and some applications. J Biochem Biophis Methods 6:317-339

Constans J, Cleve H (1988) Identification of group specific component/vitamin D-binding protein (GC/DBP) mutants by isoelectric focusing in immobilized pH gradients. Electrophoresis 9:599-602

Righetti PG, Chiari M, Gelfi C (1988) Immobilized pH gradients: Effect of salts, added carrier ampholytes and voltage gradients on protein patterns. Electrophoresis 9:65-73

4.3   Practical Application

Parentage Testing Using DBP Subtyping in South African (SA)
Populations

W. Petersen, T. Schlaphoff, R. Martell and E. du Toit

Provincial Laboratory for Tissue Immunology, Cape Town, South
Africa

INTRODUCTION

The vitamin D binding protein (DBP) of human plasma, also
referred to as group specific component (GC), was first
described by Hirschfeld in 1959. One of its major functions is
to act as a transport protein for vitamin D-3 and its naturally
occurring derivatives.

Family studies have confirmed that the DBP phenotypes are
determined by a pair of autosomal co-dominant alleles. By
using an isoelectric focusing (IEF) subtyping technique
Constans and Viau (1977), distinguished six common phenotypes,
determined by 3 alleles, namely DBP*1S, DBP*1F and DBP*2.
Using various techniques, more than 120 allelic variants of the
DBP system have been identified to date.

MATERIALS AND METHODS

This study analysed the results of serum samples collected from
238 SA Caucasoids, 515 Cape Coloureds and 465 SA Negroes
(Xhosa), all of whom were the parents in disputed paternity
cases. Samples were frozen at -70°C or -20°C until used.

The technique involved IEF subtyping in ultrathin
polyacrylamide gel using a narrow ampholyte range pH 4.5-5.4.
Visualisation of the bands was by immunofixation, using a
monospecific antiserum on cellulose acetate followed by
staining with Coomassie Brilliant Blue. An agarose gel using a
barbital buffer was used to confirm the DBP*AM and DBP*AB
variants. For the purpose of paternity testing the old
nomenclature, DBP*AM and DBP*AB, was used, since it was found
unneccessary to further identify them (personal correspondence,
Cleve, H).

The frequencies of the DBP alleles were determined by direct
counting. The power of exclusion (PE) was calculated by
dividing the number of cases with a DBP exclusion by the total
number of excluded cases, using 14 genetic systems, namely,
HLA, ABO, RH, MNSs, FY, KEL, ACP1, ESD, PGM1(IEF), CA2, GLO1,

Advances in Forensic Haemogenetics 4
Edited by Ch. Rittner and P. M. Schneider
© Springer-Verlag Berlin Heidelberg 1992

DBP(IEF), HP and BF. The cumulative power of exclusion (CPE) using the 14 genetic systems was established by using the formula:

$$CPE = 1-(1-PE_1)(1-PE_2)...(1-PE_n).$$

RESULTS

Table 1. Observed and expected DBP phenotype frequencies

Pheno-types	SA Caucasoids			Cape Coloureds			SA Negroes (Xhosa)		
	Obs.	Exp.	x^2	Obs.	Exp.	x^2	Obs.	Exp.	x^2
1S	68	68.84	0.01	44	39.72	0.58	0	2.56	2.56
1F	10	7.24	1.05	153	142.06	0.84	312	313.81	0.01
2	18	19.14	0.07	17	13.27	1.05	3	1.69	1.02
AM	0	0	0	0	0.26	0.26	0	0.26	0.26
AB	0	0	0	0	0.02	0.02	0	0.11	0.11
Var	0	0	0	0	0.04	0.04	0	0.01	0.01
1S-1F	42	44.65	0.11	140	150.22	0.70	60	56.69	0.19
2-1S	78	72.60	0.40	50	45.82	0.38	3	4.15	0.32
1S-AM	0	0	0	4	6.38	0.89	4	1.63	1.45
1S-AB	0	0	0	1	1.66	0.26	1	1.04	0
1S-Var	0	1.08	1.08	3	2.52	0.09	1	0.37	1.07
2-1F	20	23.54	0.53	75	86.66	1.57	46	45.99	0.
1F-AM	0	0	0	14	12.06	0.31	17	18.03	0.06
1F-AB	0	0	0	3	3.14	0.01	13	11.54	0.19
1F-Var	1	0.35	1.21	3	4.76	0.65	4	4.13	0.00
2-AM	0	0	0	3	3.68	0.13	1	1.32	0.08
2-AB	0	0	0	2	0.96	1.13	0	0.85	0.85
2-Var	1	0.57	0.32	1	1.45	0.14	0	0.30	0.30
1F-AM	0	0	0	0	0.13	0.13	0	0.33	0.33
AM-Var	0	0	0	2	0.20	0.20	0	0.12	0.12
AB-Var	0	0	0	0	0.05	0.05	0	0.08	0.08
Total	238	238.01	4.78	515	515.06	9.43	465	465.01	9.01

Table 1 shows the observed and expected DBP phenotype frequencies in the three populations studied. As shown in Table 2 DBP*1S is more common in the SA Caucasoids and DBP*1F is more common in the SA Negroes (Xhosa). The Cape Coloureds, who are of mixed ancestry, have DBP allele frequencies which are intermediate between those of the SA Caucasoids and SA Negroes. According to this study, some of the DBP alleles are population specific, for example the DBP*AM and DBP*AB alleles appear to be Negroid genes. These populations are in Hardy-Weinberg equilibrium, as estimated from these gene frequencies.

Table 2.   Distribution of DBP gene frequencies

	SA Caucasoids n = 238	Cape Coloureds n = 515	SA Negroes (Xhosa) n = 465
1S	0.5378	0.2777	0.0742
1F	0.1744	0.5252	0.8215
2	0.2836	0.1602	0.0602
AM	0.0	0.0223	0.0236
AB	0.0	0.0058	0.0151
variants	0.0042	0.0088	0.0054

The results in Table 3 indicate the usefulness of including DBP subtyping by IEF, in paternity testing, especially in the Cape Coloureds.

Table 3.   Power of exclusion (PE) using the DBP system

Exclusions	SA Caucasoids	Cape Coloureds	SA Negroes (Xhosa)
DBP	6	37	19
Total[*]	28	115	122
PE%	21.4	32.2	15.6

*using 14 genetic systems.

CONCLUSION

Vitamin D binding protein subtyped by isoelectric focusing, is useful in conjunction with other genetic systems for excluding a falsely accused father of parentage especially in the Cape Coloured population.

REFERENCES

Constans J and Viau M (1977) Group-specific component: evidence for two subtypes of the Gc1 gene.   Science 198:1070-1071
Hirschfeld J (1959) Immuno-electrophoretic demonstration of qualitative differences in human sera and their relation to the haptoglobins.   Acta Pathol Microbiol Scand 47:160-168

ISO-ELECTRIC FOCUSING STUDY OF SERUM PROTEINS (GC, TF, PI AND ORM) IN FOUR ENDOGAMOUS GROUPS OF MAHARASHTRA, WESTERN INDIA: APPLICATION IN PATERNITY TESTING

S.S. MASTANA[1], V. RAY[2], S.S. BHATTACHARYA[3] & S.S. PAPIHA[3]

1. DEPARTMENT OF HUMAN SCIENCES, LOUGHBOROUGH UNIVERSITY OF TECHNOLOGY, LOUGHBOROUGH, UK
2. KEM HOSPITAL BLOOD BANK, BOMBAY, INDIA
3. DEPARTMENT OF HUMAN GENETICS, SCHOOL OF PATHOLOGICAL SCIENCES, NEWCASTLE UNIVERSITY, NEWCASTLE UPON TYNE, UK

INTRODUCTION

Iso-electric focusing (IEF) has become an important and powerful technique to discriminate genetic variability for several single gene systems. For example, Transferrin system was found to be monomorphic in most populations with starch gel electrophoresis, but analysis with IEF have clearly shown further microheterogeneity in this system, which makes TF a useful marker for population genetics and paternity determination. Several other serum protein systems HP, PI, GC and BF have shown similar microheterogeneity.

Considerable genetic diversity which exists in human populations has its origins due to different ecological environments, settlements, mating and migration patterns. So it has become increasingly important to collect genetic data on various population groups of the world for its possible use in studies in human biology. The essential knowledge about the variation of IEF polymorphisms in different populations of the third world is still limited. In this investigation we have analysed four serum proteins (GC, PI, TF and ORM) by IEF, in four endogamous groups from the state of Maharashtra, Western India. Caste is an important element which influences the structure of Indian populations, it is therefore important to investigate various genetic polymorphisms in different caste groups to study genetic differentiation in the populations of the Indian subcontinent. Several population groups from India have migrated to the West and are now permanently settled in Europe, United States and Canada. More and more cases are being encountered in which the immigrant individuals are involved in paternity disputes. The data on highly polymorphic genetic systems in immigrant groups is warranted to provide an accurate probability of exclusion.

MATERIALS AND METHODS

Four endogamous groups (BRAHMIN, MARATHA, GUJURATI & PARSEE) from Maharashtra were sampled in Bombay, India. These groups form the major part of population of Maharashtra. A battery of genetic markers have been analysed for these groups and the results will be discussed elsewhere. In this presentation, we report results of GC, TF and PI subtypes and ORM1 and ORM2 phenotypes analysed by IEF technique. Standard methods for IEF were followed as described by Papiha et al (1987); Papiha et al (1989); Constans et al (1980) and Yuasa et al (1986), with minor modifications for better resolution. The allele frequencies were calculated using Maximum Likelihood methods ad population affinities were evaluated by R Matrix (Harpending and Jenkins, 1973). Heterozygosity was estimated from allele frequencies. The theoretical average Probability of Exclusion (PE) was calculated as given by Garber and Morris (1983).

RESULTS AND DISCUSSION

The allele frequencies of various systems are given in Table 1. For all systems, populations were in Hardy Weinberg Equilibrium. ORM2 locus was monomorphic in all populations. Pair-wise comparisons between different populations showed marked allele frequency differences, however, the allele frequencies are well within the gene frequency range already reported from the Indian region. The overall heterogeneity amongst four populations for several alleles is also statistically significant (Table 1). These marked differences are likely to be due to their population structure. R (Kinship) matrix calculated from gene frequency data suggest the least relationship of Parsees (negative values) with any of the other populations studies (Table 2). Two dimensional dendrogram representation of the four populations show distinct position of Parsee and Gujurati while the two caste groups Brahmin and Maratha cluster together (Fig. 1).

Heterozygosity estimated from gene frequencies shows a marked increase in GC, PI, and TF systems when analysed with IEF technique. Mean IEF heterozygosity ($\bar{H}$) is more than doubled (range 40-48%) compared to mean heterozygosity estimate calculated by using conventional technique (range 19-20).

The PE value for each system calculated from the gene frequencies using conventional electrophoresis and IEF are given in Table 3. IEF technique provides better PE values for most of the systems. These PE estimates are

Advances in Forensic Haemogenetics 4
Edited by Ch. Rittner and P. M. Schneider
© Springer-Verlag Berlin Heidelberg 1992

approximately one to twenty times higher than the conventional electrophoresis values. There is a marked difference in PE estimates in different populations indicating that it would be wrong to use the gene frequency data on any one or pooled Indian population for calculation of Paternity Index. Chakraborty and Roychoudhry (1975) reported exclusion levels for a number of genetic systems on the basis of 4 regional populations of India, but they failed to take into account the variation within the sub-populations of the Indian subcontinent. The Indian populations also differ from English population with respect to gene frequencies and PE estimates, though differences are statistically non significant.

The relative usefulness of a genetic marker in paternity dispute analysis depends upon the level of its polymorphism. These four serum proteins can be used in routine paternity work as their genetics have been formally worked out and they provide better cumulative probability of exclusion (CPE), which averages around 60%. The individual PE values reported here are better than many blood groups and serum proteins listed by Chakraborty et al (1974).

In conclusion, serum protein analysis by IEF showed high level of heterozygosity and are very informative to study the genetic differentiation in various sub-populations It is imperative that genetic information should be collected from a number of populations, especially from the third world countries as well as the immigrant populations in the West to provide better understanding of gene frequency variation and their usefulness in paternity and forensic work.

REFERENCES

Chakraborty R, Roychoudhry AK (1975). Paternity exclusion by genetic markers in Indian populations. Ind J Med Res 63: 162-169

Chakraborty R, Shaw MW, Schull, WJ (1974). Exclusion of paternity: The current state of the art. Am Hum Genet 26: 477-488

Constant J, Kühnl P, Viau M, Spielmann W (1980). A new procedure for the determination of tranferrin (TFC) subtypes by isoelectric focusing: existence of two additional alleles, TF4 and TF5. Hum Genet 55: 111-114

Harpending H C, Jenkins T (1973). Genetic distance among southern African populations. In: Crawford MH and Workman PL (eds), Methods and Theories of anthropological genetics. University of New Mexico Press, pp 177-199

Graber RA, Morris JW (1983). General equations for Average power of exclusion for genetic systems of n codominant allele in one parent and no parent cases of disputed parentage. In: Walker RH (ed), Inclusion probabilities in parentage testing. Am Ass Blood Banks. Arlington (Virg) pp 277-280

Papiha SS, White I, Roberts DF (1983). Some genetic implications of isoelectric focusing of human red cell phosphoglucomutase (PGM1) and serum protein group specific component (GC). Genetic diversity of the populations of Himachal Pradesh, India. Hum Genet 63: 67-72

Papiha SS, Pal B, Walker D, Mangion P, Hossain MA (1989). Alpha 1 antitrypsin (PI) phenotypes in two rheumatic diseases: a reappraisal of the association of PI subtypes in rheumatoid arthritis. Ann Rheu Dis 48: 48-52

Yuasa I, Umsetu K, Suenaga K, Robinet-Levy M (1986). Orosomucoid (ORM) typing by isolelectric focusing: evidence for two structural loci ORM1 and ORM2. Hum Genet 74: 160-161

Table 1. Subtype Allele frequencies in four endogamous groups

SYSTEM/ ALLELE		BRAHMIN 119	MARATHA 147	GUJURATI 84	PARSEE 53	HETERO-GENEITY χ^2
GC	1S	0.680±0.031	0.615±0.029	0.556±0.039	0.686±0.046	8.20*
	1F	0.092±0.019	0.108±0.018	0.130±0.036	0.078±0.027	2.27
	2	0.228±0.028	0.227±0.026	0.314±0.036	0.236±0.042	4.43
PI						
	M1	0.640±0.032	0.741±0.026	0.671±0.037	0.651±0.046	7.06
	M2	0.259±0.029	0.143±0.021	0.183±0.030	0.236±0.041	11.83*
	M3	0.101±0.020	0.115±0.019	0.146±0.028	0.113±0.031	2.00
TF	C1	0.789±0.027	0.874±0.020	0.825±0.031	0.710±0.058	12.09*
	C2	0.158±0.024	0.085±0.017	0.110±0.025	0.258±0.056	15.98*
	C3	0.039±0.013	0.041±0.012	0.052±0.018	0.016±0.016	1.42
	D	0.014±0.008	-----	0.013±0.009	0.016±0.016	3.64
ORM1						
	1	0.681±0.031	0.715±0.027	0.804±0.031	0.696±0.045	4.62
	2	0.310±0.030	0.275±0.010	0.196±0.031	0.304±0.045	4.62
	3	0.009±0.006	0.010±0.006	-----	-----	

*Significant at 5% level.

Table 2. R matrix of 4 Maharashtrian populations

1. BRAHMIN	0.006			
2. MARATHA	0.001	0.007		
3. GUJARATI	-0.002	0.001	0.008	
4. PARSEE	-0.005	-0.008	-0.007	0.019
	1	2	3	4

Fig. 1. Dendogram of four populations

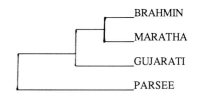

Table 3. Average Probability of Exclusion (PE)

SYSTEM	BRAHMIN		MARATHA		GUJURATI		PARSEE		ENGLISH	
	CON.	IEF	CON.	IEF	CON.	IEF	CON.	IEF	CON.	IEF
GC	0.145	0.243	0.160	0.273	0.169	0.299	0.147	0.234	0.162	0.303
PI	NI	0.261	NI	0.256	NI	0.266	NI	0.263	0.058	0.279
TF	0.012	0.176	NI	0.156	0.012	0.159	0.016	0.196	0.003	0.173
ORM	NI	0.170	NI	0.162	NI	0.133	NI	0.170	NT	NT
Cumulative PE	0.155	0.612	0.160	0.599	0.179	0.623	0.161	0.623	0.212	0.584

CON. - CONVENTIONAL   NI - NOT INFORMATIVE   NT - NOT TESTED

PGM1 SYSTEM: A RARE ALLELE AND AN INTRAGENIC RECOMBINATION IN TWO CASES OF DISPUTED PATERNITY

M. L. Pontes, M. F. Pinheiro, A. C. Gomes

Medico-Legal Institute of Oporto
Jardim Carrilho Videira
4000 PORTO, PORTUGAL

INTRODUCTION

The PGM1 system polymorphism was first studied by Spencer et al in 1964. There are at least 30 rare variants already described (Dykes and Polesky 1981; Bertrams et al 1988). In cases of disputed paternity, unexplained maternity and single paternity exclusions have been observed (Martin 1981; Wetterling 1986). Some of these can be explained by the occurrence of a null allele (Brinkmann et al in 1973; Raczek 1990). Carter et al (1979) proposed a phylogeny theory of the PGM1 locus that was developed by Takahashi et al (1982) that explains the remain exclusions. This theory has been verified since 1988, namely by Wetterling. In this report we have found a maternity exclusion corresponding to an intragenic recombination between one of the only genotypes capable of generating recombinant gametes (1B2A) carried by the mother. This study was completed by RFLP analysis. We also have found a rare allele, considered here as W12.

MATERIALS AND METHODS

Isoelectric Focusing (PAGIF)

Blood samples from 378 trios, involved in paternity cases during 1990 and the first 7 months of 1991, were collected in heparinized tubes and stored at -20ºC until tested (a few weeks later). Haemolysates were obtained by freezing and thawing and by adding an equal volume of 0.05 $\underline{M}$ dithiotreitol (DTT). The PGM1 phenotype determinations were carried out by isoelectric focusing. The PGM1 phenotypes were visualized by an agar overlay method described by Sutton and Burgess (1978). Additionally, blood samples were examined in other conventional markers including HLA.

RFLP Analysis

From the 199 trios studied during 1990, 19 were analysed using RFLP's. Blood samples were collected in EDTA-K3 tubes. DNA was isolated by haemolysis of erythrocytes and digestion in Proteinase K. Extraction was carried out using phenol (Brinkmann 1991). High molecular weight DNA samples were digested with restriction enzyme Pst I. Restriction fragments were separated in a 1.2% agarose gel(Gomes et al1991). Following electrophoresis DNA was transfered to Hybond-N membranes (Amersham), by southern blotting.

Advances in Forensic Haemogenetics 4
Edited by Ch. Rittner and P. M. Schneider
© Springer-Verlag Berlin Heidelberg 1992

The probe 3'HVR (Kindly donated by Dr. Carracedo, Faculty of Medicine, University of Santiago de Compostela, Spain), was labelled with 32P using the multiprime method (Multiprime Labelling System, Amersham). Following hybridization, radioactive bands were visualized by auto radiography carried out at -70ºC, in x-ray film, 1-4 days with intensifying screens.

RESULTS AND DISCUSSION

During 1990 and 1991, 378 trios were typed for various systems, including PGM1. In one case we have found a mother-child imcompatibility only by PGM1, according to the first rule of heredity. This result was verified at least three times with identical results by PAGIF "Fig. 1". The phenotypes presented by the putative father, the mother and the child are 1A2B, 1B2A and 2B, respectively. Many maternity exclusions and isolated paternity exclusions have been reported within the PGM1 system in other populations (Martin 1981; Bertrams et al 1988; Wetterling 1988). This is in agreement with an intragenic recombination theory developed by Takahashi et al (1982) and recently verified by Wetterling (1990). In order to complete the study of this family, we have made RFLP analysis. We used the probe 3'HVR labelled with 32P "Fig. 2". This is a preliminary study, but it shows that one of te child's band is inherited from the alleged father and other from the mother.

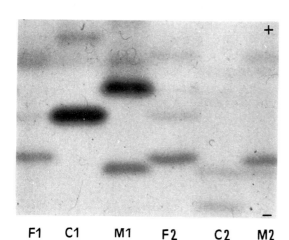

Fig. 1. PGM1 phenotyping of two paternity trios (F-father; C-child; M-mother) on polyacrylamide gel by isoelectric focusing. From left to right: 1A2B (F1); 2B (C1); 1B2A (M1); 1A2B (F2); 1BW12 (C2); 1A1B (M2)

F1   C1   M1   F2   C2   M2

Here we also report a case of a paternity exclusion where there is a rare allele involved, located cathodically to allele 1B "Fig. 1", that we think is allele W12 (personal information given to us by Dr. Weidinger). There have been reported many rare variants in the PGM1 system (Dykes and Polesky 1981; Lin-Chu et al 1991), but it was not possible to compare this rare allele with others in order to confirm if it really corresponds to W12. Further analysis of this allele is needed.

Kb

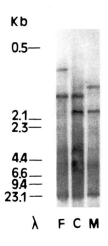

0.5—

2.1—
2.3—

4.4—
6.6—
9.4—
23.1—

λ **F C M**

Fig. 2. Auto radiogram of DNA samples from 1 paternity trio, digested to completion with the enzyme Pst I and hibridized with the probe 3'HVR labelled with 32P (λ=molecular weight marker digested with Hind III; F=father; C=child; M=mother)

REFERENCES

Bertrams J, Weber W, Höher PG (1986) On the significance of isolated exclusions in the PGM1 subtype system. In: Advances in Forensic Haemogenetics 2, Springer-Verlag, Berlin Heidelberg

Brinkmann B, Rand S and Wiegand P (1991) Population data of RFLP's using selected single- and multi-locus systems. J Leg Med 104:81-86

Carter ND, West CM, Enes E, Parkin B, Marshall WH (1979) Phosphoglucomutase polymorphism detected by isoelectric focusing: gene frequencies, evolution and linkage. Ann Hum Biol 6:221-230

Dykes DD and Polesky HF (1981) Comparison of rare PGM1 variants by isoelectric focusing and conventional electrophoresis: Identification of five new variants. Electrophoresis 2, 323-326

Gomes AC, Sunkel C, Pinheiro MF, Carracedo A (1991) Paternity study: RFLP analysis and traditional tests. In: Actas of the XVth Congress of the International Academy of Legal Medicine and Social Medicine, Zaragoza

Lin-Chu M, Loo JH, Hayward MA (1991) Phosphoglucomutase-1 polymorphism among chinese in Taiwan. Hum Hered 41:22-25

Martin W (1981) Red cell enzyme groups in paternity testing. In: Lectures 9th International Congress of the Society for Forensic Haemogenetics, Bern, p 221

Raczek E (1990) Demonstration of incompatible Mother-Child pairs in PGM1 and Duffy systems in a three generation family from the upper Silesia (Poland). Forensic Science International 44:143-149

Sutton IG and Burgess R (1978) Genetic evidence for four common alleles at the PGM locus detectable by IEF. Vox Sang 34:97-103

Takahashi N, Neel J, Satoh C, Nishizaki J, Masunari N (1982) A philogeny for the principal alleles of the human phosphoglucomutase-1-locus. Proc Nat Acad Sci USA 79:6636-6640

Wetterling G (1988) Discrepancy between gene and protein products within PGM1 system shown by improved resolution on immobiline gels. In: Advances in Forensic Haemogenetics 2, Springer-Verlag, Berlin Heidelberg

Wetterling G (1990) Intragenic recombination within the PGM1 locus. In: Advances in Forensic Haemogenetics 3, Springer-Verlag, Berlin Heidelberg

Genetic markers (HP, TF, GC and PI) in two Polish population samples
Preliminary report

H. Walter, H. Danker-Hopfe, M. Lemmermann and M. Lorenz

Dept. of Human Biology, University of Bremen, D-2800 Bremen 33, Germany

INTRODUCTION

Our knowledge on the variability of genetic serum protein markers (HP,TF,GC, PI) in Central and East European populations is so far rather limited. We therefore started several research projects in CSFR (especially in Slovakia), in East Germany (especially in Thuringia: Jena, Erfurt, Suhl) and in Poland. The results of our studies in two population samples from this country – Poles from Central Poland and Kashubes from Northern Poland – are presented here. They are compared with those obtained in some populations samples from Hungary and Slovakia in order to estimate the extent of variation of these genetic markers among Central and East European populations.

MATERIALS AND METHODS

Serum samples of 198 unrelated male and female Poles from Ostrów Wielkopolski (Central Poland) and 228 Kashubes from Kościerzyna (Northern Poland) have been collected by us in 1990 at the blood transfusion centers of these two places. The serum samples were transported deep-frozen to Bremen, where the HP typing, and the TF, GC and PI sub-typings were done.

RESULTS AND DISCUSSION

Observed and expected phenotype frequencies do not differ significantly so that genetic equilibrium can be assumed for all the four polymorphic systems under study. The allele frequencies runs as follows:

	Poles	Kashubes
n	196	225
HP*1	0.3699	0.4289
HP*2	0.6301	0.5711
	1.0000	1.0000

Advances in Forensic Haemogenetics 4
Edited by Ch. Rittner and P. M. Schneider
© Springer-Verlag Berlin Heidelberg 1992

n	198	227
TF*C1	0.7677	0.8128
TF*C2	0.1641	0.1233
TF*C3	0.0631	0.0551
TF*B	0.0051	0.0088
	1.0000	1.0000

n	194	224
GC*1F	0.0876	0.1674
GC*1S	0.5722	0.5000
GC*2	0.3402	0.3326
	1.0000	1.0000

n	195	228
PI*M1	0.6897	0.6711
PI*M2	0.1359	0.1930
PI*M3	0.1359	0.0899
PI*S	0.0103	0.0219
PI*Z	0.0128	0.0153
PI*Var	0.0154	0.0088
	1.0000	1.0000

Considering corresponding date for Slovakians (Siváková et al. 1990) and Hungarians, Matyos and Gypsies (Goedde et al. 1987) we computed standard genetic distances according to Nei (1972). The results of a UPGMA clustering of these distances are shown in Fig. 1. Hungarians and Matyos as well as Poles and Slovaks are found in two subclusters, which are linked up to one cluster. Gypsies and especially Kashubes exhibit a distinct position from this cluster, which can be explained considering the ethnohistory of these two populations. This genetic distance pattern will be analyzed and discussed in more detail elsewhere.

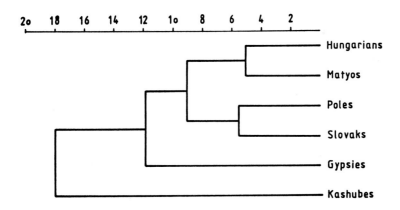

Genetic distances (d × 100)

Fig. 1 Genetic distances based on four loci (HP, TF, GC, PI) among six Central and East European population groups

Summing up we can point out that within the populations of Central and East Europe one has to consider a marked genetic heterogeneity concerning HP, TF, GC and PI polymorphisms. This is not only of considerable interest to population genetics, but also with regard to the application of Essen-Møller values in cases of disputed paternity, when Central and East Europeans are involved.

REFERENCES

Goedde HW, Benkmann HG, Kriese L, Bogdanski P, Czeizel A, Beres J (1987) Genetic markers among three population groups of Hungary. Gene Geography 1:109–120
Nei M (1972) Genetic distance between populations. Amer Nat 106:283–292
Siváková D, Sieglová Z, Walter H (1990) Serum protein polymorphisms in Slovakia. Int J Anthrop 5:359–362

Haptoglobin Subtypes in Lower Saxony (Germany)

M. Basler, G. Lang, and K.-S. Saternus

Institute of Legal Medicine, Georg-August-University, Windausweg 2, D-3400 Göttingen

INTRODUCTION

The two-allelic polymorphism of the haptoglobin system has been used in cases of disputed paternity for more than thirty years. A lack of methods suitable for routine subtyping of the Hp α-chains hindered it from being commonly used in paternity testing. Today various methods, based on somewhat different principles, have been established. Patzelt and Schröder (1985), inspired by the work of Shibata (1982), developed a time-saving procedure of Hp subtyping by isoelectric focussing of haptoglobin cleavage products. We are performing this technique with slight modifications in routine paternity testing. The aim of this study is to present the distribution of the Hp polymorphism in 431 unrelated adults from Lower Saxony.

MATERIALS AND METHODS

Sera:
Sera were obtained from probands involved in paternity testing.

Hp purification:
60 μl (in some cases 100 μl) of non-hemolytic serum were mixed with 2 ml DEAE SS-cellulose suspension (sodium acetate buffer 0.01 M, pH 4.7) and incubated for at least 40 min. After short centrifugation, the pellet was washed twice with sodium acetate buffer. The pellet was resuspended with 50 μl of 0.125 M acetic ammonium solution and centrifuged again to elute the hemoglobin molecules.

Reductive cleavage:
40 μl of the haptoglobin-containing supernatant were mixed with 20 μl of the reductive reagent (8 M urea in 0.1 M boric acid, 0.04 M sodium hydroxide, pH 8.8, 1.5 M dithiothreit), incubated for at least 30 min at 37°C, and alkylated with 8 μl 0.5 M iodoacetamide solution.

Isoelectric focussing and staining:
IEF was performed in polyacrylamide gels (T=5.5%, C=3%; 260x125x0.5 mm) containing carrier ampholytes (Ampholine LKB; 0.6 ml of pH 5-7, 0.2 ml of pH 6-8, 0.2 ml of pH 3.5-5, and 0.1 ml of pH 3-10 in 16 ml gel volume). IEF was performed for 105 min at a maximum power supply of 1600 V, 10 mA, 15 W without prefocussing. Fixation, staining and destaining of the gels were performed according to Steck et al. (1980).

RESULTS

The Hp phenotype distribution among 431 unrelated individuals and the corresponding gene frequencies were investigated (Tab. 1). The Hp phenotype distribution as well as the allele frequencies obtained are in agreement with those expected according to the Hardy-Weinberg law. Furthermore, the Hp phenotypes in 171 mother-child pairs were analysed. No mother-child exclusion was observed. The calculated Hp allele frequencies were compared to published data of different studies (Tab. 3). The evaluated data of the allele frequencies correspond to those obtained by investigators for other parts of Germany. However, in the investigated popu-

Advances in Forensic Haemogenetics 4
Edited by Ch. Rittner and P. M. Schneider
© Springer-Verlag Berlin Heidelberg 1992

lation of Lower Saxony, Hp 1F and Hp 2SS show slightly higher values, whereas Hp 1S and Hp 2FS are slightly decreased as compared to the corresponding values in the other regions of Germany.

Tab. 1: Hp phenotype distribution

Hp subtype	Observed		Expected	Allelic frequencies
	n	%		
1F	6	1.392	10.102	
1F-1S	36	2.353	31.867	
1S	22	5.104	24.846	Hp ˙1F = 0.153
1F-2FF	-	-	0.306	˙1S = 0.240
1F-2FS	79	18.329	75.013	˙2FS = 0.568
1F-2SS	5	1.160	4.751	˙2SS = 0.036
1S-2FF	-	-	0.482	˙2FF = 0.002
1S-2FS	117	27.146	117.640	
1S-2SS	10	2.320	7.451	Σ = 0.999
2FF	-	-	0.002	
2FF-2FS	2	0.464	1.137	Chi² = 5.877
2FF-2SS	-	-	0.072	df = 10
2FS	138	32.018	139.678	p = 0.825
2FS-2SS	16	3.712	17.639	
2SS	-	-	0.559	
	431	99.999	431.545	

Tab. 2: Hp phenotypes in 171 mother-child pairs

child / mother	1F	1F-1S	1S	1F-2FS	1F-2SS	1S-2FS	1S-2SS	2FS	2FS-2SS
1F	-	1	-	-	-	-	-	-	-
1F-1S	-	4	1	7	-	2	-	-	-
1S	-	-	3	-	-	7	-	-	-
1F-2FF	-	-	-	-	-	-	-	-	-
1F-2FS	3	3	-	11	-	3	-	10	1
1F-2SS	-	-	-	-	-	-	-	-	-
1S-2FF	-	-	-	-	-	-	-	-	-
1S-2FS	-	7	6	4	-	17	-	12	2
1S-2SS	-	-	2	-	-	3	1	-	-
2F-2FS	-	-	-	1	-	-	-	-	-
2FF-2SS	-	-	-	-	-	-	-	-	-
2FS	-	-	-	13	-	7	-	34	-
2FS-2SS	-	-	-	-	2	-	1	1	2
2SS	-	-	-	-	-	-	-	-	-
Total	3	15	12	36	2	39	2	57	5

Tab. 3: Hp allele frequencies of different studies

	n	1F	1S	2FS	2SS	2FF
Patzelt and Schröder (1985) Berlin	1275	0.1471	0.2502	0.5753	0.0251	0.0020
Bertrams et al. (1987) Rhine-Ruhr	1035	0.1387	0.2538	0.5864	0.0196	0.0015
Zischler et al. (1987) South-Germany	182	0.144	0.254	0.574	0.024	0.0004
Rothämel et al. (1989) Lower Saxony	1500	0.1537	0.2523	0.5620	0.0290	0.002
This study	431	0.153	0.240	0.568	0.036	0.002

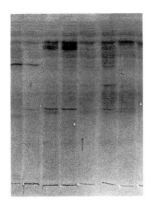

Fig. 1: Haptoglobin subtypes from left to right:
1S, 1S-2FS, 1F-2FS, 2FS, 1F-2SS, 2FS-2SS, 1F-2FS

REFERENCES

Bertrams J, Müller B, Luboldt W (1988) Haptoglobin (Hp) subtypes in the German Rhine-Ruhr area. In: Mayr WR (ed) Advances in Forensic Haemogenetics 2, p. 158-162

Patzelt D, Schröder H (1985) Haptoglobin subtypes in Berlin, GDR. Z Rechtsmedizin 94: 207-212

Rothämel T, Krüger H-J, Tröger HD (1989) Haptoglobin subtyping by isoelectric focusing in ultrathin-layer polyacrylamide gels. Population genetic data for Hanover and Lower Saxony. Z Rechtsmedizin 102: 391-397

Shibata K, Constans J, Viau M, Matsumoto H (1982) Polymorphism of the haptoglobin peptides in isoelectric focusing electrophoresis and isoelectric point determination. Hum Genet 61: 210-214

Steck G, Leuthard D, Bürk RR (1980) Detection of basis proteins and low molecular weight peptides in polyacrylamide gels by formaldehyde fixation. Anal Biochem 107: 21-24

Zischler H, Kömpf J, Ritter H (1978) IEF of Hp-subtypes: presentation of population genetic data and variants. Ärztl Lab 33: 85-87

C4 PHENOTYPE AND GENE DISTRIBUTION IN A POPULATION OF EASTERN LOMBARDY (ITALY)

N.Cerri*, F.De Ferrari*, G.Carella**, A.Malagoli**, R.Cattaneo** – *Cattedra di Medicina Legale, **Cattedra di Immunologia Clinica – Università degli Studi di Brescia - P.le Ospedale,1 - 25100 Brescia, Italy

INTRODUCTION

The fourth component of complement (C4) is a ß1-globulin (mol.wt. 200 KB) that acts in the classical pathway of complement activation. C4 molecules are encoded by two closely linked loci, C4A and C4B, located with the genes for the steroid 21-OHase in the vicinity to the HLA-DR locus, in the MHC on chromosome 6p. (Campbell et al,1986).

It is characterized by a high polymorphism; the first genetic study to define its pattern dates back to 1969 (Rosenfeld et al.) with agarose gel electrophoresis in plasma or serum. Teisberg et al. in 1976 used similar methods to define one rare and two common structural alleles at a single locus and, in 1977, employed a discontinous buffer to describe the presence of two common and two rare variants and define their allele frequencies.

O'Neill et al. in 1978 observed that the C4 pattern could not be produced by alleles at single locus but C4S and C4F were the product of two different, but closely linked loci. Subsequent electrophoretic methods have been developed (Awdeh and Alper,1980) with the confirm that the C4 system is characterized by a large number of alleles, more than 35, included the null alleles (Mauff et al,1983; Braun et al,1990), encoded by two different loci, with a distinct electrophoretic mobility, chemical reactivity and hemolitic activity.

In literature (Hobart et al,1984; Kemp et al,1987), C4 complement factor has been examined for its association with various diseases, in particular with autoimmune conditions, but it is not commonly investigated in forensic haemogenetics, especially in Italy. The aim of this work is to present a contribution to a better knowledge of the distribution of C4 polymorphism in Italy through the study of a population sample from the Brescia area (Lombardy, Northern Italy).

MATHERIAL AND METHODS

Fresh serum sampleswere obtained from 254 healthy and unrelated blood donors from the Transfusion Centre Of Brescia. Samples were stored at -80°C prior analysis and incubated with Carboxypeptidase and/or Neuraminidase overnight. C4 phenotyping was performed by high voltage agarose gel electrophoresis using Tris/Glycine/Barbital buffer, according to Awdeh and Alper (1980) with minor modifications. Electrophoresis was carried out on 0,45% agarose gel, at the condition of 500V, 100mA and 50W, until a human HbS marker band had migrated 7 cm. After separation, C4 phenotypes were identified by immunofixation. 1ml. of diluted 1:1 anti human C4 antiserum (ATAB) was applied evenly over the gel. The plate was incubated in a humid chamber, pressed with absorbent paper, washed in isotonic saline

Advances in Forensic Haemogenetics 4
Edited by Ch. Rittner and P. M. Schneider
© Springer-Verlag Berlin Heidelberg 1992

solution, dried and stained with CBB-R250. Some plates were not immunofixed but, in order to distinguish the C4A and the C4B overlapped alleles, they were developed with a functional overlay consisting of 2% sheep erytrocytes sensibilized with rabbit antibody, in 0,1% agarose in barbital buffer and C4 deficient guinea-pig serum.

RESULTS AND DISCUSSION

The distribution of the C4 alleles observed and their frequencies in the population of Brescia are given in Table 1. Good correlation was found between the observed and the expected phenotype distribution, assuming Hardy-Weinberg conditions (Locus A: $X^2 = 18,76$ for 15 d.f.; $0,2 < p < 0,3$. Locus B: $X^2 = 13,17$ for 15 d.f.; $0,5 < p < 0,7$).

Table 1: C4 alleles and their frequencies

	Alleles observed	Number	Allele Frequencies
Locus A	A3	240	C4*A3 = 0.7652
	A2	26	C4*A2 = 0.0525
	A1	2	C4*A1 = 0.0039
	A13	2	C4*A13 = 0.0039
	A4	4	C4*A4 = 0.0079
	A6	12	C4*A6 = 0.0239
	AQO	3	C4*AQO = 0.1086
Locus B	B1	241	C4*B1 = 0.7737
	B2	44	C4*B2 = 0.0907
	B3	4	C4*B3 = 0.0079
	B5	5	C4*B5 = 0.0098
	B51	2	C4*B51 = 0.0039
	B6	2	C4*B6 = 0.0039
	BQO	6	C4*BQO = 0.1536

No significant differences have been found between our allele frequencies and the others previously published in literature. Particularly, by a comparison between our frequencies and the data obtained in Pavia (De Paoli et al,1987; Abbal et al,1988), a population near geographically but with a different historical past, it results that the values of the commonest alleles are superimposed but, in Brescia, the rare alleles A5, A7 and B4 are not obtained; furthermore a higher value of QO is observed, similar to that found in Central Europe population (Kühnl et al,1988) and in accordance with other studies in Caucasians (Awdeh and Alper,1980).

In conclusion, from our observation, it appears C4 is a useful genetic marker, not only for population studies, but, for its apreciable polymorphism and the easy and simply-reproducible method, also for the application to parentage testing.

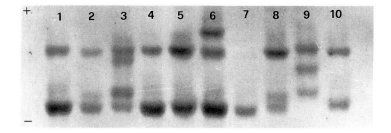

Fig. 1. C4 phenotypes after electrophoresis and immunofixation. From left to right: 1)A3,B1; 2)A3,B1; 3)A3A2,B1B2; 4)A3,B1; 5)A3,B1; 6)A3A6,B1; 7)AQ0,B1; 8)A3,B1B2; 9)A4,B2B5; 10)A3,B1. Anode at the top

REFERENCES

Abbal M, De Paoli F, Cuccia Belvedere M, Martinetti M (1988) C4A7: A new variant of human complement C4. Hum Hered 38: 363-366

Awdeh Z, Alper CA (1980) Inherited structural polymorphism of the fourth component of human complement. Proc Natl Acad Sci 77: 3576-3580

Braun L, Schneider PM, Giles CM, Bertrams J, Rittner C (1990) Null alleles of human complement C4. Evidence for pseudogenes at the C4A locus and for gene conversion at the C4B locus. J Exp Med 171: 129-140

Campbell RD, Carrol MC, Porter RR (1986) The molecular genetics of component of Complement. Advances in Immunology 3: 203-244

De Paoli F, Cuccia Belvedere M, Martinetti M, Abbal M (1987) Human MHC class III genes, Bf and C4. Polymorphism, complotypes and HLA class I and II association in Lombardy population (Italy). Gene Geography 1: 121-129

Hobart MJ, Walport MJ, Lachman PJ (1984) Complement polymorphism and disease. Clinics in Immunology and Allergy 4: 647-664

Kemp ME, Atkinson JP, Skanes VM, Levine RP, Chaplin DD (1987) Delection of C4 genes in patients with systemic lupus erytematosus. Arthritis Rheum 30: 1015-1022

Kühnl P, Specht R, Böhm BU, Seidl S, Spielmann W (1988) Vebesserte C4--typisierung durch IAGE Neuraminidase und Carboxypeptidase B-beandelt EDTA plasmen. In Mayr WR (ed) Advances in Forensic Haemogenetics vol 2, Springer, Berlin, Heidelberg, New York, pp. 145-149

Mauff G, Alper CA, Awdeh Z et al. (1983) Steatment on the nomenclature of human C4 allotypes. Immunobiology 164: 184-191

O'Neill GJ, Yang SY, Dupont B (1978) Two HLA-linked loci controlling the fourth component of human complement. Proc Natl Acad Sci 75: 5165-5169

Rosenfeld SF, Ruddy S, Auster KF (1969) Structural polymorphism of the fourth component of complement. J Clin Invest 48: 2283-2292

Teisberg P, Akesson I, Olaisen B, Gedde-Dahl T Jr, Throsby E (1976) Genetic polymorphism of C4 in man and localization of a structural C4 locus to the HLA gene complex of chromosome 6. Nature 264: 253-254

Teisberg P, Olaisen B, Jonassen R, Gedde-Dahl T Jr, Thorsby E (1977) The genetic polymorphism of the fourth component of human complement methodological aspects and a preservation of linkage and association data relegant to its localization in the HLA region. J Exp Med 146: 1380-1389

DISTRIBUTION OF TRANSFERRIN (TF), RED CELL ACID PHOSPHATASE (EAP), ESTERASE D (ESD) AND GROUP SPECIFIC COMPONENT (GC) PHENOTYPES IN CHINA

Guo Da wei, Xui Xiao li, Xing Xiao ping and Wang lin

Forensic Serology Department, Shanxi Medical College, Taiyuan, China

INTRODUCTION

Population data on electrophoretic genetic markers are necessary for a statistical evaluation of forensic evidence. Since the heterozygosity of Tf, EAP, EsD and Gc polymorphism in population is high, they are very useful in paternity testing and identification. The purpose of this work is to present the databases of Tf, EAP, EsD and Gc that are phenotypes and gene frequencies in unrelated adult Chinese; to provide the probability of discrimination and the probability of excluding paternity in four polymorphisms mentioned above; and to compare the databases in Chinese with that in other populations.

MATERIALS AND METHODS

Erythrocytes were washed three times in physiological saline solution and subsequently hemolyzed by freezing and thawing for EAP, EsD analysis; serum without additive was prepared for Tf, Gc analysis. The methods of phenotyping these four polymorphisms was according to references 1-4. The population data were analyzed using the chi-square statistic. The discriminating probability (Dp) and probability of excluding paternity (Qn) were based on the following formula:

$$Dp = 1 - \sum_{i=1}^{n} pi^2$$

$$Qn = \sum_{i=1}^{n} pi\,(1 - pi)^2\,(1 - pi + pi^2) + \sum_{i=1}^{n-1} \sum_{j=i+1}^{n} pi\,pj\,(pi + pj)\,(1 - pi - pj)^2$$

RESULTS AND DISCUSSION

The number of observed phenotypes, expected phenotypes and allelic frequencies for Tf, EAP, EsD and Gc are shown in Tables 1-4. The distributions of the phenotypes for each of the genetic markers are in Hardy-Weinberg equilibrium. Furthermore, a comparison between our data and other geographical locations are shown in Tables 5-8. It is obvious that the data for this paper (Asian) are not the same to the Causasoid and Negroid races. There is no obvious statistical difference among the Asian populations. However, pooled different population data would produce an improper statistical value, for inividuals of either geographical location's population. The Dp and Qn for each marker for Chinese are shown in Table 9. For individual identification and paternity testing purpose, the first markers to type would be EsD, then Tf or Gc, and finally, EAP would be typed according to Dp and Qn.

Advances in Forensic Haemogenetics 4
Edited by Ch. Rittner and P. M. Schneider
© Springer-Verlag Berlin Heidelberg 1992

Table 1: Distribution of Tf Subtypes in Taiyuan (China)

Subtypes	Observed	(%)	Expected	(%)	χ^2	Gene Frequencies
Tf *C1*	119	(58.05)	117.19	(57.17)	0.0279	TfC1=0.7561
Tf *C2-1*	64	(31.22)	69.56	(33.93)	0.4444	
Tf *C2*	14	(6.83)	10.32	(5.03)	1.3122	TfC2=0.2244
Tf *C1D*	7[b]	(3.41)	5.30	(2.59)	0.5453	TfD=0.0171
Others[a]	1	(0.0041)	2.63	(1.28)	1.0102	
Totals	205	(99.51)	205.00	(100.00)	3.34	

a: Tf *DD*, Tf *C1B*, Tf *C2D*, Tf *C2B*, Tf *BB* and Tf *Bd*; b: Tf *C1B*;
df = 6; 0.75 < P < 0.9; based on the Hardy-Weinberg equilibrium.

Table 2: Distribution of EAP Phenotypes in Taiyuan (China)

Phenotypes	Observed	(%)	Expected	(%)	χ^2	Gene Frequencies
EAP *B*	266	(66.86)	220	(65.28)	0.1636	Pb=0.0876
EAP *BA*	94	(27.81)	104	(30.86)	0.9615	
EAP *A*	18	(5.33)	13	(3.86)	1.9231	Pa=0.1920
Totals	338	(100.00)	337	(100.00)	3.0482	

df=1; P > 0.05; based on the Hardy-Weinberg equilibrium.

Table 3. Distribution of EsD Phenotypes in Taiyuan (Chinese)

Phenotypes	Observed	(%)	Expected	(%)	χ^2	Gene Frequencies
EsD *1*	118	(38.61)	112	(36.84)	0.3214	EsD1=0.6065
EsD *2-1*	134	(43.93)	145	(47.69)	0.8345	
EsD *2*	53	(17.38)	47	(15.46)	0.7659	EsD2=0.3934
Totals	305	(100.00)	304	(99.99)	1.9218	

df=1; P > 0.1; based on the Hardy-Weinberg equilibrium.

Table 4: Distribution Gc of phenotypes in Taiyuan (China)

Phenotypes	Observed	(%)	Expected	(%)	χ^2	Gene Frequencies
Gc *1*	219	(57.48)	217	(57.11)	0.0184	Gc1=0.7559
Gc *2-1*	138	(36.22)	140	(36.84)	0.0286	
Gc *2*	24	(6.29)	43	(6.05)	0.0435	Gc2=0.2441

df=1; P > 0.5; Based on the Hardy-Weinberg equilibrium.

Table 5: Tf gene frequencies in some populations

Population	No.	TfC1	TfC2	TfC3	TfD	χ^2	P
Germany	1108	0.79	0.13	0.07		9.1733	< 0.01
France	250	0.78	0.13	0.05		10.7915	< 0.025
White (USA)	947	0.77	0.16	0.05		3.7189	> 0.05
Black (USA)	232	0.84	0.11		0.05	16.6589	<< 0.005
Japanese	342	0.76	0.23		0.01	0.5590	> 0.5
this paper	205	0.75	0.22		0.071	./.	./.

Table 6: EsD gene frequencies in some populations

Population	No.	EsD1	EsD2	EsD5	χ^2	P
White (USA)	208	0.8490	0.1213	0.0297	96.9241	<< 0.005
Black (USA)	181	0.9365	0.0635		163.5002	<< 0.005
White (GB)	4611	0.8820	0.0973	0.0207	120.5355	<< 0.005
Black (GB)	1149	0.9019	0.0870	0.0039	135.3659	<< 0.005
Indian (GB)	309	0.8074	0.1764	0.0162	60.8244	<< 0.005
this paper	305	0.6065	0.3934			

Table 7: EAP gene frequencies in some populations

Population	No.	AcpB	AcpA	AcpC	Others	χ^2	P
White (USA)	208	0.6130	0.3389	0.0481		43.1285	<< 0.005
Black (USA)	181	0.7845	0.1934	0.0138	0.0083	1.7258	> 0.5
Britain	367	0.60	0.36	0.04		52.3520	<< 0.005
Oriental	77	0.805	0.195			1.7029	> 0.5
this paper	338	0.8076	0.1920			./.	./.

Table 8: Gc gene frequencies in some populations

Population	No.	Gc1	Gc2	χ^2	P
Sweden	3394	0.75	0.25	0.1363	> 0.90
Britain	100	0.73	0.26	0.7460	> 0.50
Germany	1523	0.74	0.26	65.0892	<< 0.005
France	256	0.67	0.31	9.6090	< 0.01
White (USA)	7274	0.71	0.27	1.9677	> 0.25
Black (USA)	540	0.85	0.10	45.7269	<< 0.005
Japanese	531	0.72	0.24	0.1304	> 0.90
this paper	381	0.7559	0.2441	./.	./.

Table 9: The discriminating probabilities and probabilities of excluding paternity of Tf, EAP, EsD and Gc for Chinese

| Discriminating Probabilities | | Excluding Paternity Probabilities | |
Marker	Dp	Marker	Qn
EsD	0.6270	EsD	0.1817
Tf	0.5579	Tf	0.1650
Gc	0.5245	Gc	0.1505
EAP	0.4727	EAP	0.1312

REFERENCES

Guo Da wei et al. (1988) Human serum transferrin polymorphism in population of Guangdong, China, and its application in forensic science. Academic Journal of Sun Yet-sen University of Medical Sciences, 9(4):25

Terence Rendall W. et al. (1980) A method of phenotyping EAP by isoelectric focusing. Med. Sci. Law 20(1):43

G.B. Divall. The Esterase D polymorphism as revealed by isoelectric focusing in ultra-thin polyacrylamide gels. Forensic Sci. Inter. 16:255

Wu Xin yao et al. (1987)　广州地区人群血清 Gc 型的测定
Human serum Gc typing in population of Guangdang, China. Chinese Journal of Forensic Medicine 1(4):233

Null and Rare Alleles in Paternity Testing

A.C. Gomes, M.F. Pinheiro, M.L. Pontes, A. Santos, J. Pinto da Costa

Medico Legal Institute
Jardim Carrilho Videira
4000 Porto, Portugal

INTRODUCTION

The iron-binding protein of human plasma transferrin (Tf) was discovered in 1946 by Schade and Caroline and the polymorphism of human red esterase D was first demonstrated by Hopkinson et al. (1973). But only recently was an extensive genetic polymorphism revealed due to the high resolving power of protein separation by isoelectric focusing (IEF).

The purpose of this work is to present the evidence of rare alleles in Tf and EsD systems in the population of North of Portugal.
An apparent maternity exclusion found in the Duffy system due to a silent allele will also be present. The frequency of this allele in a large number of trios tested in Medico Legal Institute of Oporto because of disputed paternity was determined.

MATERIALS and METHODS

Blood samples were obtained by venopuncture from healthy individuals involved in paternity cases in the North of Portugal.
Phenotyping of Tf and EsD was performed by IEF using polyacrilamide gels with pH 5-8 Ampholines and with Pharmalyte carrier ampholytes pH 4.5-5.4, respectively.
Duffy typing was done using indirect Coombs test.

RESULTS and CONCLUSION

The analyse of 873 blood samples of unrelated persons typed for Tf showed the common C subtypes C1, C2, and C3 as well as the rare C6 and B variants. The frequencies of those alleles are: C1 = 0.7697, C2 = 0.1723, C3 = 0.0532, C6 = 0.0011, B = 0.0034.

EsD was typed in 502 blood samples. The following frequencies were observed: EsD1 = 0.8256, EsD2 = 0.1623, EsD5 = 0.0079, EsD7 = 0.0039.

Advances in Forensic Haemogenetics 4
Edited by Ch. Rittner and P. M. Schneider
© Springer-Verlag Berlin Heidelberg 1992

Of interest was the observation of a mother child pair with apparent maternity exclusion in the Duffy system. However, the analyses of 20 markers indicated a very high probability for maternity, so that the presence of a "null" allele was assumed in the child and mother. The allele frequencies obtained after typing 992 blood samples are: Fya = 0.3462, Fyb = 0.6486, Fy = 0.0050.

The results of this study underline the usefulness of these systems for population studies and paternity testing. IEF with immobilized pH gradients is a supplementary method for identification and delineation of newly observed Tf and EsD subtypes.

ACKNOWLEDGEMENT

We are grateful to Dr. S. Weidinger, Institute of Anthropologie and Human Genetics, University of Munich, for his kind cooperation in the compilation of the references used in this poster and for his interest in this project.

REFERENCES

Bar W, Bierdermann V (1986) Electrophoretic "Subtyping" of Rare EsD Variants. Adv in Forensic Haemogenetics 1:179-180

Gradl W, Weidinger S, Clever H, Schwartzfisher F (1986) Genetic Study of Red Cell Esterase D Polymorphism by Isoelectric Focusing. Adv in Forensic Haemogenetics 1:175-178

Kamboh MI, Kirk RL (1983) Distribution of Transferrin (Tf) Subtypes in Asian, Pacific and Australian Aboriginal Populations: Evidence for the Existence of a new Subtype TfC6. Hum Hered 33:237-243

Polesky HF, Souhrada JM, Dykes DD (1983) The Frequency of "Null" Genes Calculated From Trios in Disputed Parentage Cases. Proceedings in the 10th International Congress of the Society for Forensic Haemogenetics, Munich, p 161-166

Souhrada JM, Polesky HF (1986) Apparent Exclusion of Maternity by Both Duffy and Kidd. Adv in Forensic Haemogenetics 1:423-426

Weidinger S, Cleve H, Schwarzfischer F, Postel W, Weser J, Gorg A (1984) Transferrin Subtypes and Variants in Germany; Further Evidence for a Tf Null Allele. Hum Genet 66:356-360

Weidinger S, Henke J (1988) Two New Esterase D (EsD) Variants Revealed by Isoelectric Focusing in Agarose Gel. Electrophoresis 2:237-243

COMPARATIVE SUBTYPING OF ACP-1, PGM-1 AND ESD IN HUMAN PLACENTA AND CORD BLOOD BY ISOELECTRIC FOCUSING: PRACTICAL CONSIDERATIONS OF FORENSIC SIGNIFICANCE

M. J. Iturralde*, M. Montesino*, A. Alonso*, I. Montesino**, M. Sancho*

* Instituto Nacional de Toxicología. Madrid. Spain
** Servicio de Obstetricia, Hospital General de Galicia. Santiago de Compostela. Spain

INTRODUCTION

Human red cell enzymes with genetic polymorphism (ACP-1, PGM-1, ESD...) were previously analyzed in placenta and other tissues by conventional starch electrophoresis (Blake et al. l973; Harris and Hopkinson 1976). However, to our knowledge, analysis of these enzymes from human placenta by isoelectric focusing (IEF) have not been performed hitherto.

In this study, the genetic polymorphism of ACP-1, PGM-1 and ESD was analyzed in placental extracts and red cell lysates from the corresponding cord and maternal bloods by IEF using miniaturized polyacrilamide gels.

MATERIALS AND METHODS

98 samples of human placenta (maternal and fetus sides) and the corresponding cord and maternal bloods were collected after delivery. Small pieces of placenta were homogenized with a glass/glass homogenizer in 100 µl of distilled water, centrifuged at 3000g for 5 min. and stored at -40°C until use. The red cells were washed three times with saline and stored at -40°C until use. Placental extracts were diluted with 0.05 M DTT (1:1 for ACP-1 and ESD typing and 1:60 for PGM-1 typing). Red cell hemolysates were diluted 1:4 with 0.05M DTT. ACP-1 typing was performed by IEF in miniaturized polyacrylamide gels as previously described (Alonso and Gascó l987) with the following modifications: 12% Glycerol was used as a density agent instead of sucrose and the pH gradient was created with a mixture of Ampholine pH 5-7 and Pharmalyte pH 6-8 (3:1 v/v). The ACP-1 patterns were detected using 4-methylumbelliferyl phosphate (MUP) as substrate, while the specific detection of the ACP-2 and ACP-3 bands was done by enzyme blotting using α-Naphthyl phosphate (α-NP) as substrate (Harris and Hopkinson 1976). PGM-1 typing was also carried out by IEF in miniaturized polyacrylamide gels using the Ampholine pH 5-7. The PGM-1 phenotypes were revealed by the overlay technique previously described (Sutton and Burgess 1978). ESD typing was done by IEF under reducing (0.05M DTT) and mild denaturing (1.5M Urea) conditions using a narrow pH gradient (Pharmalite pH 4.5-5.4) in combination with two separators (HEPES and ACES) according to Alonso et al. (1991).

RESULTS AND DISCUSSION

Figures 1A and 1B show the ACP band patterns from cord bloods and the corresponding placental extracts after IEF followed by MUP staining, respectively. As can be seen, the most striking difference between these two tissues was the presence of three monomorphic bands in

Advances in Forensic Haemogenetics 4
Edited by Ch. Rittner and P. M. Schneider
© Springer-Verlag Berlin Heidelberg 1992

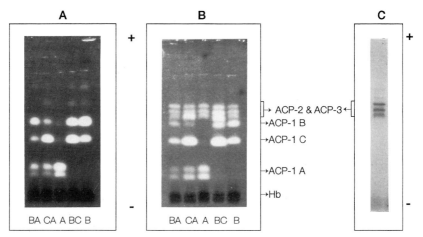

Fig. 1. Analysis of ACP by IEF: A) ACP-1 phenotypes from cord bloods, B) the corresponding placental extracts and C) ACP-2 and ACP-3 from placenta, stained with α-NP

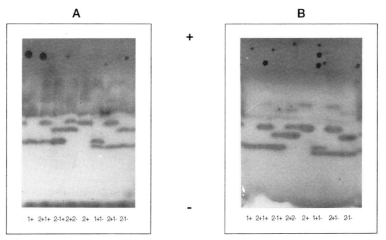

Fig. 2. PGM-1 phenotypes analyzed by IEF: A) cord bloods and B) the corresponding placental extracts

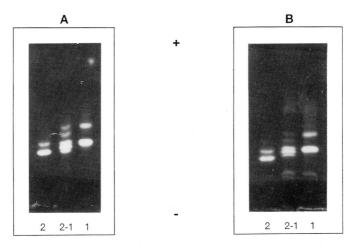

Fig. 3. ESD phenotypes analyzed by IEF: A) cord bloods and B) the corresponding placental extracts

placenta that were absent in cord blood. These monomorphic extrabands were demonstrated to be the genetic products of the ACP-2 and ACP-3 loci, since they were detected with α-NP that specificaly stains this tissue isoenzymes (Blake et al. 1973) (Fig. 1C). On the other hand, the analysis of the ACP-1 allele products from these tissues (Figs. 1A and 1B) revealed that the ACP-1 phenotypes from placenta could be assigned to the corresponding phenotypes from cord blood, making possible a genetic interpretation of the polymorphism displayed by the placental ACP-1 enzyme. However, a more detailed comparison between these two tissues showed a high staining intensity of the placental ACP-1 C band, specially in the B, BC and BA phenotypes. In spite of this difference, that must be taken into account for a correct interpretation of the genetic polymorphism of this enzyme, each phenotype can be differenciated from each other by a particular staining pattern as is shown in Fig. 1B.

The PGM-1 patterns from placenta and the corresponding cord blood as analyzed by IEF are shown in Fig. 2B and Fig. 2A, respectively. As can be seen, the genetic variability of this enzyme from placental extracts diluted 1:60 corresponded to the allelic variation that this enzyme displayed in cord blood. The placental extracts were diluted 1:60 with DTT since less diluted samples exhibited overstained tissue bands with impaired resolution as well as the presence of maternal PGM-1 bands due to blood contamination, making difficult the interpretation of the new born phenotypes in placenta.

Finally, it has been shown (Figs. 3A and 3B) that the three ESD common phenotypes analyzed in this study displayed the same band patterns and staining intensity in placenta and in the corresponding cord blood.

The results presented here clearly show that ACP-1, PGM-1 and ESD fetal phenotypes can be studied from placenta samples, using a fast and reliable IEF methodology. Therefore, we suggest the applicability of these conventional markers in the preliminary genetic analysis of forensic cases (illegal abortions and infanticides) in which fetal fragments are mixed with placental tissue.

ACKNOWLEDGMENTS

We wish to express our gratitude to Dr. José María Guerra Flecha from the Instituto de Obstetricia y Ginecología, Hospital Gregorio Marañón, Madrid for kindly providing bloods and placental tissue samples. Thanks are also due to Mrs. A. Zamora for the photographic work.

REFERENCES

Alonso A , Gascó P (1987) The use of separator isoelectric focusing in micro-ultrathin polyacrylamyde gels in the characterization of some polymorphic proteins of forensic science significance. J For Sc 32; 1558-1564

Alonso A, Visedo G, Sancho M, Fernández-Piqueras J (1991) Identification of human esterase D subunits from the homodimeric and heterodimeric forms of five phenotypes by a new two-dimensional isoelectric focusing method. Electrophoresis 12: 348-351

Blake N M, Kirk R L, Barnes K R, Thompson J M (1973) Expression of human red acid phosphatase activity in placenta and other tissues Jap J Hum Genet 18: 10-23

Harris H, Hopkinson D A (1976) Handbook of enzyme electrophoresis in human genetics. North Holland, Amsterdam

Sutton I G, Burgges R (1978) Genetic evidence for four common alleles at the phosphoglucomutase-1 locus (PGM-1) detectable by isoelectric focusing. Vox Sang 34: 97-103

Distribution of Adenosine Deaminase (EC 3.5.4.4) Phenotypes in a Series of HIV-Seropositive Patients

W. Huckenbeck, B. Jacob, B.M.E. Kuntz, H.T. Brüster

Institute of Legal Medicine, Heinrich-Heine-University Düsseldorf,FRG*

INTRODUCTION

Adenosine deaminase (ADA) takes its role in physiological pathway in deamination of adenosine to inosine. The enzyme was found in human erythrocytes and tissues. Three common phenotypes – ADA*1, ADA*2-1, ADA*2 – can be separated by electrophoresis. Rarer alleles (ADA^0, ADA^3, ADA^4, ADA^5, ADA^6) have also been described. The ADA* polymorphism is coded by chromosome 20. This enzyme seems to be of interest for immunology, too. The homocygous ADA0 type is associated with the SCID syndrome (severe combined immune defiency) [8,9]. Several authors reported on increased ADA levels in HIV-infected patients [1,2,3,4,7,13,14].

MATERIAL & METHODS

Blood samples were taken from 226 HIV-seropositive patients treated in the Institute of Blood Coagulation and Transfusions Medicine at the Heinrich-Heine-University. This series thus includes individuals that were only HIV-seropositive, patients with ARC (AIDS related complex), with full blown AIDS and with Kaposi-sarcoma. We compared this group with obviously healthy persons spot checked otherwise..
Electrophoresis was carried out on Cellogel electrophoresis membranes using electrophoresis buffer Biotest (dilution 1:10): 250 Volt, 15 mA, 50 min. Staining was performed with 15mg Adenosine, 5 mg MTT, 5 mg PMS, 25 μl nucleoside and 25 μl xanthine oxidase.

RESULTS & DISCUSSION

The ADA system takes a role in immunological reactions. The silent ADA gene ADA 0 is associated with the SCID syndrome. Several authors reported increased ADA levels in HIV-infected patients [1,2,3,4,7,13,14]. For this study we examined the distribution of the ADA*phenotypes in a series of 226 HIV-infected persons. The distribution found is shown in table 1. We observed only the common three phenotypes ADA*1, ADA*2-1 and ADA*2. The results provide a satisfactory correlation to the Hardy-Weinberg-equilibrium
(Chi2: $0.045 < 3.841; df=1; a=0.05$).
In table 2 the results of other studies on ADA*polymorphism in Germany are listed. Small differences between the gene frequencies may be due to the small volume and to the heterogeneity of the HIV-group – large clinical catchment area.
The differences are not significant and there is no association between the ADA*system and HIV-infection detectable.

* and Institute of Blood Coagulation and Transfusion Medicine

Advances in Forensic Haemogenetics 4
Edited by Ch. Rittner and P. M. Schneider
© Springer-Verlag Berlin Heidelberg 1992

TAB.1   ADA-PHENOTYPES IN HIV-SEROPOSITIVE PATIENTS

Phenotype	observed		expected	
	n	%	n*	%*
1-1	195	86.28	194.21	85.93
2-1	29	12.83	30.63	13.55
2-2	2	0.89	1.21	0.54
total	226	100	226	100

* values rounded up

gene frequencies: ADA1 : 0.9269 ; ADA2 : 0.0731

TAB.2   OTHER STUDIES ON ADA-POLYMORPHISM IN GERMANY

Country	ADA*1	ADA*2	n	Reference
Lower Rhine region	0.9447	0.0553	262	Scheil et al.
Düsseldorf region	0.9366	0.0634	500	Scheil et al.
South Western	0.9238	0.0762	302	Tariwerdian et al.
Hamburg	0.9355	0.0645	861	Goedde et al.
Hessen	0.9499	0.0501	579	Renninger et al.
Berlin	0.9420	0.0580	500	Lefevre and Niebuhr
This study	0.9269	0.0731	226	

REFERENCES

1) Casoli, C., Magnani, G., Barbuti, S., Barchi, E.(1989) Erythrocyte Adenosine Deaminase (ADA) Expression in AZT-treated Aids Patients.Abstract, V. International Conference on AIDS, June 4-9, Montreal
2) Clotet, B., Sirera, G., Pastor, C., Romeu, J., Tural, C., Jou, A., Foz, M.(1989)Adenosine Deaminase (ADA) Values in Cerebrospinal Fluid of Asymptomatic HIV Infected Patients.Abstract, V. International Conference on AIDS, June 4-9, Montreal
3) Eto, K., Tsuboi, I, Saneyoshi, Y., Yoshioka, H., Yokoyama, M.M.(1989)Adenosine Deaminase (ADA) Levels in Tears of AIDS Patients and AIDS Carriers.Abstract, V. International Conference on AIDS, June 4-9, Montreal
4) Ferrazzi, M., De Rinaldis, M.L., Pezzella, M., Caprilli, F., Bozzi, A., Strom, R.(1989)Determination of Erythrocyte Adenosine Deaminase Activity in Anti-HIV Seronegative Homosexual Men with Latent HIV Infection.Abstract, V. International Conference on AIDS, June 4-9, Montreal
5) Goedde, H., Benkmann, H.G., Christ, I., Singh, S., Hirth, L.(1970)Gene frequencies of red cell adenosine deaminase, adenylate kinase, phosphoglucomutase, acid phosphatase and serum α1-antitrypsin (Pi) in a German population.Humangenetik 10: 235-243
6) Levevre, H., Niebuhr, R.(1970)Polymorphismus der Adenosindesaminase. Untersuchung an einer Stichprobe aus der Berliner Bevölkerung.Humangenetik 10: 88-90
7) Palomba, E., David, O., Gabiano, C., Tovo, P.A.(1989)Increased ADA Activity in Children with Perinatal HIV Infection.Abstract, V. International Conference on AIDS, June 4-9, Montreal
8) Prokop, O., Göhler, W.(1986)Die menschlichen Blutgruppen
Gustav Fischer Verlag Jena

9)   Spielmann, W., Kühnl, P.(1982)Blutgruppenkunde.Georg Thieme Verlag Stuttgart New York

10) Renninger, W., Bimboese, C.(1970)Zur Genetik der Erythrocyten-Adenosin-Desaminase.Humangenetik 9: 34-37

11) Scheil, H.G., Fiedler, K.P., Huckenbeck, W.(1991) Untersuchungen zur Phänotypen-Häufigkeit einiger hämogenetischer Polymorphismen am Niederrhein (Bereich Kleve, Goch, Kalkar).
Anthrop. Anz. 1/2: 137-144

12) Tariwerdian , G., Ritter, H.(1969)Population genetics of adenosine deaminase (EC:3.5.4.4): gene frequencies in Southwestern Germany.Humangenetik 7: 179

13) Valls, V., Ena, J., Figueredo, I., Roca, V. De Salamanca R.E.(1989)Adenosine Deaminase (ADA) Levels in Sera of Patients with HIV-1 Infection.Abstract, V. International Conference on AIDS, June 4-9, Montreal

14) Yokoyama, M.M., Tsuboi, I.(1989)Adenosine Deaminase in Retrovirus Infected Diseases.Abstract, V. International Conference on AIDS, June 4-9, Montreal

DETERMINATION OF C1R TYPES IN BLOODSTAINS

A. Kido, N. Komatsu, Y. Kimura and M. Oya

Department of Legal Medicine, Yamanashi Medical University, Yamanashi-ken, Japan

Introduction

Genetic polymorphism of the C1R subcomponent was first discovered by Kamboh and Ferrell (1986). Using isoelectric focusing and immunoblotting, they described 2 common alleles C1R*1 and C1R*2 in native plasma samples from US whites and US blacks. Besides these 2 common alleles, several further variant alleles have been detected in a variety of ethnic groups by treating plasma samples with neuraminidase (Kamboh et al. 1988, 1989; Nakamura et al. 1988).

We have recently reported that the Japanese population has a large genetic variation in C1R as compared with other ethnic groups, carrying 3 common alleles C1R*1, C1R*2 and C1R*5 (Kido et al. 1991).

In the present study the distribution of C1R allele frequencies was examined in desialylated plasma samples from a rather large size of Japanese population and phenotyping of C1R was investigated in bloodstains for medicolegal purpose. We have followed the C1R nomenclature proposed by Kamboh et al. (1989).

Materials and Methods

Blood samples were collected from 1000 unrelated Japanese individuals in Yamanashi Prefecture, a central part of Japan. EDTA plasma samples were separated by centrifigation at 2000 rpm for 5 min and stored at -20°C until use. Ten µl of plasma was treated with 2 µl 1 M potassium phosphate buffer (pH 7.0) containing 50 U/ml neuraminidase from *Clostridium perfringens* (type V, Sigma, USA) for 24 h at 4°C. The samples were applied to the gel using 5 x 6 mm filter paper strips (Whatman No. 3, UK).

Venous blood from 29 donors with known phenotypes was dropped on filter paper (Whatman No. 3) and dried at room temperature. The bloodstains thus made were stored in a thermostatic chamber at 37°C, at room temperature and in a refrigerator at 4°C and examined after different time intervals. The stains were cut in 5 x 5 mm pieces and soaked in 20 µl 1 M potassium phosphate buffer (pH 7.0) containing 10 U/ml neuraminidase (type V, Sigma) for 24 h at 4°C. The extracts were

Advances in Forensic Haemogenetics 4
Edited by Ch. Rittner and P. M. Schneider
© Springer-Verlag Berlin Heidelberg 1992

absorbed onto 10 x 5 mm filter paper strips (Whatman No. 3) and
applied to the gel.

Isoelectric focusing and electroblotting were performed as
described previously (Kido et al. 1991). C1R patterns were
detected by the method of Kamboh and Ferrell (1986) with minor
modifications.

Results and Discussion

In our population sample 6 phenotypes associated with 3
common alleles, C1R*1, C1R*2 and C1R*5, and 5 variant types
were observed (Fig. 1). Table 1 shows the distribution of C1R
types and allele frequencies in 1000 Japanese individuals. The
population data fitted the Hardy-Weinberg equilibrium.

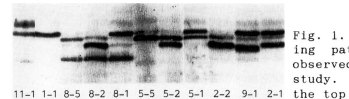

Fig. 1. Isoelectric focusing pattern of C1R types
observed in the present
study. The anode is at

11-1 1-1 8-5 8-2 8-1 5-5 5-2 5-1 2-2 9-1 2-1 the top

Table 1. Distribution of C1R types in a Japanese population

Phenotype	No. observed	%	No. expected
1-1	229	22.9	226.6
2-1	305	30.5	307.0
2-2	102	10.2	104.0
5-1	178	17.8	184.2
5-2	133	13.3	124.8
5-5	37	3.7	37.4
8-1	9	0.9	6.7
8-2	3	0.3	4.5
8-5	2	0.2	2.7
8-8	0	0	0.0
9-1	1 } 2	0.2	1.0
11-1	1		
Others	0	0	1.0
Total	1000	100.0	999.9

Allele frequencies: C1R*1 = 0.4760, C1R*2 = 0.3225, C1R*5
= 0.1935, C1R*8 = 0.0070, C1R*R (the combined frequency of
C1R*9 and C1R*11) = 0.0010. χ^2 = 4.299; d.f. = 10;
0.95 > p > 0.90

Comparison of C1R allele frequencies in different populations indicates that the Japanese population was a large
genetic variation in C1R in the following respects: (1) the C1R
polymorphism in Japanese is controlled by 3 common alleles
C1R*1, C1R*2 and C1R*5; (2) the C1R*2 allele frequency in

Japanese is considerably higher than that in other ethnic groups; (3) ClR*8 is observed at an almost polymorphic level exclusively in Japanese. Our results disagree with the geographical cline in the Japanese main islands postulated by Nakamura et al. (1990).

By the present isoelectric focusing and subsequent electroblotting, fairly clear ClR patterns were observed also from dried and stored bloodstains (Fig. 2). Our sample included 8 ClR 1-1, 8 ClR 2-1, 3 ClR 2-2, 6 ClR 5-1 and 4 ClR 5-2. All the bloodstains examined were correctly typed for ClR at 37°C for up to 3 weeks, at room temperature for up to 5 weeks and at 4°C even over 10 weeks. The products of ClR*5 stained fainter and more indistinct than those of the other 2 common alleles.

The present method permits ClR phenotyping from dried bloodstains for at least 3 weeks of storage. The ClR would therefore provide a new useful genetic marker for the medicolegal grouping of bloodstains.

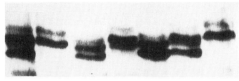

2-1 1-1 5-2 5-1 2-2 2-1 1-1

Fig. 2. Isoelectric focusing pattern of ClR types in bloodstains stored at room temperature for 1 week. The anode is at the top

References

Kamboh MI, Ferrell RE (1986) Genetic studies of low abundance human plasma proteins. III. Polymorphism of the ClR subcomponent of the first complement component. Am J Hum Genet 39: 826-831

Kamboh MI, Lyons L, Ferrell RE (1988) Genetic studies of low-abundance human plasma proteins. IX. A new allele at the complement subcomponent ClR structural locus. Hum Genet 81: 93-94

Kamboh MI, Lyons LA, Ferrell RE (1989) Genetic studies of low-abundance human plasma proteins. XIII. Population genetics of ClR complement subcomponent and description of a new variants. Am J Hum Genet 44: 148-153

Kido A, Komatsu N, Kimura Y, Oya M (1991) ClR subcomponent polymorphism in Japanese: Description of a new allele. Hum Hered 41: 129-133

Nakamura S, Ohue O, Akiyama K, Abe K (1988) Genetic polymorphism of human ClR subcomponent of the first complement component in the Japanese population. Forensic Sci Int 39: 71-76

Nakamura S, Omoto K, Ohue O, Yamashita K, Ochi J, Akiyama K, Sawaguchi A (1990) ClR polymorphism in the Japanese population. Proceedings of the First International Symposium Advances in Legal Medicine pp 438-440

COAGULATION FACTOR XIIIB PHENOTYPING IN A JAPANESE POPULATION AND IN BLOODSTAINS

N. Komatsu, A. Kido, Y. Kimura and M. Oya

Department of Legal Medicine, Yamanashi Medical University, Yamanashi-ken, Japan

Introduction

Human coagulation factor XIII B subunit (FXIIIB) exhibits genetic polymorphism with 3 codominant alleles FXIIIB*1, FXIIIB*2 and FXIIIB*3 (Board 1980). Up to the present time, a number of rare alleles have been identified, and in Japanese FXIIIB*13, FXIIIB*14 and FXIIIB*15 have been described (Nakamura et al. 1986). In the present study the distribution of FXIIIB types in a Japanese population was investigated and the phenotyping was attempted from bloodstains for medicolegal purpose.

Materials and Methods

Blood samples were collected from 555 unrelated Japanese individuals. Ten µl plasma was treated with 4 µl 40 U/ml neuraminidase (Sigma, USA) in 1 M potassium phosphate buffer (pH 7.0). After incubation for 18 h, the mixture was absorbed on 5 x 6 mm filter paper strips (Toyoroshi No. 2, Japan).

Twenty bloodstains with known phenotypes were made on filter paper (Toyoroshi No. 2) and stored at 37°C, room temperature and 4°C for different time intervals. The stains were cut in 5 x 6 mm pieces, treated with 10 µl 20 U/ml neuraminidase (Sigma) in 1 M potassium phosphate buffer (pH 7.0) for 18 h and directly applied onto the gel surface.

Isoelectric focusing was performed by the method of Sebetan and Azadeh (1989) with slight modifications. Following electrofocusing, proteins were transferred onto a sheet of nitrocellulose membrane (Bio-Rad, USA) using a Trans-Blot Cell (Bio-Rad) as described by Kido et al. (1991).

Immunologic detection of FXIIIB was performed as follows:
-brief rinse in 20 mM tris/500 mM sodium chloride buffer, pH 7.5 (TBS).
-immersion in TBS containing 3 % gelatine for 20 min.
-wash in TBS for 15 min.
-incubation in rabbit anti-human factor XIII-S serum (Behringwerke, Germany) diluted 1:500 in TBS containing 0.05 % Tween 20

Advances in Forensic Haemogenetics 4
Edited by Ch. Rittner and P. M. Schneider
© Springer-Verlag Berlin Heidelberg 1992

(TTBS) for 120 min.
-2 washes in TTBS for 15 min.
-incubation in goat anti-rabbit IgG serum conjugated with alkaline phosphatase (Sigma) diluted 1:750 in TTBS for 120 min.
-2 washes in TTBS for 15 min.
-development with a freshly-prepared reaction mixture (125 mg
β-naphtyl phosphate, 12.5 mg Fast Blue BB salt and 30 mg magnesium sulfate dissolved in 25 ml 60 mM boric acid/45 mM sodium
hydroxide buffer, pH 10.4) at 37°C for 30 min.

Results and Discussion

Figure 1 shows FXIIIB types in desialylated plasma samples
from 555 Japanese.   In our sample 5 common phenotypes FXIIIB
1-1, 2-1, 3-1, 3-2, 3-3 and a rare variant type FXIIIB 15-3
were observed.   As the FXIIIB*15 allele has been detected
exclusively in the Japanese population (Nakamura et al. 1986,
Sebetan et al. 1990), it may be unique to Japanese.
The results for the distribution are given in Table 1.   The
population data fitted the Hardy-Weinberg equilibrium.

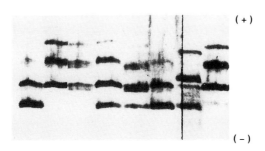

(+)

(-)

3-3 1-1 2-1 3-1 3-2 3-3 15-3 1-1

Fig. 1.   Isoelectric focusing pattern of FXIIIB

Table 1. Distribution of FXIIIB types in a Japanese
population

Phenotype	Observed	%	Expected
1-1	51	9.19	52.07
2-1	6	1.08	5.51
2-2	0	0.00	0.15
3-1	232	41.80	230.04
3-2	12	2.16	12.17
3-3	253	45.59	254.07
15-3	1	0.18	0.68
Others	0	0.00	0.33
Total	555	100.00	555.02

Allele frequency: FXIIIB*1 = 0.3063, FXIIIB*2 = 0.0162,
FXIIIB*3 = 0.6766, FXIIIB*15 = 0.0009.
χ^2 = 0.71, d.f. = 6, P > 0.99

The FXIIIB types were well demonstrated also from dried and stored bloodstains (Fig. 2). Our sample included 4 FXIIIB 1-1, 2 FXIIIB 2-1, 6 FXIIIB 3-1, 2 FXIIIB 3-2 and 6 FXIIIB 3-3. Reliable phenotyping was possible from bloodstains stored at 37°C for up to 4 months and from bloodstains stored at room temperature and at 4°C for over 6 months. The above results for the determination limits indicate that this system is stable enough to be used in medicolegal practice and quite suitable to be used even in summer or under tropical conditions. The FXIIIB system can be a new powerful genetic marker for the grouping of bloodstains.

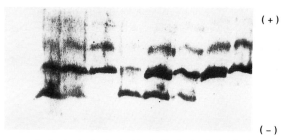

(+)

(-)

3-3 3-1 1-1 3-3 3-2 3-1 2-1 1-1

Fig. 2. Isoelectric focusing pattern of FXIIIB in bloodstains stored at room temperature for 3 months

REFERENCES

Board PG (1980) Genetic polymorphism of the B subunit of human coagulation factor XIII. Am J Hum Genet 32: 348-353

Kido A, Komatsu N, Kimura Y, Oya M (1991) C1R subcomponent polymorphism in Japanese; Description of a new allele. Hum Hered 41: 129-133

Nakamura S, Ohue O, Abe K (1986) Genetic polymorphism of coagulation factor XIII B subunit in the Japanese population: Description of the three new rare alleles. Hum Genet 73: 183-185

Sebetan IM, Azadeh B (1989) Genetic polymorphism of the B subunit of coagulation factor XIII in Libyans: Occurrence of a fourth common allele, FXIIIB*6. Z Rechtsmed 103: 125-128

Sebetan IM, Aoki Y, Sagisaka K, Oshida S (1990) Genetic polymorphism of the B subunit of coagulation factor XIII in a Japanese population. Res Pract Forensic Med 33: 55-57

FORMAL GENETIC DATA ON ORM1 SUBTYPES

C Luckenbach*, J Kömpf*, H Ritter*, J Rocha**, A Amorim**

* Inst.Anthropologie und Humangenetik 7400 Tübingen F.R.Germany

**Inst.Antropologia, Univ.Porto, 4000 Porto, Portugal

INTRODUCTION

Human plasma orosomucoid has been demonstrated to be coded by two autosomal structural loci, ORM1 and ORM2 (Dente et al., 1985; Yuasa et al., 1986; Escallon et al., 1987). At protein level ORM2 is not polymorphic in European populations while ORM1 reveals two common gene products (Johnson et al., 1969). Later, by isoelectric focusing, 'subtypes' were reported for the anodal gene product (Thymann and Eiberg, 1986; Eap et al., 1988; Krüger et al., 1989; Luckenbach et al., 1989)

Evidence for the duplication of the ORM1 locus was presented by Yuasa et al. (1987, 1988). In this work we present formal and population genetics results on the subtypes of ORM1 obtained in families from SW Germany and NW Portugal which are compatible with this duplication hypothesis.

MATERIAL AND METHODS

Blood samples were obtained by venipuncture and sera or EDTA plasmas were stored at -20°C until use. Sample treatment and phenotyping were performed as previously described (Luckenbach et al., 1989).

RESULTS AND DISCUSSION

Description of phenotypes

Common ORM1 phenotypes present either a single band – interpreted as homozygous – or two (presumable heterozygotes). However some three-banded patterns were also found (Fig.1), showing in the same individual gene products corresponding to ORM1*S, ORM1*F1 and ORM1*F2 or to ORM1*S, ORM1*F1 and ORM1*F3.

Formal genetics and segregation analysis

As stated above, common phenotypes are consistent with the hypothesis that orosomucoid is coded by two autosomal structural loci, ORM1 (with two common alleles) and ORM2.

The appearance of individuals with three gene products suggests, on the contrary, that – at least in some cases – the ORM1 locus can be duplicated, in accordance with the interpretation of Yuasa et al. (1987, 1988). Therefore, a duplication was postulated for segregation analysis. Using the evidence available in both our samples two 'haplotypes' are required: F1F2 and F1F3.

Advances in Forensic Haemogenetics 4
Edited by Ch. Rittner and P. M. Schneider
© Springer-Verlag Berlin Heidelberg 1992

TABLE 1. ORM1 Mating type distribution in SW Germany and NW Portugal

Type		SW Germany observed	expected	NW Portugal observed	expected	Allele/haplotype frequencies
F1	x F1	17	15.74	15	16.12	SW Germany:
F1	x F1F2	3	2.10	3	2.02	F1 0.578
F1	x F1F4	2	0.55	0	–	F1F2 0.019
F1	x F1F5	1	0.44	0	–	F1F3 0.004
F1	x F1S	36	42.47	40	39.60	F4 0.005
F1	x S	13	14.33	11	12.14	F5 0.004
F1F2	x F1S	3	2.84	4	2.52	S 0.390
F1F2	x F1F2S	1	0.09	0	0.08	
F1F2	x S	0	0.96	1	0.77	NW Portugal:
F1F3	x F1S	1	0.59	0	–	F1 0.608
F1F4	x F1S	1	0.73	0	–	F1F2 0.019
F1F5	x F1S	1	0.59	0	–	S 0.373
F1S	x F1S	34	28.66	24	24.28	
F1S	x F1F2S	2	1.88	2	1.52	
F1S	x S	23	19.34	13	14.89	
F1F2S	x S	1	0.64	3	0.47	
F1F3S	x S	1	0.13	0	–	
S	x S	1	3.26	2	2.28	
Others		0	5.66	0	1.31	
Total		141		118		

In Table 1 we show the mating type distribution found in SW Germany and NW Portugal. It is worth to mention that the research in the two labs, although independent, was carried out using the same techniques and produced homogeneous results, and we underline the fact that in all individuals with F2, F1 was also present.

Both distributions agree well with Hardy-Weinberg expectations; in the first case expected values were calculated according to a 6-allele/haplotype model: F1, S, F1F2, F4, F1F3 and F5, while in the Portuguese sample only F1, S and F1F2 are needed to explain the results; *S, *F4 and *F5 frequencies were estimated by gene counting; while F1F2 and F1F3 'haplotypes' were estimated using F1F2S and F1F3S heterozygotes.

We analysed the accordance of offspring phenotype distributions with mendelian expectations in both samples (totalling 407 and 315 for German and Portuguese, respectively) and we found no significant segregation distortions or unexpected phenotypes (except when F1F2 or F1F3 were involved). In Table 2, for brevity reasons, only the results concerning these matings are shown. Expected segregation ratios were calculated according to the previous hypothesis; for instance, in the first mating type, F1xF1F2, we assumed that the last phenotype can be genotypically F1F2/F1F2 or F1/F1F2.

TABLE 2. Segregation analysis of informative mating types giving evidence for duplicated ORM1 genes; families from SW Germany (G) and NW Portugal (P).

mating type	sample	offspring phenotypes						
		F1	F1F2	F1F3	F1S	F1F2S	F1F3S	S
F1 x F1F2	G	4	3					
		3.45	3.55					
	P	10	4					
		6.89	7.12					
F1F2 x F1S	G	0	3		3	2		
		1.97	2.03		1.97	2.03		
	P	7	2		2	5		
		3.93	4.07		3.93	4.07		
F1F2 x F1F2S	G		0		1	2		
			1.50		0.74	0.76		
F1F2 x S	P				0	3		
					1.48	1.52		
F1F3 x F1S	G	0		1	1		0	
		0.5		0.5	0.5		0.5	
F1F2S x S	G					2		1
						1.5		1.5
	P					3		4
						3.5		3.5
F1S x F1F2S	G		2		0	5		2
			2.25		2.25	2.25		2.25
	P		3		4	2		3
			3.0		3.0	3.0		3.0
F1F3S x S	G			2				1
				1.5				1.5

In conclusion, the results clearly support both qualitatively and quantitatively the formal hypothesis for ORM1 locus: two common alleles (*F1, *S) and rarer ones (*F1F2, *F1F3, *F4, *F5) of which two (*F1F2, *F1F3) behave like tandem duplications.

Although we have performed experiments with increasing amounts of alkylating reagents, to confirm that the appearance of three-banded patterns was not resulting from an incomplete reaction (Fig.2), an alternative hypothesis can not be ruled out: *F2 and *F3 are true, non-duplicated, alleles for which the corresponding gene products behave in a similar manner as the ORM2 product fixed in our population, i.e., producing always two bands. More formal, biochemical and molecular results are needed to clarify this issue.

REFERENCES

Dente L, Ciliberto G, Cortese R (1985) Structure of the human alpha 1-acid glycoprotein gene: sequence homology with other human acute phase protein genes. Nucleic Acids Res 13: 3941-3952

Eap CB, Cuendet C, Baumann P (1988) Orosomucoid (alpha-1 acid glycoprotein) phenotyping by use of immobilized pH gradients with 8 mol/l urea and immunoblotting. Hum Genet 80: 183-185

Escallon MH, Ferrell RE, Kamboh MJ (1987) Genetic studies of low-abundance human plasma proteins. V. Evidence for a second orosomucoid structural locus (ORM2) expressed in plasma. Am J Hum Genet 41: 418-427

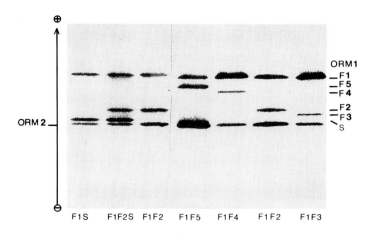

Fig. 1. ORM1 phenotypes. F1F2 sample is a pretyped reference (S Weidinger); for the other variants the nomenclature is tentative, due to the different methods used by previous reports

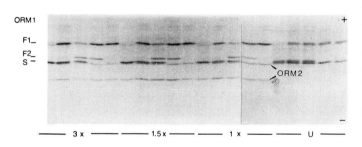

Fig. 2. ORM1 phenotypes after treatment with various amounts of alkylating reagent (iodacetamide). The same set of five samples, by the same order, was untreated (U), treated as described previously (1x) and with increasing amounts of the reagent (1.5x and 3x)

REFERENCES (cont.)

Johnson AM, Schmid K, Alper CA, Bisset L (1969). Inheritance of human alpha-1 acid glycoprotein (orosomucoid) variants. J Clin Invest 48: 2293-2299

Krüger HJ, Edler M, Keil W, Tröger HD (1989) ORM1 subtypes in Hannover and Lower Saxony, FRG, by PAG SIEF and immunoblotting (N=1934); 11 variants. Adv Forens Haemogenet 3: 308-312

Luckenbach C, Kömpf J, Ritter H (1989). Improved subtyping of orosomucoid 1 (ORM, alpha-1 acid-glycoprotein). Ärztl Lab 35: 192-193

Thymann M, Eiberg H (1986) Orosomucoid polymorphism: determination by separatory isoelectric focusing and demonstration of ORM*F subtypes. Adv Forens Haemogenet 1: 162-166

Yuasa J, Umetsu K, Suenaga K, Robinet-Levy M (1986) Orosomucoid (ORM) typing by isoelectric focusing: evidence for two structural loci ORM1 and ORM2. Hum Genet 74: 160-161

Yuasa J, Umetsu K, Suenaga K, Ito K, Robinet-Levy M (1987) Orosomucoid (ORM) typing by isoelectric focusing: evidence for gene duplication of ORM1 and genetic polymorphism of ORM2. Hum Genet 77: 255-258

Yuasa J, Umetsu K, Suenaga K (1988) Orosomucoid (ORM) typing by isoelectric focusing: evidence for an additional duplicated ORM1 locus haplotype and close linkage of two ORM loci. Am J Hum Genet 43: 165-169

ACKNOWLEDGEMENTS: This research was partially supported by DAAD.

Species identification from tissue particles using lectin- and immuno-histochemical methods

K. Nishi, T. Fukunaga, Y. Yamamoto, M. Yamada, M. Kane, N. Ito* and S. Kawahara*
Department of legal medicine, Shiga university of medical science,
Ohtsu 520-21, Shiga, Japan
*Department of legal medicine, Nara medical university,
Kashihara 634, Nara, Japan

INTRODUCTION

Many kinds of forensic biological materials found at scenes of murder and traffic accidents are brought to forensic scientists for identification. Although various immunological methods and DNA techniques for the species identification from blood and bloodstains are now available, there are few investigations for blood grouping and species identification from tissue particles or tissue debris(Fechner et al 1989). In this study we report a method for species identification from tissue particles using lectin- and immuno-histochemical techniques.

MATERIALS AND METHODS

Tissue specimens from vertebrate species including fishes, frogs, saurians, chickens , mammals and primates were used in this study. The tissue specimens from primate species including 2 chimpanzees and 3 gibbons and non-primate mammals were obtained from the Primate Institute of Kyoto University and Institute for Experimental Animals of Shiga University of Medical Science. The human tissue specimens were obtained from routine autopsies. The specimens were fixed in 10% formalin, embedded in paraffin and sectioned at a thickness of 4 μm. After deparaffinizing, the sections were incubated for lectin staining and immunostaining with monoclonal antibodies, as described previously (Ito et al 1986, Nishi et al 1989). Hoseradish-peroxidase labelled Ulex europaeus agglutinin I (UEA), blood goup H specific lectin, and Griffonia simplicifolia aggulutinin I-B4(GSAI-B4), blood group B specific lectin, were purchased from E. Y. Laboratories (San Mateo CA, USA). Anti A and B antibodies were purchased from Biotest Diagnostic (Frankfurt, Germany). Anti-type II chain H antibody were obtained from Dako (Santa Barbara, USA). Sections stained with lectins or monoclonal antibodies were counterstained with hematoxylin, dehydrated and mounted in balsam .

RESULTS AND DISCUSSION

GSAIB4 and UEA used in the present study bind specifically to non-reducing terminal αGAL and αFUC residue showing blood group B and O specificity respectively (Wood et al 1979, Pereira et al 1978). Alroy et al(1987)reported that vascular endothelia from various mammalian species are selectively stained with GSAIB4 which does not usually react with human endothelia and the vascular endothelial cells of humans are consistently stained with UEA which does not bind to other mammalian endothelial cells. In the previous report(Ito et al 1990) we showed that ABO blood group antigens and UEA reactivity appeared and GSAIB4 reactivity disappeared in endothelial cells and red blood cells directly corresponding to the stage in primate evolution.

The results obtained in this study, as shown in Tab. 1, suggest that the expression of ABH antigens and carbohydrate epitopes on erythrocytes membrane and vascular endothelial cells is closely related to the evolutionary stage of vertebrate species, although epithelial cells of gastrointestinal tract and secretory cells of tissues from various vertebrate species tested in this study expressed ABO antigens.

Advances in Forensic Haemogenetics 4
Edited by Ch. Rittner and P. M. Schneider
© Springer-Verlag Berlin Heidelberg 1992

Red blood cells and endothelia of non-mammalian vertebrates such as saurel, yellow-tail, saurians and chickens, except those cells of frogs, showed no reactivity with GSAIB4, UEA and ABH antibodies. Epithelial cells from the gastrointestinal tract from edible frogs and bullfrogs showed good reactivity with monoclonal anti B antibody. Vascular endothelial cells also reacted with monoclonal anti A antibody and red blood cells from these frogs showed weak reactivity with anti B antibody. The erythrocytes of frogs are morphologically different from those of mammals, since the erythrocytes of frogs are nucleated cells.

Epithelial cells from the gastrointestinal tract from mice, rats and rabbits showed good reactivity with ABH antibodies. Secretory cells of the salivary glands , acinar cells of the pancreas , epithelial cells of gastrointestinal tract and biliary duct epithelium from cats, dogs, prosimians (common tupai, grand galagoand, ring-tailed lemur) and new world monkeys (common marmoset, cotton-top tamarin, common squirred monkey and central american spider monkey) showed good reactivity with monoclonal A, B or H antibody. The blood group of individuals of these animals could be determined , according to the reactivity of these cells with the antibodies. UEA and GSAIB4 showed various reactivity with secretory cells and characteristic of blood group specific lectins. Vascular endothelial cells and erythrocytes from non-primate mammals, such as cow, deer, pig, wild boar and other mammals described above showed no reactivity with monoclonal ABH antibodies. In the evolutionary stage of non-primate mammals and lower primate species, such as prosimians and new world monkeys, GSAIB4 binding to erythrocytes and endothelial cells appears irrespective of animal species. These results suggest that α-galactosyl epitopes consititute a substantial proportion of carbohydrate residues on those cells of non-primate mammals and lower primates. The reactivity of GSAIB4 to these cells is not due to terminal αGal residues of the B antigen, since blood group ABH antigens are not expressed in these cells of non-primate mammals and lower primate species.

In old world monkeys (japanese monkey, crab-eating monkey, rhesus monkey, savanna monkey and hamadryas baboon) ABH antigens are expressed in secretory cells, as in non-primate mammals and lower primate species, in endothelial cells but not yet in erythrocytes. Usually, UEA and GSAI-B4 did not react with endothelial cells from old world monkeys except those individuals whose endothelial cells reacted with anti H or B antibody.

In anthropoid apes(chimpanzee and gibbon), both red blood cells and endothelial cells expressed ABH antigen as in humans. The secretory cells also showed good reactivity with ABH antibodies. Although UEA reacted with endothelial cells from two chimpanzees, which were both typed as blood group A, as found in of humans, UEA did not show reactivity with the cells of 3 gibbons which were typed as blood group AB. These results indicate that the ability of endothelial cells to show reactivity with UEA seems to be possessed only at the stage of the highest primates such as chimpanzee and humans.

In humans and chimpanzees UEA reactivity is recognized on erythrocytes and endothelial cells irrespective of the ABO group of the individuals. Although Petryniak and Goldstein(1986) demonstrated that UEA showed good affinity for the type II chain H antigen, the UEA reactivity with erythrocytes and endothelial cells is not due to αFuc of type II chain H antigen, because monoclonal anti type II chain H antibody used in this study hardly reacted with erythrocytes and endothelial cells from blood group A, B and AB individuals except blood group A $_2$ individuals(Nishi et al 1989).

It seems that both the changing of carbohydrate epitopes and the development of ABH antigen expression on red blood cells and endothelial cells are regarded as an important evolutionary event in vertebrate species.

We reported(Fechner et al 1989) that ABH antigens and human hemoglobin antigen can be reliably detected in the mummified tissues particles for a long period of time by means of immunohistochemical methods using ABH antibodies and anti human hemoglobin. Since blood vessels are present in all tissues and are expected to be found in putrified and/or mummified tissues, the histochemical method described in this study seems to be useful for the forensic practice.

Table 1.
The expression of ABH antigens and lectin binding in red blood ells, endothelial cells and body secretions of various animal species

| | Red Blood Cells | | | Endothelial Cells | | | Secretions |
	A, B, H	GSAIB4	UEA	A, B, H	GSAIB4	UEA	A, B, H
Humans	+	–	+	+	–	+	+
Anthropoid apes							
Chimpanzee	+	–	+	+	–	+	+
Gibbon	+	–	–	+	–	–	+
Old world monkeys	–	–	–	+	–/+*	–/+*	+
New world monkeys	–	+	–	–	+	–	+
Prosimians	–	+	–	–	+	–	+
Nonprimate mammals	–	+	–	–	+	–	+
Nonmammalian Vertebrates							
chicken	–	–	–	–	–	–	n. d
saurian	–	–	–	–	–	–	n. d
frog	+	+	–	+	–	–	+
fish	–	–	–	–	–	–	+

*: Cells from B and 0 typed individuals reacted with the blood group B and H specific lectins respectively. n. d: not done.

CONCLUSION

The results obtained in this study show that the species identification from tissue particles can be reliably performed by lectin- and immuno-histochemial methods using GSAIB4, UEA and blood group ABH antibodies.

REFERENCES

Alroy J, Goyal V, Skutelsky E (1987) Lectin histochemistry of mammalian endothelium. Histochemistry 86;603-607

Fechner G, Rand S, Nishi K, Brinkmann B (1989) Immunohistochemische Antigennachweise an eingetrockneten Gewebspartikeln. Z. Rechtsmed 102; 241-246

Ito N, Nishi K, Nakajima M, Ishitani A, Mizumoto J, Hirota T (1986) Localization of blood group antigens in human pancreas with lectin-horseradish peroxidase conjugates. Acta Histochem Cytochem 19;205-218

Ito N, Nishi K, Nakajima M, Okamura Y, Hirota T (1990) Relationship between lectin binding properties and the expression of blood group ABH antigens in vascular endothelia and red blood cells from 18 primate species. Histochem J 22; 113-118

Nishi K, Fechner G, Rand S, Brinkmann B (1989) Light-microscopic examination of ABH and Lewis antigens in human tracheal and epiglottic glands using the avidin-biotin-peroxidase complex technique. Z. Rechtsmed 102;256-262

Pereira MEA, Kislius EC, Gruezo F, Kabat EA (1978) Immunochemical studies on the combining site of the blood group H-specific lectin I from Ulex europeus seeds. Arch Biochem Biophys 185;108-115

Petryniak J, Goldstein, IJ (1986) Immunochemical studies on the interaction between synthetic glycoconjugate and α-L-fucosyl binding lectins. Biochemistry 25;2829-2838

Wood C, Kabat EA, Murphy LA, Goldstein IJ (1979) Immunochemical studies of the combining sites of the two isolectins, A4 and B4 isolated from Banderiraea simplicifolia. Arch Biochem Biophys 198;1-11

Polymorphism of Plasminogen in Sardinia (Italy)

R. Domenici, I. Spinetti

Department of Biomedicine - Section of Legal Medicine
University of Pisa - Via Roma 55
I-56126 Pisa (Italia)

INTRODUCTION

Plasminogen (PLG), a plasma protein of the beta globulin fraction with a molecular weigth of about 92000 and a constant portion of 2-3% carbohydrate, is the precursor of the fibrinolytic enzyme plasmin.

Plasminogen polymorphism was first independently described by Hobart (1979) and Raum et al. (1979). Several methods demonstrating PLG phenotypes have been reported. Skoda et al. (1986) recommended to use desialized serum samples, IEF for separation and subsequent functional and/or immunological methods for the detection of PLG phenotypes. Plasminogen polymorphism comprises two common, codominant autosomal, alleles and a number of rare variants, including a silent allele PLG*Q0. The common alleles are designated PLG*A and PLG*B, while the rare variants are differentiated into three groups according to their electrophoretic mobility: PLG A, PLG B and PLG M variants (for a review see Asmundo 1990).

We report the frequencies of PLG system in a population from Sardinia. This region is genetically highly differentiated, for its peculiar ethno-geographical situation, as compared to Continental Italy. This has to be taken into account considering the choice of allele frequencies for probability of paternity calculation (Domenici et al. 1988).

MATERIALS AND METHODS

Sera were collected from 495 unrelated blood donors originating from Cagliari, Sardinia (all their parents and grandparents were born in Cagliari province).
PLG typing was performed as elsewere described (Spinetti et al. 1990).

RESULTS AND DISCUSSION

PLG phenotype pattern obtained from neuraminidase-treated serum, by IEF on agarose gels followed by immunofixation with monospecific antiserum, is shown in Fig.1. The distribution of phenotypes and extimated gene frequencies in our population sample are reported in Table 1. The uncommon allotypes A-A3, A-M4 and B-M4 were seen. The observed phenotypes do not present any meaningful deviation from the Hardy-Weinberg equilibrium. The theoretical exclusion rate in cases of disputed paternity is 18.12% (I class = 9.66%, II class = 8.46%).

Advances in Forensic Haemogenetics 4
Edited by Ch. Rittner and P. M. Schneider
© Springer-Verlag Berlin Heidelberg 1992

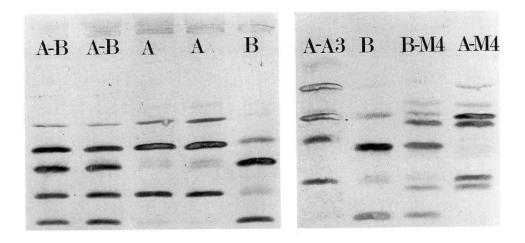

Fig.1 PLG phenotypes observed by isoelectric focusing on agarose gel and immunofixation

Table 1. Phenotype distribution and allele frequencies in a sample from Cagliari (Italy)

Phenotype	Observed	Expected	Allele frequencies
A	227	235.60	PLG*A = .6899 ±.015
A-B	218	203.52	
B	38	43.95	PLG*B = .2980 ±.014
A-A3	8		
A-M4	3	8.28 (*)	PLG*A3 = .0081 ±.003
B-A3	0		
B-M4	1	3.58 (*)	PLG*M4 = .0040 ±.002
A3	0		
M4	0	0.07 (*)	
Total	495	495.00	

$\Sigma\chi^2 = 4.73$, df = 3, P > .10   (*) A3+M4 pooled

Table 2 shows a comparison between our results and previous data about some other italian population samples. It appears that the Sardinia frequencies are very close to those of Tuscany reported by Spinetti *et al.* (1990), but very different from all the others (χ^2 heterogeneity of Sardinia against Venetia + Venetia Julia + Lombardy [pooled] = 134, P<.0001 for 1 df).

Table 2. PLG allele frequencies in Italy

Region	n	PLG*A	PLG*B	PLG*rare	References
Venetia	1325	.840	.159	.001	Cortivo *et al.* (1986)
Venetia Julia	716	.858	.140	.001	Foi *et al.* (1988)
Lombardy	877	.840	.158	.002	Cerri *et al.* (1989)
Tuscany	(*)	.830	.160	.010	Pascali *et al.* (1984)
Tuscany	383	.675	.322	.003	Spinetti *et al.* (1990)
Latium	(*)	.810	.180	.010	Pascali *et al.* (1984)
Campania	(*)	.810	180	.010	Pascali *et al.* (1984)
Lucania	(*)	.780	.210	.010	Pascali *et al.* (1984)
Sardinia	495	.690	.298	.012	This study

(*) Tuscany + Latium + Lucania + Campania: n = 2116

REFERENCES

Asmundo A (1990) I progressi e le conoscenze del polimorfismo del plasminogeno (PLG) e la sua applicazione ai casi di paternità controversa. Riv It Med Leg 12:1019-1037

Cerri N, De Ferrari F, Licenziati S (1989) Il polimorfismo del plasminogeno (PLG) nella popolazione della provincia di Brescia. Arch Med Leg Ass 11:49-55

Cortivo P, Caenazzo L, Crestani C, Scorretti C, Benciolini P, Pornaro E (1986) The polymorphism of plasminogen (PLG) by ultrathin-layer isoelectric focusing. Distribution in the Veneto population. Z Rechtsmed 96: 275-278

Domenici R, Giari A, Bargagna M (1988) Distribution of Gc, Pi and Tf subtypes in Sardinia (Italy). Adv Forens Haemogenet 2:561-565

Foi A, Michelon C, Scalettaris U (1988) Determinazione delle frequenze geniche e dei fenotipi del plasminogeno (PLG) nella provincia di Udine mediante isoelettrofocalizzazione su gel di poliacrilamide. Riv It Med Leg 10: 545-549

Hobart MJ (1979) Genetic polymorphism of human plasminogen. Ann Hum Genet 42:419-423

Pascali VL, Ranalletta D, Gentile V, Fiori A (1984) Plasminogen allotypes and their use in paternity investigation. J Forensic Sci Soc 24:437

Raum D, Marcus D, Alper CA (1979) Genetic control of human plasminogen. Clin Res 27:458A

Skoda U, Bertrams J, Dykes D, Eiberg H, Hobart M, Hummel K, Kühnl P, Mauff G, Nakamura S, Nishimukai H, Raum D, Tokunaga K, Weidénger S (1986) Proposal for the nomenclature of human plasminogen (PLG) polymorphism. Vox Sang 51:244-248

Spinetti I, Domenici R, Giari A, Bargagna M (1990) Polymorphism of plasminogen in Tuscany (Italy). Z Rechtsmed 103:163-167

HAPTAGLOBIN SUBTYPES IN A POPULATION FROM SOUTH WEST GERMANY

U. Härle[1], W. Reichert[1], R. Mattern[1] and G. Pfaff[2]

[1] Institute of Forensic Medicine, University of Heidelberg
Voßstr. 2, 6900 Heidelberg (Germany)

[2] Institute of Internal Medicine, University of Heidelberg

INTRODUCTION

Haptoglobin (HP) is a polymorphic marker whose main three phenotypes HP 1, HP 2-1, and HP 2 were first separated by Smithies (1955) using starch gel electrophoresis. Subtyping of haptoglobin by isoelectric focusing has been shown to lead to an isolated exclusion rate of up to 33 % in paternity assessment (Thymann et al 1990). Despite this high value of the HP subtype polymorphism it is still rarely included in routine testing because of the time consuming steps in HP purification.

The substitution of an immunoprecipitation technique (Scherz et al. 1990) for the more laborious ion exchange chromatographic methods overcomes this limitation. Using this technique we have determined the frequencies of HP subtypes in a large population sample from South West Germany.

MATERIAL AND METHODS

1487 sera from a random population sample of unrelated adult German nationals who had participated in a 1985 cardiovascular health survey in the city of Stuttgart were examined. Prior to analysis, samples had been stored at -20° C for five years. HP subtypes were determined by the method of Scherz et al. (1990). For a cross-validation of the new technique HP phenotypes were determined by starch gel electrophoresis according to Smithies (1955).

RESULTS AND DISCUSSION

Haptoglobin subtypes could be identified for 1485 out of 1487 samples (99,9 %). In two samples, the HP subtype could not be determined due to irregular band patterns which did not match commen subtypes. In one case sample deterioration was the likely cause. The second sample was classified as HP 2 in conventional HP typing. According to its band pattern in HP subtyping, we cannot rule out the possibility of an alpha-2-variant not yet described.

In eight other samples, initial discordance between the two methods could upon repeat analysis be traced to inferior resolution of starch gel electrophoresis.

Advances in Forensic Haemogenetics 4
Edited by Ch. Rittner and P. M. Schneider
© Springer-Verlag Berlin Heidelberg 1992

All common HP subtypes except the heterozygous HP 2FF-2SS and the both homozygous HP 2FF and HP 2SS were observed in our sample. Expected and observed frequencies of HP subtypes (Tab. 1) were in good agreement as to be expected under the Hardy-Weinberg law.

Table 1: Expected and observed frequencies of HP subtypes (n=1485)

HP SUBTYPE	OBSERVED		EXPECTED
	n	percent	n
1F	29	1.95	37.19
1F-1S	102	6.87	101.91
1S	70	4.71	69.82
1F-2FF	3	0.20	2.06
1F-2FS	299	20.13	282.16
1F-2SS	8	0.54	9.49
1S-2FF	4	0.27	2.82
1S-2FS	386	25.99	386.62
1S-2SS	12	0.81	13.01
2FF	0	0.00	0.03
2FF-2FS	6	0.40	7.80
2FF-2SS	0	0.00	0.26
2FS	526	35.42	535.20
2FS-2SS	40	2.69	36.02
2SS	0	0.00	0.61
Total	1485	100.00	1485

χ^2 goodness of fit 5,96 with 14 degrees of freedom, p = 0,97

Calculated frequencies for HP alleles were: HP*1F=0.1582, HP*1S=0.2168, HP*2FF=0.004, HP*2FS=0.60, HP*2SS=0.0202.
Table 2 contrasts the observed frequencies with reports from the literature.

Table 2: Comparison of observed HP allele frequencies with reports from the literature

POPULATION	N	HP*1F	HP*1S	HP*2FF	HP*2FS	HP*2SS	REFERENCE
NORWAY	3318	0.16	0.226	0.004	0.572	0.037	Teige et al. 1988
SWEDEN	564	0.156	0.231	0.001	0.571	0.041	Hjalmarsson 1988
DENMARK	2184	0.151	0.241	0.002	0.565	0.040	Thymann et al. 1990
GERMANY							
Berlin	1275	0.1471	0.2502	0.002	0.5753	0.0251	Patzelt a.Schröder 1985
Lower Saxony	1500	0.1537	0.2523	0.003	0.562	0.029	Rothämel et al. 1989
Rhine-Ruhr	1035	0.1391	0.2575	0.0014	0.5831	0.0188	Bertrams et al. 1988
Stuttgart	1485	0.1582	0.2168	0.004	0.6	0.0202	own data
Southwest	182	0.144	0.254	0.004	0.574	0.024	Zischler et al. 1987
SWITZERLAND							
Berne	1266	0.126	0.2389	0.0099	0.5829	0.0423	Scherz et al. 1990
Lausanne	500	0.147	0.249	0.003	0.567	0.034	Dimo-Simonin et al.1990
FRANCE							
Southwest	202	0.139	0.245	0.012	0.547	0.045	Shibata et al. 1982
SPAIN	317	0.142	0.238	0.006	0.621	0.002	Moral and Panadero 1983
HUNGARY	675	0.1185	0.2207	0.0037	0.6555	0.0015	Hevér and Hajpál

To our experience, haptoglobin isolation by immunoprecipitation and isoelectric focusing as proposed by Scherz et al.(1990) is a fast, easy, and reliable technique for HP subtyping. The possibility to process large sample sizes rapidly renders this method into a valuable tool for population studies as well as for forensic investigations. Even smaller laboratories have now the opportunity to include this marker system in the routine paternity testing. The storage of sera over an extended period of up to five years at -20° C does apparently not grossly affect sample quality for Hp subtyping.

The allele frequencies for haptoglobin observed in a population from South West Germany are in close agreement with the frequencies reported for other European populations.

REFERENCES

Bertrams J, Müller B, Luboldt W, in Mayr WR (ed):
  Advances in Forensic Haemogenetics 2, Springer
  Verlag Berlin, 1988, pp 158-162

Dimo-Simonin N, Brandt-Casadevall C, Gujer HR, in Polesky HF,
  Mayr WR (eds): Advances in Forensic Haemogenetics 3,
  Springer Verlag Berlin, 1990, pp 239-242

Hevér Ö, Hajpál A, Hum Hered 1978; 28: 100-103

Hjalmarsson K, in Mayr WR (ed): Advances in Forensic
  Haemogenetics 2, Springer Verlag Berlin, 1988, pp 179-183

Moral P, Panadero AM, Hum Hered 1983; 33: 192-194

Patzelt D, Schröder H, Z Rechtsmed 1985; 94: 207-212

Rothämel T, Krüger HJ, Tröger HD, Z Rechtsmed 1989; 102: 391-397

Scherz R, Reber B, Pflugshaupt R, in Polesky HF, Mayr WR
  (eds): Advances in Forensic Haemogenetics 3, Springer Verlag
  Berlin, 1990, pp 236-238

Shibata K, Constans J, Viau M, Matsumoto H, Hum Genet 1982;
  61: 210-214

Smithies O, Biochem J 1955; 61: 629-641

Teige B, Olaisen B, Pedersen L, Lie H, in Mayr WR (ed):
  Advances in Forensic Haemogenetics 2, Springer Verlag
  Berlin, 1988, pp 179-183

Thymann M, Svensmark O, Masumba G, Brokso H, Skibsby LB,
  Electrophoresis 1990; 11: 61-65

Zischler H, Kömpf J, Ritter H, Ärztl Lab 1987; 33: 85-87

Plasma Protein Polymorphism in HIV-Seropositive Patients: GC- and TF*C-Subtypes and PI-System

W. Huckenbeck, V. Stancu, B.M.E. Kuntz, H.T. Brüster

Institute of Legal Medicine, Heinrich-Heine-University
Düsseldorf, FRG*

INTRODUCTION

Blood samples were taken from 279 patients of the Institute of Blood Coagulation and Transfusion Medicine at the Heinrich-Heine-University. The series includes individuals only HIV-seropositive, patients with ARC (AIDS related complex), AIDS and Kaposi-sarcoma. Typing was carried out in laboratory routine use.

RESULTS & DISCUSSION

In the GC system we found the distribution shown in tab.1. Comparing the findings with two control studies (tab.2) there are no significant differences between the gene frequencies (calculated by gene counting). In the TF*C system we arrived at a similar conclusion. The distribution of the phenotypes in HIV-seropositive probands (tab.3) is comparable to those found in obviously healthy persons (tab.4).

In our pilote study (1,4,5,6) we found an unusual distribution in the PI system. The now available results do not confirm those findings. Though there are still differences between the observed and the expected values (tab.5) – especially concerning the M2 allele –, the gene frequencies are comparable to those found in other studies of PI distribution in North Rhine-Westphalia (tab.6).

At last we come to the conclusion that there is no association between the examined haemogenetic systems and HIV-infection.

TAB.1 GC-SUBTYPES IN HIV-SEROPOSITIVE PATIENTS

Phenotype	observed		expected	
	n	%	n	%
1S	107	38.35	101.76	36.47
1F1S	43	15.42	48.90	17.53
1F	7	2.51	5.88	2.11
2-1F	24	8.60	20.31	7.28
2	18	6.45	17.56	6.29
2-1S	80	28.67	84.55	30.31
total	279	100	279	100

TAB.2 OTHER STUDIES ON GC-POLYMORPHISM IN NORTH RHINE-WESTPHALIA

Country	GC*1S	GC*1F	GC*2	n	Ref.
Lower Rhine region	0.5649	0.1489	0.2824	262	(7)
Düsseldorf region	0.5471	0.1564	0.2960	1157	(7,8)
This study	0.6039	0.1452	0.2509	279	

* and Institute of Blood Coagulation and Transfusion Medicine

TAB.3   TF*C-SUBTYPES IN HIV-SEROPOSITIVE PATIENTS

Phenotype	observed		expected	
	n	%	n	%
c1	162	59.56	163.68	60.18
c2c1	73	26.84	70.59	25.95
c2	6	2.21	7.61	2.80
c3c1	25	9.19	24.05	8.84
c3	0	0	0.88	0.32
c3c2	6	2.20	5.19	1.91
total	272	100	272	100

TAB.4   OTHER STUDIES ON TF*C-POLYMORPHISM IN NORTH RHINE-WESTPHALIA

Country	c1	c2	c3	n	Ref.
Lower Rhine region	0.8111	0.1431	0.0401	262	(7)
Düsseldorf region	0.7816	0.1355	0.0711	380	(2,7)
This study	0.7757	0.1673	0.0570	272	

TAB.5   PI-PHENOTYPES IN HIV-SEROPOSITIVE PATIENTS

Phenotype	observed		expected	
	n	%	n	%
M1	153	54.84	149.89	53.72
M2M1	54	19.35	63.77	22.86
M2	13	4.66	6.78	2.43
M3M1	41	14.69	37.38	13.39
M3	2	0.72	2.33	0.84
M3M2	6	2.15	7.95	2.85
M1Var	8	2.87	8.06	2.89
M2Var	1	0.36	1.72	0.62
M3Var	0	0	1.01	0.36
Var	1	0.36	0.11	0.04
total	279	100	279	100

TAB.6   OTHER STUDIES ON PI-POLYMORPHISM IN NORTH RHINE-WESTPHALIA

Country	M1	M2	M3	Var	n	Ref.
Düsseldorf region	0.7468	0.1500	0.0906	0.0125	160	(1,4)
This study	0.7329	0.1559	0.0913	0.0197	279	

Var includes PI*S and PI*Z

REFERENCES

1) Bonte, W., Huckenbeck, W., Kuntz, B.M.E., Brüster, H.TH. (1990) Plasma Protein
   Polymorphism in HIV-seropositive Patients: GC- and TF*C Subtypes and
   PI-System. in : Polesky, H.F., Mayr, W.R. (eds.) Advances in Forensic
   Haemogenetics 3, Springer Verlag

2) Driesel, A.J., Scheil, H.-G., Pfeiffer, I.M., Röhrborn, G. (1981) Gene frequencies
   of transferrin (TF*C) subtypes in Western Germany (Düsseldorf region).
   Z.Rechtsmed. 86: 133-135

3) Eales, L.J., Nye, K.E., Parkin, J.M., Weber, J.N., Forster, S.M., Harris, J.R.W.,
   Pinching, A.J. (1987) Association of different allelic forms of group
   specific component with susceptibility to and clinical manifestation of
   human immunodeficiency virus infection. Lancet I: 999-1002

4) Huckenbeck, W., Bonte, W., Kuntz, B.M.E., Brüster, H.TH. (1989) Plasma Protein-
   Poymorphismen bei HIV-seropositiven Probanden: Gc- und TF*C-Subtypen,
   PI-, C3- und BF-System. ADLI TIP DERGESI - Journal of Forensic
   Medicine 5(3-4): 103-116

5) Huckenbeck, W., Kuntz, B.M.E., Brüster, H.TH., Bonte, W., Wehr, A. (1990)
   Distribution of C3 and BF Phenotypes in HIV-seropositive Patients
   in : Polesky, H.F., Mayr, W.R. (eds.) Advances in Forensic Haemogenetics 3
   Springer Verlag

6) Huckenbeck, W., Kuntz, B.M.E., Bonte, W., Brüster, H.TH., Wehr, A. (1990)
   Plasma Protein Polymorphism in HIV-seropositive Patients: Allotype
   Frequencies in the Gm- and Km-System
   in : Polesky, H.F., Mayr, W.R. (eds.) Advances in Forensic Haemogenetics 3
   Springer Verlag

7) Scheil, H.-G., Fiedler, K.-P., Huckenbeck, W. (1991) Untersuchungen zur
   Phänotypen-Häufigkeit einiger hämogenetischer Polymorphismen am
   Niederrhein (Bereich Kleve, Goch, Kalkar). Anthrop.Anz. 49,1/2: 137-144

8) Scheil, H.-G., Driesel, A.J., Röhrborn, G. (1980) Distribution of Gc-subtypes in
   Western Germany (Düsseldorf region). Z.Rechtsmed. 84: 95-97

DETERMINATION OF PGM, EsD, GLO (1) AND EAP POLYMORPHS FROM HUMAN DENTAL PULP

Arun Sharma*,   V.K. Arora,**   V. Bhalla ***

*Scientific Officer, (Biology & Serology), State Forensic Science Laboratory, Police Complex, Bharari, Himachal Pradesh, Shimla (India). ** Deputy Advisor, Education, Planning Commission, Govt. of India, New Delhi-1 .(India)

INTRODUCTION

Genetic manifestations (blood groups, polymorphic enzymes) in biological evidences have extensively been utilized in forensic investigations. The last decade or so has witnessed a large amount of research work especially on the stability studies from blood stains. But the literature is sparse so far as the studies of enzyme typing in human dental pulp is concerned (Petersen and Heide, 1974; Turowska and Trela, 1977; Whittaker and Rothwell 1981; Henke et al., 1982 and Imai et al., 1984). The studies especially when the dental evidence could be used assume considerable significance in case of mass disasters, bride burning and general cases of arson where bodies are received either burnt, charred or badly mutilated and need to be identified. Whittaker and Rothwell (1981) observed that in some air disasters dental evidence alone has been responsible for the identification upto 40 percent of victims. Further, when a dead body is in advance stage of decomposition and only skeleton is left, teeth (with pulp) can still serve as a standard in place of blood (Petersen and Heide, 1974 and Lele et al., 1977).

MATERIALS AND METHODS

All types of teeth namely incisors, canines and molars were collected from fresh extractions carried out in the dental clinics alongwith the donors blood. However, only complete or intact teeth were selected for analysing genetic markers. At the same time, blood stains were made on cotton cloth pieces. These were put into separate envelopes, and stored at room temperature during different ambient conditions. Haemolystates were prepared and treated with an equal volume of β-mercaptoethanol (diluted 1:40 with distilled water) for PGM, GLO (1) typing and 0.05M Cleland's reagent for EsD and EAP typing.

Human teeth samples were broken and dental pulp picked up with the help of forceps in each case and treated like lysates before being applied on to origin slits already made in the gel (Sharma et al., 1988). Further, these samples were analysed for different enzyme systems as per earlier reports: PGM, EsD (Wraxall and Stolorow, 1978), GLO (1) (Scott. and Fowler, 1982) and EAP (Wraxall and Emes, 1976).

RESULTS AND DISCUSSIONS

The results of various polymorphic forms observed in human teeth are given in table (1)

***Professor, Department of Anthropology, Panjab University, Chandigarh-14,(India)

Advances in Forensic Haemogenetics 4
Edited by Ch. Rittner and P. M. Schneider
© Springer-Verlag Berlin Heidelberg 1992

All teeth samples tested for phosphoglucomutase variants gave positive results. All the three common polymorpohic forms were detected and there was a complete agreement between the phenotypes expressed in blood and dental pulp. The zymogram revealed intense band patterns in dental phenotypes. The stability studies carried out in the months of (April-July) showed that human teeth could be typed up to three months whereas the enzymatic activity in blood stains lasted for 14-16 days only under similar conditions.

Three common occurring polymorphic forms of glyoxalase 1 enzyme were detected. The zymogram demonstrated better resolution of bands in some heterozygous samples where three distinct bands were seen. The intensity of band patterns in human dental pulp was found to be similar to that in blood indicating thus a good amount of enzyme activity. Stability studies showed that the teeth samples could be typed up to 5 months (Oct. to Feb.) and against this typability of blood stains was restricted upto 6-7 weeks only.

Esterase D Phenotypes observed in dental pulp matched completely with donors lysates. However, heterozygous samples showed three distinct bands in zymogram. When subjected to identical conditions of storage, dental pulp showed typable activity upto 2 months in summer periods (May & June) and blood stains remained typable for 6-7 days only.

Tests for erythrocyte acid Phosphatase isozymes showed its presence in dental pulp. Although, the zymogram obtained did not show intense band patterns, this could not be improved either on applying greater quantity of dental pulp. Apparently, there seems to be less quantity of enzymatically active material associated with dental pulp tissue. Hence, stability studies were not performed on this enzyme system.

Table-1. Distribution patterns of Isoenzymes in Human Blood lysates and Dental Pulp

Sr. No.	Name of Enzyme system	Phenotypes	Haemolysate	Dental Pulp
1.	PGM	1-1	46	46
		2-1	36	36
		2-2	10	10
2.	EsD	1-1	78	78
		2-1	36	36
		2-2	4	4
3.	GLO (1)	1-1	6	6
		2-1	53	53
		2-2	47	47
4.	EAP	A	3	3
		BA	10	10
		B	35	35

The studies undertaken are indicative of the findings that the genetic markers detected in dental pulp and the donors blood are alike. However, considerable difference exists in their typable time limits. Since factors like heat humidity and bacterial contamination has bearing on stability of genetic markers but are unable to affect directly the dental pulp (by virtue of its insitu position) thus could be the reason for prolonged typable activity. With the rise in periods of storage, steady decrease in enzyme activity was observed in both cases.

REFERENCES

Henke J., Baur L. and Schweitzer H. (1982) Gm-, Km- Und EsD - Bestimmungenan der Zahnpulpa menschlicher Leichen. Z. Rechtesmed. 88: 271

Imai T., Nakasono I., Ohya I. and Suyama H. (1984) An identification of bloodgroups and isozymic phenotypes from teeth. Act. Criminaol, Med. Leg. Japan. 50: 196

Lele M.V., Malwankar A.G., Dange A.H. and Mediwale M.S. (1977) J. Ind. Acad. Forens. Sci. 16:3

Petersen N. and Heide K.G. (1974) Nachweis Von genetischen merkmalen in der zahnpulpa, Archiv fur Kriminologie 153:106

Scott A.C. and Fowler J.C.S. (1982) Electrophoretic typing of glyoxalase 1 (GLO 1) isoenzymes using a mixed starchagarose gel. Forens. Sci. Int. 20:287

Sharma Arun, Arora V.K. and Bhalla V. (1988) Studies on glyoxalase 1 isoenzymes in semen stains: Polymorphhism in Himachal (India) Population. Forens. Sci. Int. 37 :201

Turowska B. and Trela F. (1977) Studies on the isoenzymes PGM, ADA and AK in human teeth. Forens. Sci. 9:45

Whittaker D.K. and Rothwell T.J.(1981) Blood group substances in tooth dentine. 9th Internationale Tagung der Gessellschaft fur Forensische Blutgruppenkunde, Bern. 29-9 to 3.10.1981 , .151

Wraxall B.G.D. and Emes E.G. (1976) Erythrocyte acid Phosphatase in blood stains. J. Forens. Sci. Soc. 16: 127

Wraxall B.G.D. and Stolorow M.D. (1978) Recent advances in electrophoretic techniques of blood stain analysis. Presented at the 30th Annual Meeting of American Academy of Forensic Sciences held in St. Louis, MO, USA

HAPTOGLOBIN SUBTYPING by POLYACRYLAMIDE GEL ISOELECTRIC
FOCUSING of SERUM, HEMOLYZED BLOOD and BLOODSTAINS

A. Correns*, D. Patzelt**, P. Otremba*, H. Schröder* and
G. Geserick*

* Inst. of Forensic Medicine, Humboldt-University, Hannoversche
Str. 06, 0-1040 Berlin, FRG
** Inst. of Forensic Medicine, Ernst-Moritz-Arndt-University,
Kuhstraße 30, 0-2200 Greifswald, FRG

INTRODUCTION

The aim of the present investigation is to compare two
alternative methods for the isolation of haptoglobin:
ion-exchange chromatography and immunoprecipitation. The
possibility of Hp-subtype determination with immunoprecipitation in hemolytic sera, blood for alcohol testing (NaF
stabilized blood) and bloodstains has been investigated too.

MATERIAL AND METHODS

Preparation of the Haptoglobin
Ion-exchange chromatographie (according to Patzelt and Schröder
1985). Absolute non-hemolytic sera are needed. We used a Serva
Cellulose-Ion-exchanger DEAE-SS.
Immunoprecipitation (according to Scherz et al. 1990 and Dimo-
Simionin et al. 1990). For the preparation from serum we dealt
with the originally quoted amounts. The double amount was used
with hemolytic sera stored up to 10 months at -18 centigrade
and blood for alcohol testing (0.08 g NaF per 8 ml blood for
stabilization) stored up to 10 weeks. The bloodstains (cotton
textile 5x5 mm in dimension soaked with blood) had been set off
with 50 µl aqua dest. at first and then treated as the
hemolyzed blood. Most of the used anti-human Hp originated from
in house production, the rest came from Atlantic Antibodies
(Cat. No. 81952 G).
Hp-cleavage (according to Pastewka et al. 1973 or Constans and
Viau 1975).

Isoelectric focusing has been carried out in polyacrylamide
flat gels, 260 x 125 x 0,5 mm in dimension, using an LKB
Multiphor set. The gel (T = 5%, C = 3%) contained the following
carrier ampholytes (LKB ampholine): 0.6 ml 5-7, 0.2 ml 6-8, 0.3
ml 5-6 and 0.1 ml 3.5-10. After 45 minutes of prefocusing the
samples were placed onto the gel surface, using 0.5 x 1.0 cm
strips of filterpaper, and allowed to stay there 1 h. Focusing
took 3 h 30 min, with maximum electric values of 1,600 V,
10 mA, 10 W. Anolyt 1M H_3PO_4, catolyt 1M NaOH.
Visualization with Serva Blue (1 g Serva Blue + 180 ml ethanol
+ 100 ml formalin + 420 ml aqua dest.).

Advances in Forensic Haemogenetics 4
Edited by Ch. Rittner and P. M. Schneider
© Springer-Verlag Berlin Heidelberg 1992

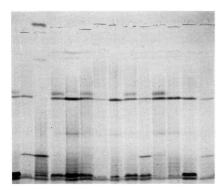

Fig. 1. Hp-subtypes prepared through ion-exchange chromatographie from sera. From left to right: 1S-2FS, 2FS, 2FS, 2FS-1F, 1S-2FS, 2FS-1F, 2FS, 2FS, 2FS-1F, 2FS, 2FS-1F, 1S-2FF, 1S-2FS, 2FS-1F. The anode is at the top

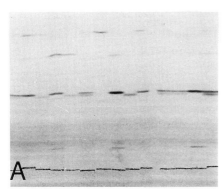

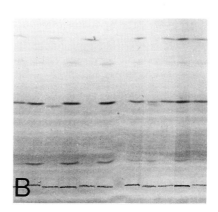

Fig. 2. Hp-subtypes prepared through immunoprecipitation
A) from sera. From left to right: 2FS-1F, 1S-2FS, 1S-1F, 2SS-2FS, 2SS-1F, 2FS-1F, 1S, 2FS, 1F, 1S-2FS, 2FS-1F, 2FS-1F, 2FS, 2FS-1F.
B) from hemolytic sera: 1S-2FS, 2FS, 1S-1F, 2FS, 1S, 2FS, 1S-2FS, 2FS-1F, 1S-2FS, 1S-2FS, 1S-2FS. The anode is at the top

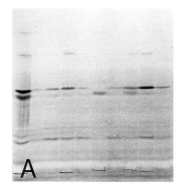

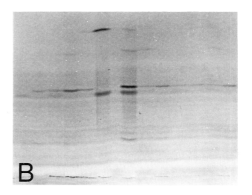

Fig. 3. Hp-subtypes prepared through immunoprecipitation
A) from NaF stabilized blood. From left to right: Control 2FS-1F 2FS, 2FS, 2FS, 2FS, 1F, 2FS, 2FS-1F, 2FS, 2FS.
B) from blood stains. From left ro right: 1F, 2FS, 2FS-1F, 2FS, 1S-2FS, control 1S-1F and 2FS-1F, 2SS-2FS, 2FS, 2FS-1F, 1S-2FS, 2SS-2FS, 2FS

RESULTS AND DISCUSSION

Figure 1 shows the visualization of the Hp-subtypes from sera using ion-exchange-chromatography, Fig. 2A using immunoprecipitation. No discrepancies between the two methods are to be observed. The cheaper method is ion-exchange-chromatography though it demands absolute non-hemolytic sera. Figure 2B shows the Hp-subtypes from hemolytic sera, Fig. 3A from blood for alcohol testing and Fig. 3B from bloodstains, all after immunoprecipitation. To prove the existence of Hp-subtypes in a bloodstain it must be considerable large and fresh according to our practical knowledge.

As result of our analyses we ascertain that the ion-exchange chromatography suits good to the routine analysis of sera. The immunoprecipitation is the method of choice for the haptoglobin subtyping of hemolyzed blood and bloodstains.

REFERENCES

Constans J, Vian M (1975) Distribution of haptoglobin subtypes in French Basques. Ham Hered 25: 156-159

Dimo-Simonin N, Brandt-Casadevall C, Gujer HR (1910) Haptoglobin subtyping by agarose isoelektric focusing. In: Polesky HF, Mayr WR (ed) Advances in Forensic Haemogenetics 3. Springer-Verlag, Berlin, p 239

Pastewka JV, Reed RA, Ness AI, Pencock AC (1973) An improved haptoglobin subtyping procedure using polyacrylamide gel electrophoresis. Anal Biochem 51: 152-162

Patzelt D, Schröder H (1985) Haptoglobin subtypes in Berlin, GDR. A simple procedure for haptoglobin purification an subtyping. Z Rechtsmed 94: 207-212

Scherz R, Reber B, Pflugshaupt R (1990) Haptoglobin subtypes in the swiss population: Phenotype and gene frequencies-description of an easy method for routine typing. In: Polesky HF, Mayr WR (ed) Advences in Forensic Haemogenetics 3. Springer-Verlag, Berlin, p 236

DETECTION OF BLOOD GROUP H ANTIGENS OF RED CELLS, BLOOD AND SALIVA STAINS, AND HAIRS BY ANTI-H REAGENTS

K. Furukawa*, T. Nakajima*, T. Matsuki*, K. Kubo**

Department of Legal Medicine, Gunma University School of Medicine*
and Police Science Investigation Laboratory, Gunma Prefecture
Police**, Maebashi, 371 Japan

INTRODUCTION

Numerous anti-H active reagents have been found in normal and
immunnized human and animal sera and the extracts of certain plant
seeds. The reagents from different sources enabled us to undertake
a study of the detection of the different nature of the human H
substances. This papers reports the specificity differences among
various anti-H reagents against red cells, blood and saliva stains
and hairs.

MATERIALS AND METHODS

Human isoagglutinins, chicken immune serum, monoclonal antibodies,
eel sera from Anguilla japonica and Ulex europaeus lectins were
used in this examinations (Matsuki et al. 1990). Determination of
agglutinating activities of red cells, agglutination inhibition
experiments were identical to that previously reported (Matsuki et
al. 1990). Absorption-elution experiments were done with O cells,
using Bombay phenotype cells as a control by the heat elution
method of Landsteiner and Miller.

RESULTS

The sera and lectins which preferentially react with group O red
cells and differentiate group O secretor salivas from nonsecretors were previously reported (Matsuki et al. 1990).

Table 1. Agglutinability of group O and A_1 red cells

Red cell		Agglutinability of red cells						
		Anti-H Bombay	Anti-H F.M.	Anti-H chicken	Anti-H mouse	Eel serum	Ulex I	Ulex II
O_h	Saline	0	0	4	0	0	0	0
O	Saline	32	32	4,096	64	1,024	32	32
A_1	Saline	8	4	2,048	0	32	8	8
O_h	Papain	2	1	16	0	2	0	0
O	Papain	128	128	16,384	128	8,192	1,024	1,024
A_1	Papain	32	32	8,192	0	1,024	256	256

Agglutinability of saline and papain-treated group O and A1 red cells with anti-H active reagents were shown in Table 1. In the saline agglutination large differences of agglutinability between O and A₁ was demonstrated in mouse monoclonal anti-H and eel serum. After the red cells were treated with papain the agglutinability of the red cells were enhanced in all of the reagents, especially in Ulex europaeus lectins. The reactivity of red cells of group A genotypes, A₁O and A₁A₁ were tested with the anti-H reagents (Table 2). Most of the reagents except chicken anti-H were agglutinated A₁O cells stronger than A₁A₁ cells. Difference of the agglutinability between A₁O and A₁A₁ was remarkable in eel serum by saline agglutination. Reactivity of BO and BB red cells were the same strength as A₁O and A₁A₁. Therefore, in the E blood groups determined by eel type II serum (Furuhata 1974), type E red cells react with the eel serum as strongly as similar to O cells may be heterozygote A₁O and BO. Type e whose red cells agglutinate very weakly or not at all by the eel serum may be homozygote of A₁ and B.

Table 2. Agglutinability of A₁O and A₁A₁ red cells

Blood group genotype	Agglutinability of red cells						
	Anti-H Bombay	Anti-H F.M.*	Anti-H chicken	Anti-H mouse*	Eel	Ulex I	Ulex II
OO	32	128	1024	128	1024	64	64
A₁O	8	32	512	16	32	16	16
A₁A₁	4	0	512	1	0	4	4

* Papain treated cells were used

Table 3. Inhibition of agglutinations by L-fucose and fucose containing oligosaccharides

Sugar	Agglutination inhibition titer					
	Anti-H Bombay	Anti-H chicken	Anti-H mouse	Eel	Ulex I	Ulex II
L-Fuc (0.5M)	2	4	0	512	256	<4
2'-FL (0.1M)	128	512	32	256	2,048	2,048
LNF I (0.1M)	256	32	32	0	32	32
LNF II (0.1M)	0	0	0	0	0	0
LNDF I (0.1M)	0	32	0	32	0	0

L-Fuc: L-fucose, 2'-FL: 2'-fucosyllactose, LNF I: lacto-N-fucopentaose I, LNF II: lacto-N-fucopentaose II, LNDF I: lacto-N-difucohexaose I

The results of inhibition of anti-H reagents by L-fucose and fucose containing oligosaccharides were shown in Table 3. The human, chicken and mouse anti-H sera were inhibited by 2'-FL and LNF I which contains α-(1→2)-fucosyl residues in the structures. L-Fucose and 2'-FL were most strong inhibitor for eel serum and

Ulex I lectin. Ulex II lectin was hardly inhibited by L-fucose while 2'-FL is the highest inhibitor against the lectin. It is demonstrated that the Ulex II lectin is inhibited by di-N-acetyl-chitobiose which has unrelated structure of H active antigen determinants (Matsumoto and Oosawa 1969).
The results of the absorption test of anti-H reagents with blood and saliva stains indicated that chicken and mouse monoclonal antibodies, Ulex I and II lectins showed powerful affinity to the stains (Table 4).

Table 4. Absorption test and Absorption-elution test of anti-H sera and lectins with group O blood and saliva stains, and hairs

Anti-H active reagent	Absoption			Agglutination of eluate from					
	Before	After with		Test cells	Blood		Hair		Saliva
		Blood	Saliva		O	Oh	O	Oh	O
Anti-H F.M.	32	2	2	Saline	+	–	(+)	–	+
				Papain	+	–	(+)	–	+
Anti-H chicken	32	0	0	Saline	++	–	(+)	–	+
				Papain	++	–	(+)	–	++
Anti-H mouse	32	0	0	Saline	–	–	–	–	–
				Papain	–	–	–	–	–
Eel	32	2	16	Saline	+	–	–	–	–
				Papain	++	–	–	–	–
Ulex I	32	0	0	Saline	–	–	–	–	–
				Papain	+	–	(+)	–	+
Ulex II	32	0	0	Saline	–	–	–	–	–
				Papain	+	–	(+)	–	+

(+): not all hairs tested showed positive reaction

When the chicken serum was used for absorption and elution test of the stains and hairs strong agglutination of O red cells with the eluate was observed (Table 4). IgM anti-H mouse monoclonal antibodies and Ulex lectins were heardly eluted by the heating. Most strong agglutination of the eluates from hair was observed when Ulex I and II lectins were used and papain treated O red cells were used as test cells. Eluates from Ulex lectins were only reactive with papain treated O red cells.

REFERENCES

Furuhata T (1974) Development of haemotypology in Japan. Tokyo Standard Serums, Matsumoto, pp 88-94
Matsuki T, Nakajima T, Furukawa K (1990) Application of anti-H active antibodies and lectins to the detection of human blood group H substances. Proc Internatl Symp Advances in Legal Medicine, Kanazawa, pp 399-401
Matsumoto I, Oosawa, T (1969) Purification and characterization of an anti-H(O) phytohemagglutinin of Ulex europaeus. Biochem Biophys, Acta, 194:180-189

Evaluation of Sperm Specific Lactate Dehydrogenase Isoenzyme C4 (LDH C4). Application to Semen Detection in Stains

R. Pawlowski (*), B. Brinkmann (**)
Inst. of Forensic Med., Medical Academy Gdańsk, Debinki 7, 80-210 Gdansk, Poland (*)
Inst. für Rechtsmedizin, Uni. Münster, 4400 Münster, Von Esmarch Str.86, Germany (**)

INTRODUCTION

Lactate dehydrogenase is present in most tissues as a series of 5 tetrameric isoenzymes, but in semen 6 isoenzymes can be found. The sixth is LDH C4 or X which is specific for semen and has never been observed in any male and female tissues other than testes and spermatozoa (Wheat and Goldberg 1983).

LDH C4 activity accounts for about 80 % of the total LDH activity in spermatozoa, and is present largely in the mitochondria but partly also in the cytosol. In previous experiments (Pawlowski et al. 1988) we observed that LDH C4 is relatively stable in liquid semen and mixtures of semen with vaginal washings incubated in vitro.

The main aim of the work was the analysis of LDH C 4 in semen, semen stains and mixtures using IEF and to establish a reliable and sensitive method of semen detection, which could be used as an alternative to microscopical searching for spermatozoa.

MATERIALS AND METHODS

Samples analysed: Fresh semen, blood, saliva, vaginal swabs. Semen stains and mixed stains were stored at room temperature for up to 8 months.

Electrophoretical methods: LDH isozymes were separated on 1% agarose gel (Shaler 1981), and on ultrathin PAGIEF, pH 3-10 and 6-8 with 0.4 M beta alanin as a separator. LDH C was determined semiquanitatively using rocket immunoelectrophoresis, with subsequent SDS electrotransfer and avidin-biotin detection system, and using a dot blot method.

Total LDH activity was detected using lactate staining. LDH C was detected specifically using alpha hydroxyhexanoate or antibody against LDH C (LeVan et al.1991).

PCR: Presence of sperm and other male cells in vaginal swabs was analysed with X and Y chromosome specific primers flanking a segment of the amelogenin gene (Nakahori 1991).

RESULTS AND DISCUSSION

Conventional agarose gel electrophoresis (Fig. 1) and PAGE of LDH isoenzymes present in semen or testicular tissue homogenates show one additional band in comparison with blood and other human fluids or tissue extracts (Goldberg 1963).

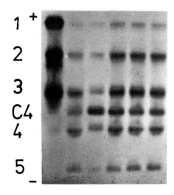

Fig. 1: Agarose gel electrophoresis of LDH isoenzymes.
From left to right: Blood, seminal fluid, lysed spermatozoa and three semen samples. Staining for total LDH activity

Advances in Forensic Haemogenetics 4
Edited by Ch. Rittner and P. M. Schneider
© Springer-Verlag Berlin Heidelberg 1992

Figure 2 presents IEF pattern of LDH pattern of LDH in semen, blood and mixtures analysed in broad pH 3-10. Multiple bands of LDH are present both in blood and semen samples with some additional bands in semen. Under these conditions it is possible to detect LDH C bands up to dilutions where semen consist of 1/50 part of the mixture.

Semen specific bands are more easily recognized in the narrow pH range from 6 to 8. The use of 0.4 M beta alanine as a separator improved separation pattern.

Figure 3 shows LDH C4 pattern obtained after immunodetection with anti LDH C. Multiple bands with different activities are present showing microheterogeneity of LDH C, indicating that LDH C subunits are able to form heterotetramers with other LDH subunits similar to the A and B homo- and heterotetramers present in fluids other than semen.

No variants were observed in 120 samples, of fresh semen lysed using mechanical or chemical methods. Pseudopolymorphism of LDH C, could be observed after 2-3 freeze-thaw cycles. Microheterogeneity of LDH A and B in blood and some tissue cytosols was found in 1988 using IEF (Romero-Saravia et al. 1988). No papers presenting microheterogeneity of LDH C have yet been presented.

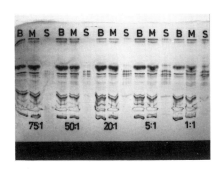

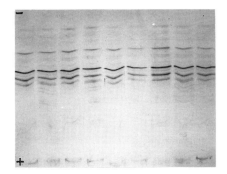

Fig. 2: IEF pattern of blood and semen LDH isozymes separated on pH 3-10 polyacryl-amide gel. Semen sample /S/ and blood /B/ were mixed /M/ in different ratios /S:B 1:1 - 1:75/ and subjected to IEF. LDH activity was detected using lactate staining

Fig. 3: IEF pattern of LDH C isozymes from human semen. Semen samples were separated on 200 μm thick PA gel at pH gradient 6-8 with beta alanin as a separator. After blotting LDH C bands were detected using specific antibody against human LDH C and biotin system

FORENSIC APPLICATION OF LDH C

The presence of semen in stains or swabs can only be documented with certainty by the microscopic detection of spermatozoa or by presence of other semen specific components such as LDH C4, p 30 etc. Because LDH C is a semen specific component it could be used as a semen specific indicator in mixtures of semen with other body fluids.

Dot blot analysis. LDH C and other LDH isoenzymes are tetramers, which in stains are usually present in a denatured form. During the extraction process special conditions are needed, to restore the tertiary and quaternary structure of the enzyme.

The best results were achieved after at least 12 hours extraction at 4°C in a buffer containing DTT, Triton X-100, BSA and potassium chloride at pH 8.0.

The stability of LDH C in semen stains as a function of storage time and sperm count is shown in Fig. 4. After 8 months about 50 % stains with normal sperm counts still gave positive reactions. It was also possible to detect LDH C in semen samples with very low sperm concentrations. Even some semen stains with no detectable sperm gave weak positive reactions.

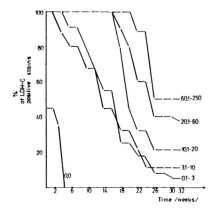

Fig. 4: Stability of LDH C in semen stains.Semen stains with different
sperm counts ranging from 0-250 mill/ml were stored at room temperature
for 8 months. LDH C was analysed using dot blot method and
avidin-biotin detection system

We also compared different methods of LDH C detection (agarose gel electrophoresis, IEF, rocket
immunoelectrophoresis and dot blot) with microscopical searching for sperm. Results from some stains
showed that dot blot and rocket immuno-electrophoresis gave better results than microscopical searching
for spermatozoa. LDH C analysis was also applied to the semen detection in vaginal swabs.The results
of microscopic searching for spermatozoa and LDH C analysis using dot blot method were similar, but
PCR amplification of a Y chromosome specific sequence was superior to both these methods.

SUMMARY

IEF analysis of semen specific LDH C reveals the microheterogenic nature of this enzyme but
    polymorphism of LDH C was not observed.
LDH C could be used as a semen indicator in stains. Sometimes LDH C analysis gave better
    results than classical sperm searching method.
The LDH C is detectable in stains over relatively long time periods but depends on sperm
    concentration.

REFERENCES

Goldberg E (1963) Lactic and malic dehydrogenases in human spermatozoa. Science 139:602-
    603
LeVan KM, Goldberg E (1991) Properties of human testis-specific lactate dehydrogenase
    expressed from Escherichia coli. Biochem J 273: 587-592
Nakahori Y, Hamano K, Iwaya M, Nakagome Y (1991) Sex identification by polymerase chain
    reaction using X-Y homologous primer. Am J Med Genet 39: 472-473
Pawlowski R, Hauser R, Raszeja S (1988) Zur Stabilität ausgewählter Spermabestandteile in
    einem Gemisch von Sperma und Vaginalsekret. Beitr Gerichtl Med 46:219-226
Romero-Saravia O, Solem E, Lorentz M (1988) High resolution of human dehydrogenase:New
    multiple forms and potential tumor markers. Electrophoresis 9: 816-819
Shaler RC (1981) A multi-enzyme electrophoretic system for the identification of seminal fluid
    from postmortem species. Am J Forensic Med Pathol 2: 315-321
Wheat TE, Goldberg E (1983) Sperm-specific lactate dehydrogenase C4: Antigenic structure
    and immunosuppression of fertility. Isozymes: Current Topics in Biological and Medical Re-
    search 7: 113-130

PGM1 Subtyping by Isoelectric Focusing (IEF) in Parentage Testing in South African (SA) Populations

V. Borrill, W. Petersen, R. Martell and E. du Toit

Provincial Laboratory for Tissue Immunology, Cape Town, South Africa

INTRODUCTION

PGM1 is an ubiquitous enzyme which is coded for by a gene situated on chromosome 1p. PGM1 reversibly catalyses the transfer of phosphate from the first to the sixth position of glucose in the glycolytic pathway. The polymorphism of PGM1 was first demonstrated by conventional starch gel electrophoresis by Spencer et al in 1964. Using IEF, later studies showed more complex band patterns due to the presence of four common alleles at the PGM1 locus, giving rise to ten possible phenotypes (Bark et al. 1976; Sutton and Burgess 1978). PGM1 is one of thirteen genetic marker systems currently used in disputed paternity testing in this laboratory. The aim of this study was to assess the usefulness of PGM1 subtyping by IEF in disputed parentage testing and compare the results with those obtained using starch gel electrophoresis.

MATERIALS AND METHODS

Acid citrate dextrose anticoagulated blood samples were obtained from 638 mother-child-alleged father trios, from SA Caucasoids, Cape Coloureds and SA Negroes (Xhosa).

Haemolysates were prepared from washed packed cells treated with 10% Triton X-100 and stored at -70°C. Polyacrylamide gels were prepared at a concentration of T=5% and C=3% with an ampholyte range pH 5.0 - 7.0. Five ul of haemolysate were applied on filter paper 2cm anodally. The anolyte was 1M phosphoric acid. The catholyte was 1M sodium hydroxide. IEF was performed at 1200V, 15mA, 20W at 10°C for 180 minutes. Enzyme activity was revealed using the electron transfer stain, as described by Sutton and Burgess (1978).

Gene frequencies were established by direct counting.
The observed power of exclusion (PE) was calculated by counting the number of men excluded by the PGM1 system, out of the total number of men excluded, using thirteen systems.

Advances in Forensic Haemogenetics 4
Edited by Ch. Rittner and P. M. Schneider
© Springer-Verlag Berlin Heidelberg 1992

RESULTS

Table 1. Observed and expected PGM1 phenotype frequencies

Pheno-types	SA Caucasoids			Cape Coloureds			SA Negroes (Xhosa)		
	Obs.	Exp.	X2	Obs.	Exp.	X2	Obs.	Exp.	X2
1A	100	102.47	0,06	242	231.47	0.48	174	176.91	0.05
1B	1	3.44	1.73	13	15.50	0.40	12	16.61	1.28
2A	10	8.55	0.25	12	11.29	0.05	18	16.04	0.24
2B	2	1.01	0.97	2	.73	2.20	0	0.21	0.21
1A1B	44	37.55	1.11	116	119.80	0.12	119	108.41	1.03
2A1A	60	59.19	0.01	93	102.24	0.84	103	106.55	0.12
2B1A	18	20.35	0.27	18	26.02	2.47	11	12.20	0.12
2A1B	8	10.84	0.75	32	26.46	1.16	31	32.65	0.08
2B1B	5	3.73	0.43	10	6.74	1.58	4	3.74	0.02
2A2B	5	5.88	0.13	8	5.75	0.88	5	3.67	0.48
Total	253	253.01	5.71	546	546.00	10.18	477	476.99	3.63

Table 1 shows the observed and expected phenotype frequencies
for the three populations studied. The gene frequencies for
the PGM1 alleles in SA Caucasoids, Cape Coloureds and SA
Negroes are shown in Table 2. The observed and expected values
of the phenotypes within each population were in accordance
with Hardy-Weinberg equilibrium.

Table 2. Distribution of PGM1 gene frequencies

	SA Caucasoids n = 253	Cape Coloureds n = 546	SA Negroes (Xhosa) n = 477
1A	0.6364	0.6511	0.6090
1B	0.1166	0.1685	0.1866
2A	0.1838	0.1438	0.1834
2B	0.0632	0.0366	0.0210

Figure 1 shows the comparison between the power of exclusion in the various South African populations using PGM1 typing by either starch gel electrophoresis or IEF.

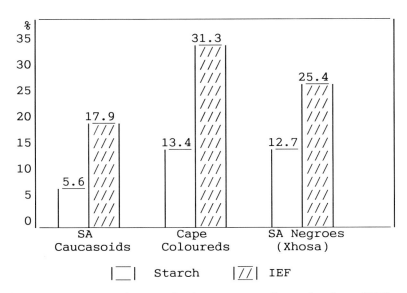

Figure 1. Comparison of the power of exclusion (PE) of PGM1 using starch gel electrophoresis and IEF

CONCLUSION

In view of the increased power of exclusion of PGM1 detected using IEF, this method is more useful than starch gel electrophoresis especially in the Cape Coloureds. Therefore PGM1 detected using IEF is recommended as an additional system for disputed parentage testing.

REFERENCES

Bark J, Harris M, Firth M (1976) Typing of the common phosphoglucomutase variants using isoelectric focusing. J Forensic Sci Soc 16:115-120
Spencer N, Hopkinson D, Harris H (1964) Phosphoglucomutase polymorphism in man. Nature 204:742-745
Sutton J, Burgess R (1978) Genetic evidence for four common alleles at the phosphoglucomutase -1 - locus (PGM1) detectable by iso-electric focusing. Vox Sang 34:97-103

Orosomucoid (ORM) Phenotyping by Isoelectric Focusing in Immobilized pH-Gradient Followed by Immunoblotting

W. Huckenbeck, S. Weidinger*, V. Stancu

Institute of Legal Medicine, Heinrich-Heine-University, Düsseldorf, FRG

INTRODUCTION

Orosomucoid or α1-acid glycoprotein is an acute phase reactant. It is coded by chromosome 9 (12) and its concentration increases in response to non-specific stimuli. The protein has a binding capacity for several drugs (2, 5, 9, 13, 17, 24, 25, 29). Clinical investigations did not lead to significant association with diseases (7,10,23). Numerous population data have been published (6, 15, 16, 22, 33, 34, 36, 37). Rare variants (11, 14, 19, 20, 21, 22, 31, 32, 36) have been reported using different improved techniques (4, 8, 14, 16, 18, 27, 28, 29, 30, 33, 38).

MATERIALS and METHODS

Serum samples had been stored at -50° C until examined.
Treatment of samples: desialyzation by neuraminidase (C. perfringens ; serum/enzyme 2:1) at 37°C overnight (20-24 hours). Adding of 30 µl reductive clearage solution 1: 0.12 g boric acid, 4.81 g urea, 0.015 g DDT ad 10 ml aqua dest. (adjusted to pH 9, NaOH). Components mixed by Vortex and incubated for 20 min. at room temperature.
Adding of 30 µl reductive clearage solution 2 : 0.12 g boric acid and 0.36 g jodacetamide ad 10 ml aqua dest. (adjusted to pH 9, NaOH). Components mixed by Vortex and incubation for 20 min. at room temperature.
Isoelectric focusing (Immobiline dry plate; LKB, pH 4.5-5.4): 3000 V, 6 mA, 12 W, 4 hours.
Immunoblotting (20 min.) by passive transfer to nitrocellulose membrane, stopped by incubating the membrane in 2% TWEEN 20 (PBS-buffer, pH 10.2) for 15 min..
Primary antibody: rabbit-antihuman ORM (DAKOPATTS), 1:300 in PBS buffer (1% bovine albumine 30%), incubation overnight.
Washing the membrane three times for 5 minutes in the same buffer.
Second antibody: peroxidase-conjugated swine-rabbit immunoglobine (DAKOPATTS) 1:1000 solution (PBS buffer, see above) for 2 hours.
Visualization: Washing the membrane in 0.05 M acetate buffer pH 5;
incubation in the staining solution: 20 mg 3-amino-9-ethylcarbazol, 2,5 ml acetone, 50 ml acetate buffer 0.05 M (pH 5), 25 µl hydrogen peroxidase(30%); staining time about 5 min.
The reaction is stopped by washing the membrane in aqua dest.

RESULTS and DISCUSSION

Figure 1 shows the banding pattern of the ORM phenotypes observed by IEF with the method described above. Five of the six common phenotypes are presented in high resolution and can be identified definetely. In case of the heterozygous ORM1*F1F2 and the homozygous ORM1*F2 the examiner has to observe different intensities. Interpreting the banding pattern of a fresh visualized blot this means no problem. In lane 3 and lane 4 two rare ORM1 variants are presented : ORM1 F1A2 and ORM1 F1F3. The additional bands anodally and cathodally from the

*Institute of Anthropology and Human Genetics, University of Munich, FRG

Advances in Forensic Haemogenetics 4
Edited by Ch. Rittner and P. M. Schneider
© Springer-Verlag Berlin Heidelberg 1992

F1 band are marked. The cathodal bands may be assigned to the ORM2 locus. The common phenotype is ORM2 A. Nevertheless the examiner has to reckon on rare variants : on this blot ORM2*AB1 and ORM2*AB2 (lane 6,8,9). The B2 variant was found in a family with putative father from Africa.

Fig.1   ORM PHENOTYPING, IEF FOLLOWED BY IMMUNOBLOTTING

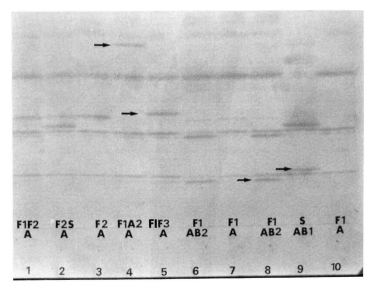

REFERENCES

1) Akeo, K., Tanaka, Y., Akiya, S., Uemura, Y.(1986)Growth Effects of alpha1 Acid Glycoprotein (Human) on Human Skin Fibroblasts in Culture.Acta Soc. Ophtalm. Jap. 90/5: 653-656

2) Alavan, G.(1986)Other protein variants with pharmacogenetic consequences albumin and orosomucoid.Pro. Clin. Biol. Res. 214: 345-355

3) Araki, F.(1985)Diagnostic Significance of the simultaneous determination of serum alpha-1-acid glycoprotein and carcinoembryonic antigen in relatively early stages of malignant status.Rinsho-Byori 33/10: 1160-1164

4) Berger, E.G., Wyss, S.R., Nimberg, R.B., Schmid, K.(1980)The Microheterogeneity of Human Plasma alpha-1-Acid Glycoprotein Hoppe-Seyler's Z. Physiol.Chem. 361: 1567-1572

5) Busby, T.F., Ingham, K.C.(1986)Thermal stability and ligand-binding properties of human plasma alpha-1-acid glycoprotein (orosomucoid) as determined with fluorescent probes.Biochim. Biophys. Acta 871: 61-71

6) Caenazzo, L., Cortivo, P., Crestani, C., Scorretti, C., Veneri, A.(1988)Genetic Study of Serum Orosomucoid (ORM) by Ultrathin Layer Isoelectric Focusing.in: Advances in Forensic Haemogenetics 2 , Mayr, W.R. (ed.),Springer Verlag

7) Candeira, S.R., Blasco, L.H., Espanol, C.S., Raja, A.G., Zaragoza, C.Z., Buades, J.S., Serrano, C.M.(1986)Utilidad clinica de los marcadores tumorales en el diagnostico de los derrames pleurales. Antigeno carcinoembrionario, alfa-fetoproteina y orosomucoide.Med. Clin (Barc.) 86: 439-443

8) Carracedo, A., Montiel, M.D., Rodriguez-Calvo, M.S., Concheiro, L., Huguet, E., Gene, M.(1988)Improved Diagnosis of Orosomucoid (ORM) Phenotypes by isoelectric focusing in immobilized pH gradients. Comparison with other phenotyping methods.in: Advances in Forensic Haemogenetics 2 , Mayr, W.R. (ed.),Springer Verlag

9) Casey, C.A., Kragskow, S.L., Sorrell, M.F., Tuma, D.J.(1987)Chronic Ethanol Administration Impairs the Binding and Endocytosis of Asialo-orosomucoid in Isolated Hepatocytes.J. Biol. Chem. 262/6: 2704-2710

10) Cleve, H., Weidinger, S., Gürtler, L.G., Deinhardt, F.(1988)
AIDS: No Association with the Genetic Systems GC (D-binding protein), ORM (Orosomucoid=Alpha-1-acid Glycoprotein), and A2HS (1Alpha-2-HS-Glycoprotein).Infection 16/1 : 31-35

11) Cooper, R., Papaconstantinou, J.(1986)Evidence for the Existence of Multiple alpha-1-acid Glycoprotein Genes in the Mouse
J. Biol. Chem. 261/4: 1849-1853

12) Eiberg, H., Mohr, J., Nielsen, L.S.(1983)Delta-Aminolevulinatedehydrase: synteny with ABO-AK1-ORM (and assignment to chromosome 9).Clin. Gen. 23: 150-154

13) Gillis, A.M., Yee, Y.G., Kates, R.E.(1985)Binding of antiarrhythmic drugs to purified human alpha-1-acid glycoprotein
Biochem. Pharmacol. 34/24: 4279-4282

14) Johnson, A.M., Schmid, K., Alper, C.A., Bissett, L.(1969)
Inheritance of Human alpha-1-Acid Glycoprotein (Orosomucoid) Variants.J. Clin. Invest. 48 : 2293-2299

15) Metzner, D., Scheil, H.G.(1988)Polymorphism of human orosomucoid in populations of Western Germany and Switzerland
Gene Geography 2: 119-122

16) Montiel, M.D., Carracedo, A., Lopez-Rodriguez, M.S., Blasquez-Caeiro, J.L., Concheiro, L.(1988)Correlation between Native and Desialyzed Forms of
Orosomucoid.Hum. Hered. 38: 353-358

17) Schley, J., Müller-Oerlinghausen, B.(1986)Investigation of the binding of various tricyclic neuroleptics and antidepressants to alpha-1-acid glycoprotein.J.
Pharm. Pharmacol. 38: 102-106

18) Schmid, K., Binette, J.P.(1961)Polymorphism of alpha-1-acid Glycoprotein.Nature 190 , May 13: 630

19) Schmid, K., Binette, J.P., Kamiyama, S., Pfister, V., Takahashi, S.(1962)Studies on the structure of alpha-1-acid glycoprotein. III. Polymorphism of alpha-1-acid
glycoprotein and the partial resolution and characterization of its variants.
Biochemistry 1/6 : 959-966

20) Schmid, K., Kaufmann, H., Isemura, S., Bauer, F., Emura, J., Motoyama, T., Ishiguro, M., Nanno, S.(1973)Structure of alpha-1-acid glycoprotein. The complete
Amino Acid Sequence, Multi Amino Acid Substitutions, and Homology with the Immunoglobulins
Biochemistry 12/14 : 2711-2724

21) Schmid, K., Tokita, K., Yoshizaki, H.(1965)The alpha-1-Acid Glycoprotein Variants of Normal Caucasian and Japanese Individuals
J. Clin. Invest. 44/8 : 1394-1401

22) Sebatan, M., Sagisaka, K.(1989)Genetic polymorphisms of orosomucoid ORM1 and ORM2 in a Japanese population: occurence of new ORM1 alleles.Z. Rechtsmed 102:
5-9

23) Serbource-Goguel Seta, N., Durand, G., Corbic, M., Agneray, J., Feger, J.(1986)Alterations in Relative Proportions of Microheterogenous Forms of Human Alpha-
1-Acid Glycoprotein in Liver Disease.J. Hepatol. 2: 245-252

24) Sluijs, P. van den, Spanjer, H.H., Meijer, D.K.F.(1987)Hepatic Disposition of Cationic Drugs Bound to Asialoorosomucoid: Lack of Coendocytosis and Evidence for
Intrahepatic Dissociation.J. Pharmacol. Exp. Ther. 240/3: 668-673

25) Soltes, L., Bree, F., Sebille, B., Tillement, J.P., Durisova, M., Trnovec, T.(1985)Study of propanolol binding to alpha-1-acid glycoprotein by high-performance
liquid chromatography.Biochem. Pharmacol. 34/24 : 4331-4334

26) Suzuki, Y., Sugiyama, Y., Sawada, Y., Iga, T., Hanano, M.(1985)Assesssment of contribution of alpha-1-acid glycoptotein to the serum binding of drugs using
serum treated with sulphosalicylic acid and DEAE-cellulose.J. Pharm. Pharmakol. 37: 712-717

27) Thymann, M., Eiberg, H.(1986)Orosomucoid polymorphism: Determination by Separator Isoelectric Focusing and Demonstration of ORM*F subtypes:in :Advances in
Forensic Haemogenetics 1 , Brinkmann, B., Henningsen, K. (eds.);Springer Verlag

28) Thymann, M., Weidinger, S.(1988)Subtyping of orosomucoid (ORM1) by isoelectric focusing in agarose and polyacrylamide gels
Electrophoresis 9: 380-383

29) Tokita, K., Schmid, K.(1963)Variants of alpha-1-acid Glycoprotein.Nature 200 , October 19: 266

30) Umetsu, K., Ikeda, N., Kashimura, S., Suzuki, T.(1985)
Orosomucoid (ORM) typing by print lectinofixation: a new technique for isoelectric focusing. Two common alleles in Japan.Hum. Genet. 71: 223-224

31) Umetsu, K., Yuasa, I., Nishi, K., Brinkmann, B., Suzuki, T.(1989)Orosomucoid (ORM) typing by isoelectric focusing: description of two new alleles in a German
population and thermostability in bloodstains.Z. Rechtsmed. 102: 171-177

32) Weidinger, S., Müller, T., Schwarzfischer, F., Cleve, H.(1987)
Three new orosomucoid (ORM) variants revealed by isoelectric focusing and print immunofixation.Hum. Genet. 77: 286-288

33) Weidinger, S., Schwarzfischer, F., Müller, T., Cleve, H.(1988)Orosomucoid (ORM) Subtyping: Application to Paternity Testing.in: Advances in Forensic
Haemogenetics 2 , Mayr, W.R. (ed.),Springer Verlag

34) Wimmer, F., Luckenbach, Ch., Kömpf, J., Ritter, H.(1988)Polymorphism of Orosomucoid (ORM). Formal genetics and population data.in: Advances in Forensic
Haemogenetics 2 , Mayr, W.R. (ed.),Springer Verlag

35) Yuasa, I., Suenaga, K., Umetsu, K., Ito, K., Robinet-Levy, M.
(1987)Orosomucoid (ORM) typing by isoelectric focusing: evidence for gene duplication of ORM1 and genetic polymorphism of ORM2.
Hum. Genet. 77 :255-258

36) Yuasa, I., Umetsu, K., Suenaga, K.(1988)Orosomucoid (ORM) Typing by Isoelectric Focusing: Evidence for an Additional Duplicated ORM1 Locus Haplotype and
Close Linkage of Two ORM Loci.Am. J. Hum. Genet. 43: 165-169

37) Yuasa, I., Umetsu, K., Suenaga, K., Robinet-Levy, M.(1986)
Orosomucoid typing by isoelectric focusing: evidence for two structural loci ORM1 and ORM2.Hum. Genet. 74: 160-161

38) Yuasa, I., Umetsu, K., Suenega, K., Robinat-Levy, M.(1986)
Isoelectric focusing of desialyzed orosomucoid.Jap. J. Legal Med. 40: 682

ABO Blood Grouping and Species Identification of Bloodstains
by Sandwich ELISA Using Monoclonal Antibody Specific for Human
Erythrocyte Band 3

A. Kimura, T. Uda, S. Nakashima, M. Osawa, H. Ikeda, S. Yasuda
and T. Tsuji

Department of Legal Medicine, Wakayama Medical College,
27 Kyuban-cho, 640 Wakayam, Japan

INTRODUCTION

Species identification and ABO blood grouping of bloodstains
constitute the main subjects in medicolegal practices. The methods
employed for species identification and ABO blood grouping, e.g.
immunodiffusion with anti-human hemoglobin antibody and absorption
-elution test using anti-ABO blood group sera, are well established and highly reliable. However, methods of distinguish between species, especially between humans and other primates, and
methods of ABO blood grouping of bloodstains contaminated by other
body fluids are not yet satisfactory. In our study of species
-specific epitopes on human erythrocyte membrane, we produced
monoclonal antibodies (mAbs) to species specific-epitopes on human
erythrocyte membrane band 3. One (P3-9H) of these mAbs could even
discriminate erythrocytes of human from those of chimpanzee
(Kimura 1990). Since erythrocyte membrane band 3 carries ABO
blood group active carbohydrate chains, the use of P3-9H may be
applicable not only to human blood identification but also to ABO
blood grouping.

In this paper, we describe the applications of P3-9H for human
blood identification and for ABO blood grouping from bloodstains
contaminated by other body fluids.

MATERIALS AND METHODS

Production of mAbs: Anti-human erythrocyte membrane band 3 mAb
(P3-9H) was produced by using human erythrocyte membrane as an
immunogen as described previously(Kimura 1990).
SDS-polyacrylamide gel electrophoresis (SDS-PAGE) and immunoblotting: SDS-PAGE was performed by method of Laemmli and immunoblotting was performed as described by Towbin.
Sandwich ELISA: A microwell plate was coated with P3-9H (10μg/ml
PBS) and blocked with 0.3% gelatin (10mM TBS, pH7.4). Erythrocyte
membrane proteins were extracted from bloodstains with PBS containing 1% Triton X-100 and 1mM EDTA and the extracts were incubated on the P3-9H coated plate. ABO blood group epitopes on
band 3 captured by P3-9H were detected with mAbs to ABO blood
group and with peroxidase conjugated goat anti-mouse IgM.

Advances in Forensic Haemogenetics 4
Edited by Ch. Rittner and P. M. Schneider
© Springer-Verlag Berlin Heidelberg 1992

RESULTS AND DISCUSSION

As shown in Fig. 1, anti-human band 3 mAb P3-9H (IgG1) bound to whole band 3, and to its 60 and 42 kDa amino-terminal fragments (N-60 and N-42) in the human erythrocyte membrane but not to that of the chimpanzee on the blot, indicating that the epitope defined by P3-9H existed on N-42 and was specific for human. P3-9H did not cross-react with the erythrocytes of other primates (spider monkey, capuchin monkey, rhesus monkey, Japanese monkey or orang-utan) or other mammals (dog, cat, cow, pig and rabbit).

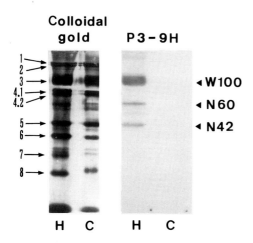

Fig. 1. Identification of the antigen defined by P3-9H by immuno-blotting. Proteins in the erythrocyte membranes of human and chimpanzee were separated by SDS-PAGE (10% acrylamide gel) and transferred onto PVDF membranes. The blots were stained with colloidal gold or P3-9H. H, human; C, chimpanzee: W100, whole band 3; N60 and N42, 60kDa and 42kDa amino-terminal fragments respectively, of band 3. Nomenclature for human erythrocyte mem-brane proteins is according to Steck (1974).

Band 3 is an integral membrane protein in erythrocytes; it acts as an anion channel in erythrocyte membrane and also carries the ABO blood group active sugar chain (Tsuji 1981). About 25% of the ABO blood group determinants in the erythrocyte membrane are distrib-uted on the sugar chain which links to an asparagine residue on band 3 (Finne 1980). Since the human-specific epitope and the ABO blood group epitopes are located apart from each other on the band 3 molecule, the binding of each antibody to each epitope is not disturbed by the binding of other antibody. Therefore, it appeared to be appropriate to apply P3-9H to a capture antibody in sandwich ELISA for the ABO blood grouping of bloodstains. ABO blood group epitopes were detected in extracts from minute blood-stains by sandwich ELISA using P3-9H. Even when bloodstains were contaminated by other body fluids (e.g., semen, saliva and sweat),

only the ABO blood group epitopes on band 3 captured by P3-9H were
detected by the ABO blood group antibodies without interference
from other body fluids. Sakata et al. reported the same sandwich
ELISA using a mAb which recognized the intramembrane domain of
band 3 and cross-reacted with only some primates, for the ABO
blood grouping of bloodstains (1988). In a blind trial, all A, B
and O bloodstains (a 1cm long thread) were precisely typed, but
some AB bloodstains were typed as blood group A (Table 1). In
general, B epitopes are detected less than A epitopes by the
present method. However, when increased amounts (a 1.5cm long
thread) of AB bloodstain specimens were used the ABO blood group
was determined precisely. Furthermore, since P3-9H is specific for
human erythrocyte band 3, it is evident that if ABO blood group
epitopes are detected on the specimens by the present method, they
are those of human blood.

Table 1. Blind trials of ABO blood grouping
of bloodstains by sandwich ELISA using P3-9H

bloodstains	number	correct
A	16	16
B	21	21
O	19	19
AB	13	11[a]

a) Two specimens were typed as blood
   group A.

REFERENCES

Finne J (1980) Identification of the blood-group ABH-active glycoprotein components of human erythrocyte membrane. Eur J Biochem
   104: 181-189
Kimura A, Osawa M, Yasuda S, Ikeda H, Uda T, Nakashima S, Ohta M,
   Tsuji T (1990) On monoclonal antibodies to epitopes specific
   for species in primates. In: Nagano T (ed) Proceeding of the
   first international symposium ADVANCES IN LEGAL MEDICINE,
   p 415-417
Sakata N, Kuwaki Y, Kawakami N, Gomi M, Kitahama M (1988) ABO
   blood group typing of bloodstain by ELISA using anti-human
   band 3 monoclonal antibody. Jpn J Leg Med (suppl) 42: 267
Steck T L (1974) The organization op proteins in human red blood
   cell membrane. J Cell Biol 62: 1-19
Tsuji T, Irimura T, Osawa T (1981) The carbohydrate moiety of
   band 3 glycoprotein of human erythrocyte membranes. J Biol Chem
   256: 10497-10502

Monoclonal Antibodies to Blood Group Substances in Vaginal Secretions

A. Kimura, M. Osawa, H. Ikeda, S. Yasuda, T. Tsuji, S. Rand[*]
and B. Brinkmann[*]

Department of Legal Medicine, Wakayama Medical College,
27 Kyubancho, 640 Wakayama, Japan
*Institut für Rechtsmedizin der Universität Münster,
Von-Esmarch-Straße 86. 4400 Münster, B.R.D.

INTRODUCTION

ABO blood grouping of an individual body fluid in a mixture of
body fluids is an extremely important problem in medicolegal practices. We are currently carrying out a series of studies to produce monoclonal antibodies (mAbs) to ABO blood group substances
(ABO-BGS) in various body fluids, since sandwich ELISA using mAbs
to ABO-BGSs in body fluids seems to be the most suitable method
for resolving the problem. Consequently, we have already produced
mAbs to ABO-BGSs in saliva and semen and we have already applied
these mAbs to ABO blood grouping of saliva or semen in a mixture
of body fluids by sandwich ELISA (Kimura 1991a,b,c). In the present study, we attempted to produce mAbs to ABO-BGS in vaginal
secretions.

MATERIALS AND METHODS

Pooled vaginal swabs (A Se) were extracted with 20mM phosphate
buffer, pH 7.4 (PB). The extract was centrifuged and then passed
through a membrane filter (0.22μ). The filtrate was applied to a
sepharose 4B column (16x200mm) equilibrated with PB and eluated
with the same buffer. The fractions carrying A blood group activity were rechromatographed on a sepharose 4B column in the presence of 0.1% SDS. SDS-polyacrylamide gel electrophoresis (SDS
-PAGE) and immunoblotting were performed in the conventional
manner. Anti-vaginal ABO-BGS mAbs were produced as described
previously except that purified vaginal ABO-BGS was used as the
immunogen (Kimura 1991a). The procedure for the immunostaining of
tissue specimens has been described previously (Ohshima 1991).
Sandwich ELISA for ABO blood grouping was performed as described
previously (Kimura 1991b).

RESULTS AND DISCUSSION

ABO-BGSs in vaginal secretions (A Se) were analyzed by sepharose
4B chromatography to obtain an immunogen for the production of
mAbs to vaginal ABO-BGS. The elution pattern of A blood group
activity showed one peak; the Le^b blood group was also found in

Advances in Forensic Haemogenetics 4
Edited by Ch. Rittner and P. M. Schneider
© Springer-Verlag Berlin Heidelberg 1992

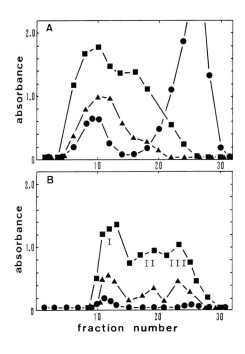

Fig.1.Chromatography of vaginal secretions on sepharose 4B. Fractionation of vaginal secretions was carried out on a sepharose 4B column (A) and then fractions carrying ABO blood group activity were rechromatographed on a sepharose 4B column in the presence of 0.1% SDS (B). Fractions were collected and aliquots were analyzed for protein (●), A blood group activity (■), and Le^b blood group activity (▲).
I, fraction I; II, fraction II; III, fraction III

this peak (Fig. 1A). A and Le^b blood group activities were found in three fractions (fraction I, II, III) on sepharose 4B rechromatography in the presence of SDS (Fig.1B), suggesting that vaginal ABO-BGS consist of at least three components which also carry Lewis blood group activity and which form a complex in vaginal secretions.

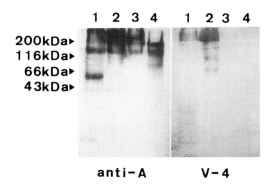

Fig.2.Immunoblotting of fractions containing A blood group activity with anti-A and V-4. whole vaginal secretions and fractions in sepharose 4B rechromatography (Fig. 1B) were separated by SDS-PAGE (5-15% acrylamide gel) and transferred onto a nitrocellulose membrane. The blots were stained with anti-A or V-4. 1, whole vaginal secretions; 2, faction I; 3, fraction II; 4, fraction III

Blood group active fractions obtained by the above chromatographic procedures were analyzed by immunoblotting with anti-A mAb (Fig. 2, left panel). Each fraction consisted of blood group active glycoproteins of over 200 kDa, and about 200kDa and 170 kDa, respectively. Anti-vaginal ABO-BGS mAbs were produced by using the highest molecular weight component (fraction I) of vaginal ABO-BGS as an immunogen. One (V-4) of the mAbs obtained bound to ABO-BGS in fraction I and to an identical position to that in fraction I in whole vaginal secretions on the blot (Fig. 2, right panel), indicating that V-4 defined the highest molecular weight component of vaginal ABO-BGS. V-4 was specific for vaginal ABO-BGS but not for ABO or Lewis blood groups. Some cells in the cervical glands and almost all the surface columnar cells in formalin fixed tissues of the uterine cervix were stained specifically by V-4, irrespective of ABO blood groups. In the preliminary results only, when V-4 was applied to sandwich ELISA to determine the ABO blood groups in mixtures of body fluids, the ABO blood group of only vaginal secretions was determined (Table 1), although some vaginal secretions derived from blood group O donors showed weak blood group A activity. Further investigations must be carried out to establish the reliability of the present method.

Table 1. ABO blood grouping of body fluids by sandwich ELISA using V-4

specimens	absorbance at 492nm	
	anti-A	anti-B
A Se vaginal secretion (A-Vag)	1.13	0.00
A Se saliva (A-sal)	0.04	0.03
B Se semen (B-sem)	0.00	0.06
A-vag + B-sem	1.20	0.00
A-vag + B-sal	1.16	0.00

REFERENCES

Kimura A, Matsumura F, Sodesaki K, Tsuji T (1991a) Production and characterization of monoclonal antibodies against epitopes on ABO blood group substances in saliva. Int J Leg Med (in press)
Kimura A, Matsumura F, Sodesaki K, Tsuji T (1991b) ABO blood grouping of saliva from mixed body fluids by sandwich methods using monoclonal antibodies to tissue specific epitopes on blood group substance in saliva. Int J Leg Med (in press)
Kimura A, Matsumura F, Sodesaki K, Osawa M, Ikeda H, Yasuda S, Tsuji T (1991c) ABO blood grouping of semen from mixed body fluids with monoclonal antibody to tissue specific epitope on seminal ABO blood group substance. (submitted)
Ohshima T, Nagano T, Kimura A, Matsumura F, Sodesaki K, Tsuji T, Maeda H (1991) Immunohistochemical study on the localization of the epitope defined by a human saliva-specific mouse monoclonal antibody (P4-5C). Int J Leg Med 104: 137-140

Gc in Human Saliva Stains

J. Lötterle, J. Bolt

Institute of Forensic Medicine, Friedrich-Alexander University,
8520 Erlangen FRG

Introduction

The best method for sub-typing the vitamin-D-binding protein Gc in stains is the isoelectric focusing on immobilised pH gradients with subsequent immunoblotting. Many authors have shown the Gc-types in dried blood with this method (THOMAS et al. 1989, ARNDT 1989, KEIL et al. 1988, KIDO et al. 1984, PFLUG 1986, RAND et al. 1987, 1990, WESTWOOD and WERRETT 1990). MILLS and CHASE (1989) described a method for Gc-typing in urin after concentration. In many laboratories the Gc-typing of seminal stains is also successfully carried out. Demonstration of Gc-types in saliva stains has not yet been reported in the accessible literature.

The identification of saliva stains is presently restricted to the bloodgroup systems ABO/Se/Lewis (IKEMOTO et al. 1990). Therefore, a better differentiation of saliva stains using more bloodgroup systems would be desirable.

Materials and Methods

Saliva stains from donors of the most common Gc-types were collected on filter paper, airdried and kept at 23 °C (for 1, 3 and 7 days), at 4 °C (for 1, 3 and 7 days) and at -24 °C (for 1, 3, 7, 12, 28 and 40 days). For determination of the Gc-phenotype small pieces of the filter paper were allowed to soak overnight in 15 μl 6 M urea. Isoelectric focusing was done on commercial 0.5 mm polyacrylamide gels pH 4,5- 5,4. More detailed information on the preparation, focusing and the blotting technique are given in table 1. Besides the experiments with dried saliva on filter paper, some experiments were performed with smoked cigarette ends.

Tab. 1: Data for preparation, focusing, blotting and staining

> **Elution**: Incubate dried saliva stains on filter paper (2 cm² cutted in several small pieces) with 15 μl 6M urea with 0,5% BSA at 4 °C overnight. Spin it [e.g. in a serum filter (Filter Sampler Porex Medical)] and place 5-6 μl on the gel 1 cm from the cathode using an applicator strip.
> **Gel**: Immobiline dry plate (Pharmacia) pH 4,5-5,4, reswelling solution 25% glycerol for 1 h.
> **Focusing**: Electrode solution aqua bidest. 5000 V, 4 mA, 10 W, 4 h.
> **Blotting**: Cellulose acetate sheet (Sartorius, Order Nr. 11200-70-400-6) equilibrated in aqua bidest and soaked with goat anti human Gc globulin (Atlantic Antibodies) 1:50. Passive blotting for 1 h. Washing with Triton X 100 buffer (0,01 M Tris/HCl pH 7,4, 0,9% NaCl, 1% Triton X 100) 3 times for 10 min. Second antibody: rabbit anti goat globulin, peroxidase conjugated (Atlantic Antibodies) 1:200, incubation time 1 h. Washing with Triton X 100 buffer 2 times for 10 min and with washing buffer (0,01 M Tris/HCl pH 7,4, 0,9% NaCl) 2 times for 5 min.
> **Staining**: Prepare staining agar (1% agar purum in destilled water, 0,25 M glycerol/NaOH buffer pH 10,4, 0,1 M $MgCl_2$, 0,1 M $ZnCl_2$, 0,1 M BCIP solution, dissolved in dimethylformamid) on Gel-Bond film (Pharmacia) and incubate the cellulose acetate sheet overnight at 37 °C.

Advances in Forensic Haemogenetics 4
Edited by Ch. Rittner and P. M. Schneider
© Springer-Verlag Berlin Heidelberg 1992

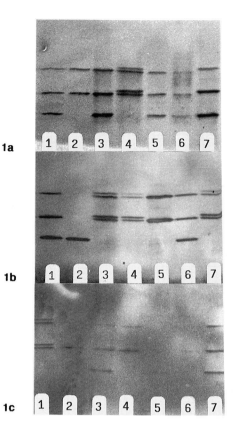

1a

1b

1c

Fig.1a-1c

Results of Gc sub-typing of 8-day old blood stains (1a, from left to right: 2-1S, 1S, 2-1S, 1F-1S, 2-1S, 2-1S, 2-1F), of fresh serum (1b, from left to right: 2-1S, 2, 1F-1S, 1F-1S, 1S, 2-1S, 1F-1S) and of 1-day old saliva stains (1c, from left to right: 1F-1S, 1S, 2-1S, 1S, 2-1S, 1S, 2-1S); anode at the top

Results

Some typical results of saliva stains, stored for one day at room temperature in comparison to results of 8-day old blood stains and serum samples are shown in figure 1a-1c. The Gc-content of the saliva stains is obviously lower than that of serum and some people secrete in their saliva so little Gc that a demonstration with the method used here is not possible. The Gc-phenotype of the saliva stains that could be determined were always the Gc-type of the donor's serum.

Figure 2 shows the demonstration of the Gc proteins' dependence on time and storing temperature. 30 different saliva stains were stored at -24 °C over a period of 40 days and examined, the remaining results refer to 10 different saliva stains respectively. It is recognised, that samples stored at room temperature for more than 1 week for the greater part could not be typed, while the keeping quality of storage at -24 °C is relatively good (66 % of the stains could be typed after 40 days). With the method used it was not possible to determine the Gc-type on smoked cigarette ends.

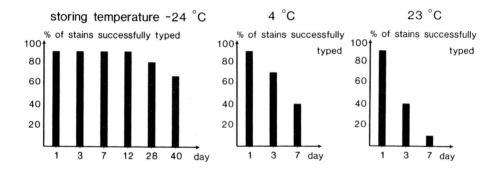

Fig. 2: Dependence of Gc proteins' demonstration in saliva stains on time and storing temperature

Discussion

The results show, that the demonstration of Gc in fresh saliva stains or saliva stains stored for days or weeks at -24 °C on filterpaper seems to be quite promising.

For the determination of the Gc-type on smoked cigarette ends, the method was not sensitive enough. Investigations on gumlack of stamps and/or envelopes have not yet been done.

Literature

ARNDT RE [1989] Group Specific Component: Isoelectric Focusing Subtyping and Immunoblot Detection. J For Sci 34: 1318-1322

IKEMOTO S, TSUCHIDA S, KAJII E, NOZAWA E and TOMITA K [1990] Distribution of Twelve Human Salivary Polymorphisms in Japanese Population. In: Polesky HF and Mayr WR (Eds) Advances in Forensic Haemogenetics 3. Springer-Verlag, Berlin Heidelberg, P 263-264

KEIL W, SEMM K und PATZELT D [1988] Darstellung der genetischen Tf-, Gc- und Pi-Subtypen in gelagerten Blutproben. Kriminal Forens Wissensch 71,72: 135-138

KIDO A, OYA M, KOMTASU N and SHIBATA R [1984] A Stability Study on Gc Subtyping in Bloodstains: Comparison by two Different Techniques. For Sci Int 26: 39-43

MILLS PR and CHASE MG [1989] The Detection of Group-Specific Component from Urine Samples. 43: 215-221

PLFUG W [1986] Sensitive Alkaline Phosphatase Linked Secondary Antibody System for Detection of Group Specific Component after Isoelectric Focusing on 250 µm Thick Reusable Immobilized pH-Gradients. Electrophoresis 7: 273-278

RAND S, RITTER P, KOHFAHL A and BRINKMANN [1987] A Comparative Study of Immuno-Blotting Techniques for the Detection of Gc-Subtypes after Isoelectric Focusing on Agarose and Polyacrylamide Gels. Z Rechtsmed 98: 175-180

RAND S, TILLMANN B, BRINKMANN B [1990] Gc in Bloodstains. Z Rechtsmed 103: 453-456

THOMAS AS, ANSFORD AJ, AASKOV JG [1989] The Application of Immununoblotting to the Phenotyping of Group-Specific Component. J For Sci Soc 29: 197-205

WESTWOOD AS and WERRETT DJ [1990] The Collaborative Study on Typing Group-Specific Component in Casework Bloodstains. J For Sci Soc 30: 33-38

Immunoblotting and Immunofixation Techniques for Subtyping Gc in
Old Bloodstains and Semen Stains

I. López-Abadía, A. Gremo, J.M. Ruiz de la Cuesta

Departamento Toxicología y Legislación Sanitaria. Sección
Biología Forense. Universidad Complutense. 28040 Madrid, Spain

INTRODUCTION

Group-specific component (Gc) is a polymorphic genetic marker
used in blood characterization. A number of isoelectrofocusing
methods have been described for separating common Gc subtypes
- Gc 1F, Gc 1S and Gc 2- (Constans 1978, Lizana 1981, Cleve 1982)

Gc polymorphism has proved to be very useful in paternity
testing, and, as stable protein, well suited for forensic
casework.

We here compare immunofixation (Baxter 1982, Westwood 1985) and
immunoblotting (Thomas 1989, Alonso 1988) techniques for
subtyping Gc in old blood and semen stains.

MATERIAL AND METHOD

The equipment used was FBE-2000 (Pharmacia) with power supply
from Pharmacia ECPS 3000/150 with volthour integrator VH-1. Gels
were made through the following mixture: PAGIEF T=6.2%, C=3.2%,
sucrose=12%; ampholytes: 4-6=0.06%, 4-6.5=0.02%, 4.5-5.4=0.02%.
Electrode gap was 95 mm. Samples consisted of bloodstains on 100%
cotton cloth stored at room temperature and semen stains on 100%
cotton cloth stored at 4°C. An urea 6M solution was used for
extraction and samples were incubated overnight at 4°C. Samples
were applied using 5×3 mm Whatman paper 1 cm from cathode.
Isoelectric focusing conditions are shown in Table 1.
Immunofixation was performed using antiGc serum + physiological
serum 1:1 30 min at 37°C in moist chamber. Overnight washing in
physiological serum. Development was carried out using silver
staining techniques. Immunoblotting was carried out through a
double antibody procedure according to Alonso (1988).

Advances in Forensic Haemogenetics 4
Edited by Ch. Rittner and P. M. Schneider
© Springer-Verlag Berlin Heidelberg 1992

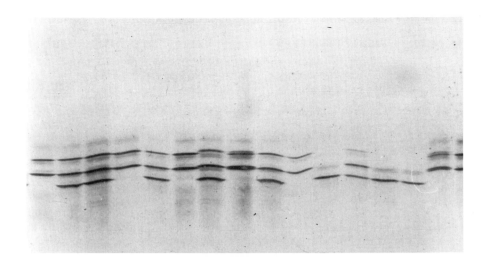

Fig 1. Gc protein. Immunofixation followed by silver staining.
Anode is at the top. Phenotypes are: Lanes 1,4,6 and 10: 1s1s;
Lanes 2,3,5,9 and 12: 2-1s; Lanes 11, 13 and 14: 2-2; Lanes 8 and
15: 1F-1S; Lane 7: 2-1F

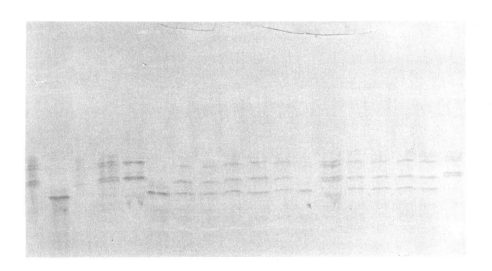

Fig 2. Gc protein. Immunoblotting. Anode is at the top.
Phenotypes are: Lanes 1,4,13 and 18: 1F1S; Lanes 2,6 and 12: 2-2;
Lanes 3: 1S1S; Lane 5: 1F-1F; Lanes 7,8,9,11,14,15,16 and 17: 2-
1S; Lane 10: 2-1F

Table 1.   Isoelectric focusing conditions

Prefocusing	1500V	150mA	8W	8°C	500vh
Samples	1500V	150mA	5W	8°C	700vh
Focusing	1500V	150mA	6W	8°C	5000vh

RESULTS AND CONCLUSIONS

Both methods showed a high reliability for Gc characterization even with very old bloodstains; Gc subtyping was possible in at least 10 months-old bloodstains mantained at room temperature. Both techniques were very sensitive and we did not find any additional band.

We consider immunofixation easier to carry out, quicker and cheaper than immunoblotting and as we did not find differences in the results obtained we advise the use of the former for routine casework involving bloodstains or semen stains.

REFERENCES

Alonso A   (1988)   Group specific component subtyping in bloodstains by separator isoelectric focusing in micro-ultrathin polyacrilamide gels followed by immunoblotting. J For Sci 33:1277-1272

Baxter M, Randall TW, Thorpe JW   (1982)   A method for phenotyping group specific component protein from dried bloodstains by immunofixation thin-layer polyacrilamide gel isoelectric focusing. J For Sci 22:367-371

Cleve H et al   (1982)   Analysis of the genetic variants of the human Gc system (VDBP) by isoelectric focusing in immobilized pH gradients. Electrophoresis 3:342-345

Constans J et al   (1978)   Analysis of the Gc polymorphism in human populations by isoelectric focusing on polyacrilamide gels. Demonstration of sub-types of Gc 1 allele and of additional Gc variants. Hum Genet 41:53-60

Lizana J, Savill B, Olsson I   (1981)   Agarose isoelectric focusing and related immunochemical techniques in the analysis of serum Gc globulin. In: Allen RC and Arnaud P (eds) Electrophoresis 81, Walter de Gruyter, Berlin (pub) p 549

Thomas AS, Ansford AJ, Aaskov JG   (1989)   The application of immunoblotting to the phenotyping of Group-specific component. J For Sci 29:197-205

Westwood SA   (1985)   Silver staining of immunofixed group specific component on cellulose acetate membranes after isoelectric focusing in narrow pH interval gels. Electrophoresis 6:498-503

Old Bloodstain and Semen stain Characterization in the Transferrin Typing System Using Minigels and PhastSystem

I. López-Abadía, A. Gremo, J.M. Ruiz de la Cuesta

Departamento Toxicología y Legislación Sanitaria. Sección Biología Forense. Universidad Complutense. 28040 Madrid, Spain

INTRODUCTION

Transferrin is the major iron binding protein in vertebrate serum. It carries ferric iron from the intestine, reticulo-endothelial system and liver parenchimal cells to all proliferating cells in the body.

Several genetic variants can be separated by polyacrilamide or agarose gel isoelectric focusing. Gene typing can give important and useful information for paternity determination and in forensic medicine.

We here describe a fast simple method for subtyping transferrin in bloodstains and semen stains. We use PhastSystem, commercial gels and immunofixation techniques. It is a very sensitive method that allows discrimination of phenotypes for the transferrin system in very old bloodstains.

MATERIAL AND METHOD

The equipment used was PhastSystem and commercial gels (PhastGel IEF 4-6.5) re-equilibrated for 1 hour in the following solution: 0.6 g. sucrose(MERCK), 0.25 ml. Nonidet P40 20% (LKB), 1 ml Servalyt 5-7 (SERVA), 5 ml. distilled water. Samples consisted of bloodstains on 100% cotton cloth stored at room temperature and semen stains on 100% cotton cloth stored at 4°c. A neuraminidase 2% solution was used for extraction and samples were incubated overnight at 4°C. Iron saturation was carried out with ferrous ammonium sulfate 0.3% 1:1 incubated at 37°C for 3 hours. Samples were applied using PhastGel Sample Applicator 8/1 in cathodal position. Isoelectric focusing conditions are shown in Table 1. Immnunofixation was used using antiTf serum + physiological serum 1:1 30 min. at 37°C in moist chamber. Coomassie Blue staining was used for bloodstains and siver staining for semen stains. In both cases we used PhastSystem protocols.

Advances in Forensic Haemogenetics 4
Edited by Ch. Rittner and P. M. Schneider
© Springer-Verlag Berlin Heidelberg 1992

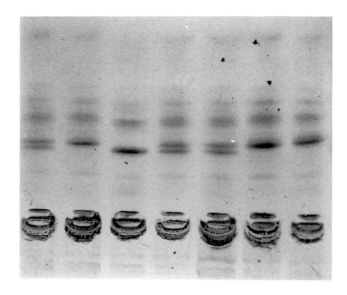

Fig 1. Transferrin phenotypes. 10 month-old bloodstains. Anode is at the top. From left to right phenotypes are: c1c2, c1c1, c2c2, c1c2, c1c2, c1c1, c1c1

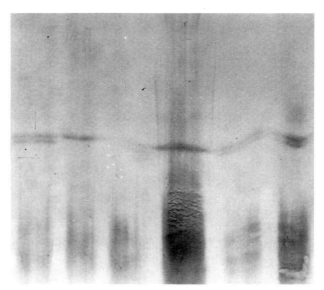

Fig 2. Transferrin phenotypes. Semen stains. Anode is at the top. From left to right phenotypes are: c1c2, c1c1, c1c1, c1c1, c1c2, c1c2

Table 1. Microprocessor program

Sample appl. down at	1.2				0vh
Sample appl. up at	1.3				0vh
Extra alarm to sound	1.1				73vh
Sep 1.1	2000V	2.0mA	2.5W	15°C	75vh
Sep 1.2	200V	2.0mA	2.5W	15°C	20vh
Sep 1.3	2000V	2.0mA	2.5W	15°C	100vh
Sep 1.4	2000V	2.0mA	3.5W	15°C	600vh

RESULTS AND CONCLUSIONS

The method reported shows simple, reliable and very sensitive.
The little amount of sample necessary made possible the
characterization of phenotypes for the transferrin system in very
old bloodstains.

Commercial gels are suitable for this technique so we avoid
homemade gels saving time and making it easier to standardize.
The use of an automated system for isoelectric focusing and
development noticeably reduced the time and cost of the
experiments.

Forensic investigations need a simple reliable method for routine
use. We believe that the method proposed here fulfills these
requirements.

REFERENCES

Aisen P, Listowsky I   (1980)   Iron transport and storage
    proteins. Ann Rev Biochem 49:357-393
Budowle B, Scott E   (1985)   Transferrin subtyping of human
    blood. For Sci Int 28:269-275
Kamboh MJ, Ferrel RE   (1987)   Human transferrin polymorfism.
    Hum Hered 37:65-81

Printing: Druckhaus Beltz, Hemsbach
Binding: Buchbinderei Schäffer, Grünstadt